Biotechnology
in Personal Care

COSMETIC SCIENCE AND TECHNOLOGY

Series Editor
ERIC JUNGERMANN
Jungermann Associates, Inc.
Phoenix, Arizona

Biotechnology in Personal Care

edited by

Raj Lad

Genencor International, a Danisco Company
Palo Alto, California, U.S.A.

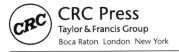

CRC Press
Taylor & Francis Group
Boca Raton London New York

CRC Press is an imprint of the
Taylor & Francis Group, an **informa** business

CRC Press
Taylor & Francis Group
6000 Broken Sound Parkway NW, Suite 3000
Boca Raton, FL 33487-2742

First issued in paperback 2019

© 2011 by Taylor & Francis Group, LLC
CRC Press is an imprint of Taylor & Francis Group, an Informa business

No claim to original U.S. Government works

ISBN-13: 978-0-8247-2534-1 (hbk)
ISBN-13: 978-0-367-39107-2 (pbk)

A CIP record for this book is available from the British Library.

Library of Congress Cataloging-in-Publication Data available on application

Visit the Taylor & Francis Web site at
http://www.taylorandfrancis.com

and the CRC Press Web site at
http://www.crcpress.com

About the Series

The *Cosmetic Science and Technology* series was conceived to permit discussion of a broad range of current knowledge and theories of cosmetic science and technology. The series is composed of books written by one or two authors and edited volumes with a number of contributors. Authorities from industry, academia, and the government participate in writing these books.

The aim of the series is to cover the many facets of cosmetic science and technology. Topics are drawn from a wide spectrum of disciplines ranging from chemistry, physics, biochemistry, and dermatology to consumer evaluations, safety issues, efficacy, toxicity, and regulatory questions. Organic, inorganic, physical, analytical, and polymer chemistry, microbiology, emulsion, and lipid technology all play important roles in cosmetic science.

There is little commonality in the scientific methods, processes, and formulations required for the wide variety of toiletries and cosmetics in the market. Products range from hair, skin, and oral care products to lipsticks, nail polishes, deodorants, body powders, and aerosols to cosmeceuticals, are quasi-pharmaceutical over-the-counter products such as antiperspirants, dandruff shampoos, wrinkle reducers, antimicrobial soaps, acne treatments, or sun screen products.

Cosmetics and toiletries represent a highly diversified field involving many subsections of science and "art." Even in these days of high technology and ever increasing scientific sophistication, art and intuition continue to play an important part in the development of formulations, their evaluation, selection of raw materials, and, perhaps most importantly, the successful marketing of new products. Fragrance, color, packaging, and product positioning often are as important to the success of a new product as delivering the promised (implied) performance. The application of more sophisticated methodologies to the evaluation of cosmetics that began in the 1980s has continued and has greatly impacted such areas as claim substantiation, safety and efficacy testing, product evaluations and testing, and development of new raw materials, such as biotechnology products (for example, products produced by microorganisms where genes are modified by recombinant DNA technologies).

Emphasis in the Cosmetic Science and Technology series is placed on reporting the current status of cosmetic science and technology, the ever changing regulatory climate, and historical reviews. The series has now grown to 29 books dealing with the constantly changing trends in the cosmetic industry, including globalization. Several of the books have been translated into Japanese and Chinese. Contributions range from highly sophisticated and scientific treaties to primers and presentations of practical applications. Authors are encouraged to present their own concepts as well as established theories. Contributors have been asked not to shy away from fields that are in a state of transition or somewhat controversial and not to hesitate to present detailed discussions of their own work. Altogether, we intend to develop in this series a collection of critical surveys and ideas covering the diverse phases of the cosmetic industry.

The twenty-ninth book in this series, *Biotechnology in Personal Care*, edited by Dr. Raj Lad comprises 17 chapters authored by 30 experts in the field. This is a forward looking book; while covering current use of biotechnology by the personal care industry, the main focus of the book will be on the future use and potential of biotechnology and of products developed by using biotechnology. To date, the major potential applications of biotechnology fall in the realm of therapeutics, which has raised difficult technical problems, as well as ethical considerations. The latter have been under study by the President's Council on Bioethics, and a major report was issued in October 2003 (www.bioethics.gov). To quote: "To advance human good and avoid harm, biotechnology must be used with ethical constraints. It is the task of bioethics to help society develop these constraints, and bioethics, therefore, must be of concern to all of us."

Chapter 6 of the above report has bearing on extending biotechnology "Beyond Therapy," including personal care applications. The new age of biotechnology is not so much about technology itself, but about *human beings empowered by biotechnology*. Some of the objectives to be achieved beyond therapy may include genetic enhancement of muscles, retardation of aging, or increased self-esteem. The section entitled "Commerce, Regulations, and the Manufacture of Desire" highlights the situation of the cosmetic industry and their application of biotechnological techniques, as illustrated by these extracts:

Progress in biology and biotechnology is now intimately bound up with industry and commerce.... The emergence of a vigorous biotech industry, growing rapidly even before it has delivered very much of its great promise, is a sign of things to come. Whatever one finally thinks about the relative virtues and vices of contemporary capitalism, it is a fact that progress in science and technology owes much to free enterprise. We have reason to expect exponential increases in biotechnologies and, therefore, in their potential uses in all aspects of human life.... Entrepreneurs ... promote public demand. The success of enterprises often turns on anticipating and stimulating consumer demand, even at times creating it where none exists. Suitably stimulated, for easier means to better-behaved children, more youthful or beautiful or potent bodies . . . is potentially enormous. If the existing cosmetic industry may be taken as a model, the sky may be the limit for a truly effective "cosmetic pharmacology" that would deliver stronger muscles, better memories, brighter moods, and peace of mind. The direct-to-consumer advertising of pharmaceutical or other companies is a harbinger of things to come. Today it is Ritalin, Botox, Rogaine, Viagara, and Prozac; could tomorrow be "Memorase," "Popeye's Potion," "Exotocon," "Self-Love," or "Soma"? Desires can be manufactured almost as effectively as pills, especially if the pills work more or less as promised to satisfy the newly stimulated desires. By providing quick solutions for short-term problems or prompt fulfillment of easily satisfied desires, the character of human longings itself could be altered, with large aspirations for long-term flourishing giving way before the immediate gratification of smaller desires. What to do about this is far from clear, but its importance should not be underestimated.

I want to thank all contributors and the editor, Dr. Raj Lad, for participating in the *Cosmetic Science and Technology Series* and Taylor and Francis Group and the many people in this organization, particularly Sandra Beberman, with whom I have worked since the inception of this series twenty-five years ago, for their support and help.

Eric Jungermann, Ph.D.
Series Editor

Preface

This book is an attempt to connect one of the newest technologies, biotechnology, to one of the oldest human needs—that of looking or staying young. The use of biological or natural ingredients in cosmetics and for personal care is ancient, known since the time of Cleopatra, who used many remedies containing natural ingredients, such as "henna" for hair color. In the twenty-first century, the application of biotechnology has begun to revolutionize the personal care industry by making novel ingredients available for fulfilling personal care needs and by providing insights into the biological processes that could be used to develop new products.

Many economists, futurists, scientists, and thought leaders refer to the twenty-first century as the century of biology, specifically of biotechnology. As our understanding of the human biology has expanded in the last few decades, the excitement around the impact of biotechnology on a range of industries has grown. Many biotechnologists believe that so far, we have only scratched the surface of the potential of biotechnology. In the coming years, biotechnology is not only poised to make an impact on health care, but is also geared toward offering breakthrough innovations for personal care. Biotechnology has passed the stage of curiosity or early discoveries and is now entering into the ascending portion of the S-curve, suggesting that the time has come for it to fulfill its promise. Such bullish enthusiasm could be ascribed to many things, such as—completion of the sequencing of the human genome; progress in information technology, which has expanded the volume of data that computers can now handle; and the increased number of tools, techniques, and instruments now available to the biotechnologist. Of course, biotechnology's biggest impact will be felt in health care, but at the same time, knowledge gained during the development of pharmaceutical products could be used to create new personal care products that would truly meet the current unmet consumer needs.

The current era is often referred to as the "knowledge-based economy" since most of the new technologies that are involved in growing the global economy are based on knowledge. And biotechnology is no exception. First, biotechnology needs discoveries in basic sciences. A number of discoveries have been made since the discovery of DNA 50 years ago, but many more are still essential to get the most out of biotechnology. Second, those discoveries need to result in accumulation of knowledge that would lead to elucidating the underlying mechanisms of healthy skin, hair, and lips such that products could be developed by the personal care industry. Finally, production processes and stable formulations need to be developed, based on the accumulation of precise knowledge about microbial physiology, scale up, and protein stability. Only then can biotechnology become a viable commercial technology for the personal care industry and make a true impact on the development of personal care products.

As a result, among many of the new technologies, biotechnology is one of the most R&D-intensive technologies. In addition, biotechnology-based ingredients need to be produced at the costs that are in line with other ingredients used in the personal care industry. This means that for biotechnology to gain a foothold in personal care, biotechnology companies have to spend money on research in a manner similar to drug development companies, but in return for a smaller reward. This hurdle can be overcome via cooperation between biotechnology and personal care companies by taking advantage of the knowledge developed by pharmaceutical companies and academic institutions. This book is an effort toward achieving that goal. Contributors represent biotechnology scientists, scientists working in the personal care industry, academics, and other supporting disciplines.

Both "personal care" and "biotechnology" encompass huge areas of science and applications. These terms have no strict definitions and are used broadly. Biotechnology means different things to different people. In addition, its meaning has evolved over time. Many thought leaders perceive biotechnology as mostly related to human genome efforts and health care and have a very broad definition for it. Here are a couple of definitions of biotechnology:

1. Biotechnology: FDA definition
   Application of biological systems and organisms to technical and industrial processes
2. Biotechnology: BIO (Biotechnology Industrial Organization) definition
   Break biotechnology into its root words and you have
   - bio—using biological processes; and
   - technology—solving problems or making useful products.

To manage the content of this book, use of the term biotechnology (and products derived from it) is restricted to: "products produced by microorganisms in which genes are modified by recombinant DNA technologies." In addition, the book addresses use of recombinant DNA technology to identify mechanisms and targets to develop new personal care products and ingredients. In this book, an attempt is made to cover as many applications as possible that fall under a broad definition of personal care, for example, skin, hair, oral, and lip care, as well as other cosmetics.

This is a forward-looking book. It covers not only biotechnology ingredients currently used in personal care, but also a significant focus is on the use of biotechnology to develop new ingredients and future personal care products. Unlike the computer industry, where new technologies make older ones obsolete, in biotechnology, scientists build on each others' knowledge so that new, efficacious products can be developed. This book, therefore, strives to emphasize this look into the future so that innovation processes and overall progress can be accelerated.

This book is divided into three sections:

    I.   Biotechnology: What It Is and Current Products
    II.   Biotechnology: Use in Personal Care Applications
    III. Biotechnology: Challenges in the Personal Care World

The first section, which includes chapters 1–4, familiarizes the readers with biotechnology and related terms. It covers the fundamentals of biotechnology and provides short descriptions of key terms like, cloning, RNA, DNA, rDNA, protein engineering, genetic engineering, genomics and proteomics, and so on. Since the discovery of the structure of DNA in 1950s, many innovations have been made, and I believe many more are coming. Therefore, this section also covers upcoming technologies based on new tools that are being developed. It also covers biotechnology-based products currently used in personal care applications. These include proteins, peptides, enzymes, and biologicals.

The second section (chaps. 5–14) looks at many personal care applications individually. Each application is represented from a biotechnology perspective. Individual chapters cover historical perspective for the application and how biotechnology is used to understand the underlying mechanisms and to develop products.

The third section, containing chapters 15–17, covers the challenges that scientists and industry could face as the use of biotechnology expands in personal care products. This is not unique, because adaptation of any new technology by the personal care or any other industry would face some key challenges. We all have to remember that the personal care industry is one of the oldest and most practiced industries; therefore, adapting to new processes will be challenging. At the same time, this book represents my strong belief that in the long term, biotechnology will change the personal care marketplace.

Pushkaraj (Raj) Lad

Acknowledgments

This book is a combined effort of many people. First and foremost, I wish to thank all the authors who contributed to the book. I recognize that they had to take time out of their busy schedules and work after hours on this project. I had to do the same; therefore, this project would not have been completed without the understanding and support from my wife Padmashri and my son Sameep.

My special thanks to my colleagues around the world at Genencor, who were available for discussions and supported the project. The manuscript could not have come together without the help of Dr. Roopa Ghirnikar, Ms. Tita Scheller, and Ms. Georgette Shintaku.

Contents

Contributors

Honnavara N. Ananthaswamy *Department of Immunology, The University of Texas, M.D. Anderson Cancer Center, Houston, Texas, U.S.A.*

William H. Bowen *University of Rochester, Rochester, New York, U.S.A.*

Fredi Brühlmann *Department of Biotechnology, Corporate R&D, Firmenich SA, Geneva, Switzerland*

Gopal Chotani *Genencor International, a Danisco Company, Palo Alto, California, U.S.A.*

Anthony J. Clark *Department of Biotechnology, Corporate R&D, Firmenich SA, Geneva, Switzerland*

Diane Cummins *Colgate-Palmolive Company, Piscataway, New Jersey, U.S.A.*

Roopa Ghirnikar *Genencor International, a Danisco Company, Palo Alto, California, U.S.A.*

Helmut Greim *Technical University of Munich, Institute of Toxicology and Environmental Hygiene, Freising-Weihenstephan, Germany*

Meng Heng *Genencor International, a Danisco Company, Palo Alto, California, U.S.A.*

Shintaro Inoue *Basic Research Laboratory, Kanebo Cosmetics Inc., Odawara, Kanagawa, Japan*

Susanne Iobst *Unilever Research U.S., Edgewater, New Jersey, U.S.A.*

James T. Kellis, Jr. *Genencor International, a Danisco Company, Palo Alto, California, U.S.A.*

Daniela Kessler-Becker *Henkel KGaA, Corporate Biological Research, Dusseldorf, Germany*

Jiro Kishimoto *Shiseido Research Center, Yokohama, Japan*

Manoj Kumar *Genencor International, a Danisco Company, Palo Alto, California, U.S.A.*

Raj Lad *Genencor International, a Danisco Company, Palo Alto, California, U.S.A.*

Yasuhiro Matsumura *Department of Immunology, The University of Texas, M.D. Anderson Cancer Center, Houston, Texas, U.S.A., and Department of Dermatology, Kansai Medical University, Osaka, Japan*

Hugh C. McDonald *Genencor International, a Danisco Company, Palo Alto, California, U.S.A.*

Louis C. Paul *Louis C. Paul & Associates, PLLC, New York, New York, U.S.A.*

Anthony V. Rawlings *AVR Consulting Ltd., Kingsmead, Northwich, Cheshire, U.K.*

Uma Santhanam *Unilever Research U.S., Edgewater, New Jersey, U.S.A.*

Michel Schalk *Department of Biotechnology, Corporate R&D, Firmenich SA, Geneva, Switzerland*

Miri Seiberg *Skin Research Center, Johnson & Johnson CPPW, Skillman, New Jersey, U.S.A.*

Wim Soetaert *Department of Biochemical and Microbial Technology, Faculty of Bioscience Engineering, Ghent University, Ghent, Belgium*

Tsutomu Soma *Shiseido Research Center, Yokohama, Japan*

Desmond J. Tobin *Department of Biomedical Sciences, University of Bradford, Bradford, U.K.*

Erick J. Vandamme *Department of Biochemical and Microbial Technology, Faculty of Bioscience Engineering, Ghent University, Ghent, Belgium*

Ronni L. Weinkauf *Unilever Research U.S., Edgewater, New Jersey, U.S.A.*

Debbie Winetzky *Genencor International, a Danisco Company, Palo Alto, California, U.S.A.*

Kiichiro Yano *Shiseido Research Center, Yokohama, Japan*

1

Overview and Fundamentals of Biotechnology

Hugh C. McDonald and Roopa Ghirnikar

Genencor International, a Danisco Company, Palo Alto, California, U.S.A.

DEFINITION AND PERSONAL CARE VIEWPOINT

What is biotechnology and how do we define and understand it in a way that is relevant to personal care? The historical definition would be the use of living organisms and their products to solve life's basic problems, such as food, shelter, health, security, and happiness. Making beer and cheese (1), for example, is a biotechnology application more than 4000 years old that used bacteria and their enzymes to ferment milk and grain into higher value foods. Personal care (2) applications are also thought to have originated more than 4000 years ago, in Egypt, when such plant extracts as henna and indigo were used as makeup to paint faces, hair, and bodies, and animal and vegetable fats and beeswax were used for skin creams and coverings.

Although true, these definitions are too broad for use in this book. Rather, we need to focus on a modern definition of biotechnology that could be applied to present and future personal care applications. With that in mind, one can define biotechnology as "products produced by microorganisms in which the genes are modified by recombinant DNA technologies." To understand that definition and its importance, we need to review historical events in the field of microbiology, because biotechnology is the grown-up, robust child of microbiology.

HISTORICAL SEEDS OF BIOTECHNOLOGY

Microbiology began (Table 1) as the study of sickness in animals and humans. There were many misconceptions about the causes of such diseases as smallpox, plague, and tuberculosis, and progress was limited to magic, medicine men, and natural remedies. During the early 1800s, Edward Jenner (3) stunned the world by injecting patients with cowpox to protect them against smallpox. Jenner didn't understand that the cowpox virus was less virulent than the human smallpox virus and thus easier for the body to build defenses against. It took Louis Pasteur (4) and others another 70 years to build the scientific understanding for the basis of food spoilage, bacteria, and the concept of sterility. Pasteur was the first to demonstrate that boiling and pasteurization—treatment of materials at high temperature under pressure could result in bacteria-free materials. Pasteur's work also was the first to explain fermentation and how this process was directly related to making beer and cheese.

Table 1   Key Events in the History of Biotechnology

Date	Who	What	Comment
1798	Edward Jenner	Smallpox prevention	First vaccine
1885	Louis Pasteur	Germs and fermentation	Sterilization
1929	Alexander Flemming	Penicillin from molds	First antibiotic
1944	Oswald Avery, Colin MacLeod, and Maclyn McCarty	Transfer of a genetic trait in pneumococcal bacteria	Bacterial DNA carried the trait
1952	Alfred Hershey and Martha Chase	DNA is the genetic molecule	DNA not protein
1957	James Watson and Francis Crick	How DNA works to replicate genes	Basis for central dogma of biology
1972	Paul Berg	First recombinant DNA molecule	Cutting and splicing DNAs
1974	Stanley Cohen and Herbert Boyer	First recombinant organism	Human gene in bacteria *E. coli*
1978	Robert Swanson and Herbert Boyer	Genentech	First recombinant company
1983	Kary Mullis	Polymerase chain reaction	Application with many uses
1990	NIH and Watson	Human genome project	A long and difficult project
1995	Craig Venter	First genome deciphered	Haemophilus influenza with 1000 genes
2001	Celera and NIH	Human genome deciphered	30,000–40,000 human genes

The revolution in thinking caused by Pasteur directly led to numerous studies during the early 1900s on immunity and how the body generated protections against microbial invaders. While this resulted in new vaccines and new strategies against dangerous pathogens, other microbiologists were attempting to characterize and understand the life cycle of various microbes. These investigations directly led to one of the greatest applications still in use today, namely, penicillin. In 1922, Alexander Fleming (5) discovered the antibacterial action of products secreted from the mold *Penicillium*. This finding initiated a long and fruitful search for other antibacterial agents and products secreted by molds and bacteria. Eventually, this became the basis for large-scale cultivation of such microbes in enormous fermenters, leading to the recovery and purification of such active agents as penicillin and streptomycin that form the basis of today's pharmaceutical industry. Coupled with environmental advances in proper sewage treatment and water handling, antibiotics like penicillin were magic health bullets and directly led to increased longevity and quality of life. With the discovery of penicillin, a small part of the dangerous world of disease came under civilization's control.

The use of antibiotics in World War II alleviated battlefield deaths and positioned bacteria and industrial fermentation as an industry with great potential for human good. While many new antibiotics were being discovered, microbiologists attempted to understand how they were made in the bacterial cell and how they worked. At this time, scientists were aware that each bacterial species was physically and metabolically different and produced different products. In 1944, working with *Pneumococcus*, the bacteria that causes pneumonia, Avery, MacLeod, and McCarty (6) showed that an extract from a pneumococcal bacteria with a large polysaccharide capsule, or surface covering, could be transferred to an organism without a capsule. Most remarkably, the capsular traits of the host would be found in the recipient organism after cultivation and continued as a part of the recipient's stable, physical characteristics, or phenotype. In 1952, Hershey and Chase (6) did a classic experiment with viruses that infect bacteria (called bacteriophage), which proved that genetic traits are associated with deoxyribonucleic acid, or DNA. Using DNA and protein, each labeled with different radioisotopes, they proved beyond doubt that DNA and not protein was the carrier of hereditary material.

These experiments were the first to move a stable, genetic trait from one organism to another by transfer of an extract containing DNA and paved the way to think about manipulating living things using laboratory procedures. Progress in the biochemistry of proteins and in new biophysical tools encouraged new thinking to understand how organisms expressed and stably maintained different characteristics. With the advent of the new tool of X-ray crystallography, which permitted the analysis of crystal structure and the structure of many biological molecules, the key biological discovery of the 20th century occurred. In 1957, Watson and Crick (7), two young Cambridge scientists using the data of many and the scientific insight of a lifetime, solved the structure of DNA, the genetic molecule of life (Fig. 1). DNA is present in every cell nucleus in a double helix and is held together by a sugar–phosphate backbone and four nucleotide bases. The bases join each other, adenine with thymine, and guanine with cytosine, in a non-covalent, hydrogen bond structure that under the proper conditions unzips and makes a complementary strand. Genes, the units of heredity, are long stretches of specific nucleotide bases that are reproduced with fidelity when new copies of DNA are made. With the solving of the DNA structure, the mystery of how living things are different and are able to reproduce those differences in their

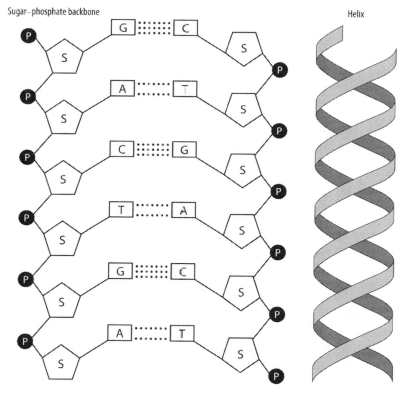

Figure 1   Model of DNA: DNA is composed of base units of nucleotides, a purine or pyrimidine attached to a sugar phosphate. There are four separate nucleotides: two purines (adenine and guanine) and two pyrimidines (thymine and cytosine). Nucleotide bases are polymerized by linking their sugar (deoxyribose) phosphates. The helix forms when two strings of polymerized phosphate polymers face each other with their phosphate backbones to the outside and their base pairs to the inside. By a noncovalent binding process, called hydrogen bonding, specific base pairs form between adenine (A) and thymine (T) and between cytosine (C) and guanine (G). The two chains intertwine around each sharing a common axis in a complementary alpha helix structure.

progeny was solved. The concept of DNA and how it works and how different animals and humans can maintain their peculiar and specific characteristics over time brought to life the concept of the genetic code. This fueled an explosion of knowledge—much of it in the bacterium *Escherichia coli*, which became the organism of choice for microbiologists and scientists working in molecular biology—and generated ideas that became the central dogma of biology (Fig. 2). In the nucleus of each cell of every organism, there is a specific string of DNA composed of long stretches of the molecule—called a gene—that are responsible for every characteristic of the organism. DNA holds the information for these traits in its sequence of nucleotide bases, the genetic blueprint. The exact order of nucleotide bases is transcribed into another molecule called mRNA, or messenger ribonucleic acid. Once information from the DNA is passed on to the messenger, it moves into the cell cytoplasm and is stabilized on structures called ribosomes, where specific proteins special to each cell are made that perform the job of structure, catalysis, and control and regulation of cellular metabolism. Depending on the type of cell, whether it's a brain cell, blood cell, or muscle cell, different genes are expressed to make different mRNAs, which make the library of proteins needed to run and maintain that particular cell. The central dogma of biology that genetic information is transferred from DNA to mRNA and that mRNA is used as a pattern to build proteins from amino acids in the cell holds today. This concept was first worked out in *E. coli* bacteria where there is a single piece of circular, double-stranded DNA that has more than 4000 different genes and generates more than 4000 to 5000 proteins.

Additional work in many other bacteria and many other cells, including human cells confirmed the central dogma and extended it. Research on *E. coli* has also provided answers to a key question in molecular biology—how are genes regulated? If a cell has 4000 genes, it doesn't need to synthesize the corresponding protein from each gene all the time. Although each human cell carries the entire human genome, each cell varies the protein it makes depending on its tissue origin and function and is capable of varying the amounts of each protein. Bacteria regulate gene expression and protein production by a control unit called the operon, the unit of transcription in bacteria. An operon is composed of a section of DNA that contains adjacent genes that code for structural genes, such as muscle protein or enzymes; regulatory genes that code for regulatory proteins, such as enzyme inhibitors or DNA or RNA binding proteins; and control elements, which are specific sites on DNA where the regulatory proteins interact. In bacteria, a gene can be turned on by an inducer molecule and turned off by a repressor molecule. In one case, the gene makes a new enzyme or set of enzymes, which the cells require to take advantage of the induction agent. In repression, the agent signals that sufficient protein has been made and synthesizing more would represent unnecessary overproduction. Human cells have more complicated regulatory strategies than the bacterial operon, but the general concept of a transcription unit under control with feedback signals from its cellular environment remains the same.

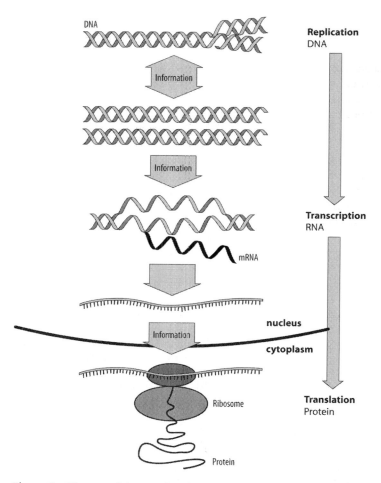

Figure 2   The central dogma of molecular biology: Genetic information flows from DNA to RNA to protein. DNA is the genetic blueprint, and the information it codes in the linear sequence of its base pairs determines what proteins get synthesized. After the DNA helix unfolds, an enzyme called RNA polymerase duplicates the DNA sequence into RNA and replaces thymidine with uracil. This process is called transcription. The mRNA molecule formed is the working blueprint copy, or messenger, that leaves the nucleus and attaches to a series of large structural proteins called ribosomes. Ribosomes exist throughout the cell cytoplasm and act as a scaffold or physical support to synthesize proteins. As the mRNA is pulled through the ribosomes, each three-base unit, or codon, is matched with molecules called transfer RNA that bring a specific amino acid related to the codon. This happens for the entire set of codons in the mRNA, and this process by which mRNA information is converted into specific proteins is called translation. Amino acids that are polymerized to form peptides and proteins fall off the ribosome into the cytoplasm and perform the specific functions of proteins.

Once the basis of gene regulation was understood, it opened the way to begin thinking about how to turn genes off and on using drugs and genetic engineering. Such terms as "upregulate," the process of making changes in genetic control elements to increase production, or "downregulate," the process of making changes to decrease production, became strategies molecular biologists could implement. But these molecular biology strategies could not be perfected until cloning, the ability to copy a gene, was developed.

Cloning

Cloning is the key procedure of molecular biology and the cornerstone of genetic engineering. Again, the groundbreaking work occurred in bacteria when it was found that there were enzymes called restriction enzymes that cut DNA at specific places and worked on many kinds of DNA from many organisms. In addition, there were other enzymes called coupling, or annealing/ligating, enzymes that could join cut pieces of DNA together to heal and link them together. Using these specific DNA enzymes, Paul Berg and Colleagues (8) in 1972 made the first recombinant DNA molecule. It was a combination of viral and bacterial DNA. The next step paved the way for the modern biotechnology industry. In 1973, Cohen and Boyer (9) created the first recombinant DNA organism by putting a mammalian gene into a growing *E. coli* culture. The vehicle for moving the recombinant gene was a plasmid. Years before, it was discovered that *E. coli* and other bacteria had small pieces of circular DNA that were distinct and not attached to the primary DNA and coded for different proteins, especially drug resistant proteins. These circular pieces of DNA acted as carriers for genetic information and were naturally transferred from one group of bacteria to another. During the 1970s, when all these biochemical reagents were in place, including restriction enzymes, annealing enzymes, plasmids, antibiotic markers, and pieces of DNA, the technique of cloning single genes was born.

Cloning works like the schematic diagram shown in Figure 3. For example, bacterial culture A makes a protein that you want to make in bacterial culture B. The first step is to grow culture A and isolate its DNA. The second step is to treat this DNA with a panel of restriction enzymes, such as Eco R1, that cut in different places. Some of these cuts will keep the DNA coding for the enzyme you want to clone intact. The cut DNA, containing the gene of interest, is then mixed with a plasmid selectively cut in places with restriction enzymes. Finally, the host DNA and plasmid are mixed together with ligating enzymes. Some of the plasmid DNA is recircularized, but it now contains a piece of foreign DNA, a piece of DNA that has recombined with a piece of the plasmid DNA. Now the plasmid is purified, and mixed with recipient cells, under the right transforming conditions, and some of the plasmid with the new genes get permanently located in the cytoplasm of the recipient cell. Using antibiotic markers that permit cells with new plasmids to live and other cells to die, only cells containing the new plasmid will survive. After screening thousands of

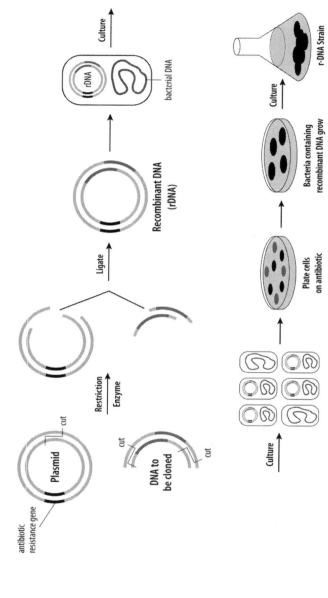

Figure 3   Cloning: This is the key process in molecular biology and the source of recombinant DNA (rDNA). A piece of DNA to be cloned and copied is cut in specific places by a DNA cleaving enzyme called a restriction enzyme. The cut DNA contains the sequence of base pairs (genes) to be cloned. A plasmid, designed to be inserted and to replicate in a host cell, is cut with the same restriction enzyme. The cut plasmid DNA and cut foreign DNA are spliced together with a DNA ligase enzyme. The plasmid containing the new DNA insert is delivered into the host bacteria through a process called transformation. Transformed host cells containing the plasmid are plated on media containing an antibiotic that permits only cells with the plasmid to survive. The surviving colonies containing the plasmid with the foreign DNA are cultured, and host cells are isolated and checked for the cloned gene. The plasmid can be purified and saved for experiments to test the new DNA or to isolate the cloned gene.

bacterial clones under the right conditions, where the gene making the desired protein can be synthesized and identified, one or many bacterial cells making the protein from the new piece of DNA inserted into the plasmid can be found.

Although the biochemical basis for the genetic code in all living organisms is the same, there is a significant difference between cloning in prokaryocytes, bacteria and other organisms without a nucleus, and cloning in eukaryocytes, mammalian and higher organisms with a nucleus. In prokaryotes, functional genes can be cloned directly from cellular DNA to produce mRNA transcripts that can be translated directly into functional proteins. This cannot be done in eukaryotes because mammalian genes contain extra nucleotide sequences that are noncoding DNA sequences called introns. Introns interrupt most mammalian genes and are sliced out of the final DNA sequences, called exons, that are translated. The role of introns in the eukaryotic genome is under study. This DNA has been referred to as nonsense or junk DNA. Clearly when the genomes of bacteria and mammalian cells are compared, eukaryotes contain hundreds of times more DNA than bacteria, although less than 5% may account for all genes. Genetic information in eukaryotes is present in a more disseminated and loose form. Direct cloning of eukaryotic DNA results in an mRNA transcript with introns that cannot be properly cut and spliced in bacterial hosts. To get around this problem, a complementary DNA (cDNA) is synthesized from functional eukaryotic DNA. One way to make cDNA is to isolate eukaryotic mRNA and use it as a template to synthesize cDNA using an enzyme called reverse transcriptase. The cDNA is a copy of the eukaryotic gene without the introns and can be used in cloning procedures. As the level of mRNAs varies in cells, making a complete copy or a cDNA library of a cell's mRNA generally requires some enrichment of the desired target mRNA. Strategies to make cDNA libraries from mammalian cells are critical to molecular biology research, and a range of cloning vectors and methods are available (10). The cloning procedure and the process to make recombinant DNA is the basis for every biotechnology company. It allows selected pieces of DNA and RNA to be made in large quantities in special host cells. Because the genetic code is so similar among bacteria, animals, and humans, the tools for cloning work in many systems, especially between humans and bacteria. This technology produced the first genetic engineering company, Genentech, in 1978. Genentech synthesized DNA for the hormone insulin, cut it, recombined it with a plasmid from bacteria, and transformed it into *E. coli* where bacterial cultures were found making the first human protein, human insulin. In 1982, Eli Lilly marketed human insulin as made in *E. coli*, called Humulin®, the first genetically engineered drug. This was remarkable, repeatable with other hormones and enzymes, and formed the basis for modern biology and the biotechnology industry. Starting with antibiotics made by specific molds and bacteria, we now had recombinant bacteria with pieces of human genes that made valuable human proteins in fermenters.

With this background our definition of biotechnology becomes clear. We define biotechnology as products produced by microorganisms in which the genes are modified by recombinant DNA technologies. It leaves out important areas, such as animal and plant cloning and major modifications of human genes. However, it includes a wide view of a technology that can deliver mechanisms to identify targets, develop fermentation strategies to produce them, and create new products and a view of the future that will produce value-added products for personal care applications.

TOOLS OF BIOTECHNOLOGY

Progress in science and development of new technologies has always been directly related to the perfection of new tools and processes. The telescope, microscope, and transistor were inventions that ushered new fields of study of astronomy, microbiology, and computers. Biotechnology is no different. There are several key tools that propelled biotechnology to its remarkable maturity and complexity in less than 50 years.

Once cloning was understood, it could be done in a high school laboratory if one had plasmids, *E. coli* bacteria, and restriction enzymes. There was an explosion of cloning experiments that resulted in new and unusual DNA, and molecular biologists needed to know three things about their experiment. One, what was the DNA sequence that was cloned? Two, was the cloned DNA expressed (i.e., cloned DNA to mRNA copy to protein sequence) in the bacteria? Three, what was the amino acid sequence of the new protein? Two biochemistry tools became the rate limiting steps in biotechnology progress—the DNA sequencer and the protein sequencer. The discovery of the structure of DNA by Watson and Crick ushered in a new urgency to understand DNA, RNA, and the interactions between these molecules and proteins. Although proteins and their building blocks, amino acids, were known and studied for years before the knowledge of DNA as the directing agent came along, their complexities were formidable. Built around the possibilities of 20 building block amino acids as their basis, proteins could be structural components, such as keratin in fingernails; large molecules that attacked invading bacteria, such as the gamma globulins in antibodies; and enzymatically active molecules with diverse properties, such as digestive proteins found in saliva or the gut or such smaller proteins as insulin, a hormone. Proteins had complicated secondary and tertiary structures, but each had a primary linear sequence that could be elucidated. In 1967, the Edman (11) degradation procedure for peptides and small proteins led the way and eventually became automated as the amino acid sequencer. In almost parallel developments, peptides and proteins up to 20 amino acids long could be synthesized by wet biochemical procedures and automated on resins designed by Merrifield (12) at Rockefeller University. Now, automated machines synthesize 100 amino acid long proteins with quality and efficiency using computer programs and (11) specialized amino acid derivatives. Insulin, the mammalian hormone used to treat diabetes, was one of the first proteins to be completely sequenced, one of the first proteins to be synthesized, and the first protein to be cloned, made in bacteria, and commercialized as a recombinant DNA product.

Machines used to sequence and synthesize proteins were critical to biochemical structure and function, but the machine directly associated with the genetic revolution and science of genomics was the DNA sequencer. Because the amino acids in proteins were ultimately coded by linear combinations of three nucleotides, knowing the direct nucleotide sequence revealed what the linear amino acid sequence would become and ultimately how the protein should fold into its correct structure. If you knew the base sequence in a piece of DNA from a particular gene, then you had direct knowledge of what kind of protein sequence the gene made. DNA sequencing was first done during the late 1970s using enzymes that cut DNA and resynthesized it after the four nucleotides were labeled with radioactive phosphorous 32 and then the pieces run on long polyacrylamide gels. The gels were developed by autoradiography, and the presence of the sequences could be read from the pattern on the film. Although this method worked, it required skill to perfect, was tedious, and generated radioactive wastes that had to be stored carefully. In 1986, at the Caltech Laboratories in Pasadena, Leroy Hood's group (13) automated the entire sequencing process by replacing radioactive bases with fluorescent nucleotides that could be distinguished by a fluorescent reader. The gels were still needed, but the machine read the gels and generated DNA sequence that could be run over and over until the operator was confident in the detailed sequence. Better and more powerful machines have been developed since then, and their speed, accuracy, and fidelity have reached a level of quality that has permitted the elucidation of the full sequence of genomes, containing 500 to 40,000 genes and 100 times that many base pairs.

Another tool in every molecular biology laboratory, and in many forensic labs, is the DNA cycler. In 1985, Kary Mullis (14), a researcher at Cetus, an early biotechnology company now defunct, invented a method to take a small amount of DNA, even 100 molecules, treat it with a DNA polymerase enzyme, and amplify the original DNA. This process, called PCR, or the polymerase chain reaction, is done by heating the DNA sample to be amplified. For separating the two strands to create single chains, new primers are added along with the four nucleotides and the DNA polymerase enzyme, resulting in additional set of copies of the original DNA but now in double the original amount. This recycling could be done for hours with fidelity, and the result would be a multiplication of the original DNA from 100 copies to five billion. Once this amount of DNA is available, it is easy to sequence it, and that knowledge decodes the sequence of the original trace DNA sample. Mullis shared the 1993 Nobel Prize for this invention. From small dried samples of blood, hair, or cells left from fingerprints, workers in forensic laboratories now use this basic technique to specifically identify genes of individuals. The PCR machine is a critical tool in the investigation and proof of criminality in both current and old cases.

As the basic science progressed, so have the cloning tools, recombinant hosts, and even strategies to modify the genomes of whole animals. Kits are available to clone, to make mutations in DNA, to find and generate peptides, to fingerprint proteins, and to express genes in many different backgrounds. *E. coli* is still important, but it is used mainly as a research tool. A wide variety of cells including insect cells, like the Baculovirus system are available for cloning and protein expression. Large-scale protein production from recombinant DNA is performed using fungi like *Aspergillus* and *Trichoderma*, bacteria like *Bacillus*, and mammalian cells, like CHO cells for human proteins and mouse cells for antibody production.

Two methods of genetic manipulation in whole animals have found widespread use in research. Methods have been developed to clone foreign genes into animals and to delete specific genes out. The first technique generates transgenic animals, animals that from birth contain a gene of another species. The new gene is inserted into the genome of a fertilized egg and the eggs are implanted into a foster mother. Offspring are tested for the new gene and positive animals are bred to establish a new strain. Examples of this technology are the production of human proteins and human antibodies in cattle and the generation of green mice, transgenic mice that contain a green fluorescent protein originally found in jellyfish.

The genetic method that deletes specific genes from animals is called "knockout" and has been used to make knockout mice. A recombinant purified gene is purposely made defective and inserted into an embryonic stem cell. The cells are cultured and screened to find those containing the altered gene and are expanded in culture, injected into an embryonic cell group called a blastocyst, and implanted in a foster mother. Offspring are selected for the altered gene and mice with the genetic alteration are bred to create a new strain. Knockout mice have been used to study the loss of a particular enzyme or receptor protein in mouse metabolism, or to delete parts of the mouse immunological system to study responses against diseases. In the personal care area, knockout mice have been used to study skin development, fur color, and hair growth modulation.

Enzyme and Protein Engineering

As the tools of cloning and DNA manipulation drove biotechnology, new strategies were developed to modify everything an organism does and to change protein and metabolite production in order to engineer new and unusual biochemical pathways in organisms. The technology that deals with mutations, host manipulations, and screening has now become the predominant technology behind product production. The best example is the practice of enzyme engineering. Twenty years ago all commercial enzymes like papain, rennet, and subtilisin detergent proteases were made by extracting plant, animal, or bacterial cultures and by purifying and concentrating the preparations sufficiently to get active ingredients that could be added to different processes. Now, more than 90% of all commercial enzymes (15) are made with the assistance of recombinant enzyme engineering to maximize production. The first application is always to increase yields because nature never intended bacteria or any organism to overproduce anything, unless by accident, and that accident would not be competitive for long. Organisms are shaped and perfected for their environment by evolution and competition to make what is needed to survive efficiently. Historically, it was known that in every million bacteria there were a few special cells or mutants that overproduced a protein or metabolite and could be isolated and purified. These special cells could be mutated, and the overproducers successively isolated and mutated again. Now, microbiologists go to all ends of the world looking for extremophiles, organisms thriving in hot springs, in arctic cold water, in acid and high salt fields, and in high radiation sites. To survive in these extreme environments, organisms make special adaptations, such as specific molecules for osmoregulation, or specialized enzymes, such as enzymes from thermophiles that are stable at high temperatures. The special enzymes from these extremophiles are then cloned into host bacteria designed to grow at high concentrations in fermenters. As a safety precaution, these host cells have built-in genetic deficiencies that do not permit them to exist in nature. These commercial strains are not only safe for the environment but also produce levels of recombinant product never observed in nature. With this strategy, relatively obscure and minor enzymes made at milligrams/ liter can be upregulated until they are secreted into the growth medium at 10 g/L. Often the cloned gene is present in multiple copies of plasmids, or the host bacteria has increased abilities to secrete proteins or has many of its natural proteases removed. The product of the cloned gene is made at high levels, secreted rapidly, and builds up to high concentrations in the culture fluid, where it can be rapidly purified and recovered.

But extraordinary increases in production are only part of how enzyme engineering is used. An enzyme gene can be rationally manipulated by mutation and cloning strategies, and with the proper screening tools, it can be continually modified to perform better in such applications as detergents, or biomass conversion processes, or in the generation of high fructose corn syrup. Most often, its pH optimum, or heat stability, or substrate specificity can be modified. This is done by making specific changes to the enzyme DNA by single base-pair changes or by whole-scale modification by incorporating cassettes of different base pairs or by mixing the genes of related but different enzymes to create new genetic variants with different diversities. Using these techniques, the gene for a protease that works in detergents can be modified and designed to be resistant to bleach, to operate at higher or lower pH optima, to hydrolyze more actively on blood or grass stains, and to be more stable to all the other detergent ingredients, especially surfactants. These new compositions of biological matter are referred to sometimes as designer enzymes (16) and represent some of the most useful applications of genetic engineering, to make products that can carry out specific industrial applications.

Pathway Engineering

Mammalian cells can also be engineered and modified by the tools of biotechnology to make and secrete antibodies, enzymes, and hormones at levels never thought possible. In fact, in many cases recombinant products from mammalian cells, such as albumins and gamma globulins, are often preferred over the same products from natural sources, especially blood-related product extracts that may contain the AIDS viruses and prions that cause Mad Cow disease. Once single products are modified to increase production or to change activity, additional changes to the host production cells (microorganisms or mammalian cells) can be made to facilitate product production and make it even more efficient. This strategy is called pathway engineering (17) and represents the techniques of total cellular manipulation to achieve a particular goal. At its simplest, it means taking bacterial or mammalian cells and adapting them to grow on inexpensive nutrients, such as glucose, to make desired end products as efficiently as possible. Pathway engineering uses all the tools of biotechnology to identify both genes that need to be added or replaced and the desired enzymes and proteins that the cells need to maintain themselves as efficiently as possible. Typical changes engineered into organisms include making bacterial cell grow rapidly on cheap nutrients, removing many biochemical side pathways, deregulating other pathways, increasing the cell's ability to secrete proteins, preventing sporulation in spore-forming organisms, or allowing growing cells to divide no more than a planned number of times. An example of pathway engineering was the production of the plant dye indigo in bacteria. To make quality indigo for textile dyeing, changes to more than 10 metabolic pathways (18) were made in *E. coli*, and once the entire biosynthetic pathway was constructed, the bacteria were able to make indigo from glucose at 17 mg/mL. Joined with cell extraction and recovery steps, indigo was produced in an environmentally friendly process identical in quality to one that was chemically synthesized.

Pathway engineering is a powerful strategy generally used to make products other than proteins. The carbon flow is streamlined to generate the desired bacterial product, remove contaminants, and make it easier to recover and purify. Recently it has been used to make both 1,2 propanediol at 135 g/L and an intermediate of vitamin C by converting 97% of the starting material glucose into product (17). Through pathway engineering, the possibility of making simple chemical products at large-scale commercial levels at costs comparable to the chemical industry shows the way to a future where manufacturing processes that sustain rather than degrade the natural environment can be designed. Using pathway engineering and recombinant technology, hyaluronic acid, a product used in personal care applications, was historically extracted from animal carcasses but can now be manufactured in *Streptococcus zooepidemicus* (19) cells and purified to pharmaceutical standards.

Genomics and the Human Genome

In the mid-1980s, with key biotechnology tools in place, scientists began thinking about the largest biology project ever imagined. The project—complete sequencing of the human genome—was a goal so beyond the ordinary that it was equivalent in space technology to going to the moon. The genome represents the total of all the genes possessed by an organism. James D. Watson, who codiscovered the double helix, was a key proponent in convincing the National Institutes of Health (NIH) of the U.S. government in 1988 to sequence the entire human genome. At first, it was criticized as a work project made only for molecular biologists and a scientific fantasy. But with rapid improvements in technology, within a few years, an international consortium of laboratories was involved in the task. Through this endeavor, several disease-related genes, such as cystic fibrosis and the Huntington disease gene, were discovered, and the project soon demonstrated the real promise of linking genes with specific human diseases. Work continued on the human genome and on the genomes of many organisms. In 1995, the genome of the bacterium *Haemophilus influenzae*, with 1000 genes, became the first complete genome to be sequenced, soon followed by the genomes of yeast, *E. coli*, the fruit fly, Drosophila, and the first plant, *Arabidopsis thaliana*. In 2001, the human genome was published by a private company, Celera Genetics, and by the public consortium led by NIH (20). Less than 50 years since the discovery of DNA, and four years earlier than originally expected, the sequencing of the human genome was essentially complete. Competition between private industry and government-supported programs was generally considered responsible for the rapid and unexpected pace of progress.

By 2004, we could step back and look at the science of genomics (21), defined as the study of all the genes in an organism and how they direct growth and development and determine biological function. All 23 human chromosomes have been sequenced. Key disease genes were assigned to each chromosome, and many new human proteins were proposed and searched for on the basis of the genetic code. The most unexpected finding was that instead of more than 100,000 human genes, there were between 30,000 and 40,000, with much of the DNA being introns, or nonsense sequences, sequences not coded into protein, sequences with no obvious functionality as far as we know. In fact, it became clear that the proteins that make up the individual cell and do the work of life were more numerous, probably 300,000 or more, and more complicated. Although we knew a finite number of genes made up the human genome, we were still a long way from understanding how everything worked and how the genes and their products interacted with the environment.

An important part of genomics is comparing DNA among humans, animals, and bacteria. The information gathered from such comparative genomic studies is very data intensive, and so analysis cannot be done manually. An entirely new science to solve this problem has emerged, called informatics, requiring specialized skills, specialized software, international data libraries, and banks of networking computers. Now (22) more than 125 bacterial genomes, 1600 viral genomes, and several mammalian genomes, including human, rat, and mouse, have been sequenced. With a network of computers, it's possible to compare one genome against all others in a short time frame of 48 hours. The results have been humbling. The DNA of humans, bacteria, and all living things, even plants is very similar All races of man share at least 99% of the same DNA. Human and chimpanzees share 98.8%, and mice and humans share 97% of DNA. Once the first primitive living cells replicated using DNA, the future direction of life on earth was set. For that reason all living things share the same genetic chemistry.

The Gene Chip

DNA knowledge will set the stage for a fundamental revolution in health care, biological processes, and individual customized medicines. Such new sciences as nutrigenomics, the understanding of interactions between nutrition and genes, and pharmacogenomics, understanding the interaction of drugs with genes, are in their developmental stages and will emerge in the future. One application of genomics is the possibility of customizing drugs, personal care products, and treatments for each person based on single, individual genomes. But, how is this done? How do biotechnologists start with the information in the human genome and derived products and treatments that will be able to cure disease and improve the quality of life?

Let's use the human genome database and tools of modern biotechnology to investigate a problem of red skin, such as that observed in rosacea or lupus. These skin problems have complicated pathologies but often have an underlying immunological basis. The first step is to take blood samples from a group of patients that shows clinical signs of these problems and ideally from patients who have a family history of these same or similar problems. Rarely is there one gene or one protein that is responsible, but many disorders are caused by multiple genetic problems resulting in deficiencies or excesses of proteins.

The first analysis is the personal genome (23) analysis. It is now possible to purchase a gene chip or DNA microarray (Fig. 4) with one copy of every piece of normal human DNA. It works like this. A one-centimeter square piece of glass is coated with special polymers, usually positively charged that will bind pieces of DNA or RNA. Pieces of oligonucleotides up to 40 base pairs or pieces of c-DNA up to 1000 bases from each chromosome that have been cloned to remove nonsense DNA segments are spotted by robots on the slide in segments corresponding to the major genes in the particular chromosome. Not every gene is included, but hundreds of genes from each chromosome can be represented on the gene chip. The DNA pieces are aligned and covalently attached to the chip

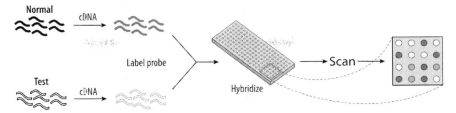

Figure 4 DNA microarrays: Microarrays permit the analysis and comparison of DNA samples by taking advantage of the property that DNA will bind to its complementary partner. DNA from a normal sample and a test sample are isolated, cut, and prepared into short pieces called probes. In the case of human DNA, this requires making cDNA copies of the samples in stable single-stranded form. These probes are labeled with a fluorescent dye so that the control and test probes have a different signal. The probes are hybridized with a glass chip, the surface of which contains an orderly arrangement of DNA pieces from all or a selected group of genes. The DNA pieces are ordered in position by chromosome number or other patterns that can be detected by the scanner. The DNA probes are reacted with the microarray containing the known DNA pieces. Probes bind to their complementary strands on the microarray. After washing and processing, the microarray is analyzed for the fluorescent signal, and a comparison is made between the control and test signals. The location of the signal on the chip identifies the specific gene.

so the molecule is basically linear and in single line arrays. To this chip is added a sample of the patient's individual c-DNA that has been isolated, purified, and cut with a variety of restriction enzymes and is in a single stranded linear, nonhelix form following a PCR reaction. In addition, the patient's c-DNA is labeled with fluorescent probe. Under different temperatures and buffer conditions, the patient's DNA pieces are permitted to hybridize to and bind their DNA partners. After the hybridization process, excess reagents are washed away, and the entire microarray is scanned for fluorescent activity. By the position of the signal in the gene chip, a readout of the genes in the patient's samples can be determined. To facilitate the analyses, the process may be done by comparing normal and test DNA samples at the same time. These experiments are done with several chips to reduce the noise and error in the analysis and often done at different times to reduce normal variability. Once this is done, a first screen of the patient's DNA can be obtained, and key information about hormones, cytokines, enzymes, and other biochemical and genetic characteristics may be estimated. For our red skin example, the analysis might show the presence of increased amounts of such immune mediators as cytokines and interferons.

The data obtained in the first gene chip is used as a screen to focus in on the problem. Now, another gene chip is used but one that is specific for immunity associated genes and peptides known to mediate skin reactions. As genetic disorders are often problems of quantity rather than outright absence or presence, another gene chip that analyzes for single nucleotide polymorphisms (SNPs) is also tried. SNPs (23) represent minute, personal variations in DNA bases that are responsible for our individuality. Often individuals have single changes in their DNA that affect the production and/or number of genes that can express a particular protein. In sickle cell anemia, a base-pair change modifies a protein that not only causes red blood cells to become less susceptible for malaria but also to have a less efficient shape to carry oxygen. A gene chip with SNPs is able to pick up mutants or individual genes that may be less likely to generate quality proteins. In fact, although we all share 99% of all DNA, the 1% of the genome that constitutes SNPs are responsible for our differences. The patient's DNA is mixed with a special SNP gene chip containing DNA strands filled with known SNPs, to give a much finer and focused version of the immunological capacity of each patient. After analysis, this secondary gene screen can reveal specific genetic deficiencies due to SNP changes that signal hormonal or cytokine problems.

Proteomics

Once a gene target is identified as a potential problem, confirmatory assays need to be done, usually by a proteomics procedure to confirm the absence or presence of the protein. As the excitement in genomics converts into routine identifications of problem genes, a new frontier, called proteomics has emerged (24). Proteomics is the study of the entire pool of protein, the proteome, that a cell or organism makes. Proteomics is a more complicated science than genomics and lags further behind it because the biochemical rules for protein folding and protein interactions are less well worked out than for DNA and RNA. In fact, although there are super computers and numerous groups working on this problem, it is still impossible to take a string of amino acids and predict how it will fold in solution and how effectively it will interact with the other protein surfaces it must interact with and recognize. The genome may show the map of possibilities, but protein interactions, including binding and catalysis by enzymes, are the forces that make all cells function. Already there are 35,000 enzymes from all organisms (25) that are tracked in databases, and this is expected to increase. If there are 30,000 human genes, there are a quarter to half a million proteins associated with those genes. The 20 amino acids involved in making proteins generate huge possibilities of different structures due to linear and conformational options. Moreover, in mammalian cells, there is a whole range of possible posttranslational changes, biochemical changes that occur beyond the normal, DNA to RNA to protein, resulting in phosphorylations, glycosylations, and many other biochemical modifications. Most occur as biochemical changes in the cytosol, in membranes, or in specialized endosomes. In addition, there are biochemical changes (26) proteins undergo just sitting in a cell and serum milieu that result in even greater numbers of different proteins, including protease clips, dimers and multimer formations, and critical combinations of specific protein amino acids with carbohydrates, metals, lipids, and salts. Recently, it has been found that plants, bacteria, and now mammals have the ability to join protein fragments present in the cytosol. This finding will further expand the total number of proteome components. Thus, in order to understand how proteins interact with each other as well as with other macromolecules to perform their function, it is important to exactly know what proteins are present in a given cell under any specific condition. Several new tools to help investigators identify the human proteome are now available.

Monoclonal Antibodies

Monoclonal antibodies are a 20-year-old genetic and protein technology that has constantly generated new products and serves as a supporting technology for many proteomic tools, including the protein chip.

Protein chips are like gene chips that analyze for individual proteins and peptides rather than genes. However, the basis for recognition of a specific protein on a chip is its specific binding with another protein. One commercially advanced concept uses monoclonal antibodies (Fig. 5), one of the first products of mammalian molecular biology and genetic engineering. In 1975, Kohler and Milstein in Cambridge invented a procedure to make highly specific antibodies, called monoclonal antibodies. Antibodies are large mammalian proteins of a molecular weight of 155,000 daltons and are key to the adaptive immune system in humans. When bacteria or viruses attack us, the body responds with a first line of

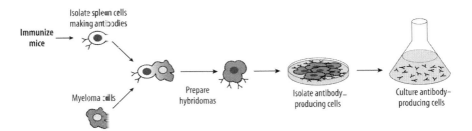

Figure 5 Monoclonal antibody production: The adaptive immune response of mammals generates a variety of antibodies to natural infections and most antigens. This is called a polyclonal response because many different antibody-producing cells are stimulated to generate populations of antibodies that have differences in specificity, in binding strength, and in cross-reactivity. Monoclonal antibody technology permits the generation of specific populations of antibody molecules that derive from one clone and thus produce one kind of antibody. Mice are immunized with an antigen. After generating an immune response, antibody-producing cells in the spleen are removed. The spleen cells are fused with myeloma cells to make hybrid cells called hybridomas that are capable of continued growth as well as secretion of the antibody made by the fused spleen cell. Hybridomas are plated on special media to reject the unfused cells and can be isolated in pure form. Individual cells are screened for secretion of specific antibody, and the best producing hybridoma clones are cultivated and the specificity of the antibody characterized.

defense with killer cells, innate binding proteins, and macrophages. After an incubation and synthesis period of three to seven days, lymphocytes make and secrete antibody proteins that are specific to the invader. The most common antibody is immunoglobulin G, IgG. It has two binding sites and reacts with invaders in the body to coat, aggregate, and sensitize them for destruction and clearance by other components of the immune systems. Each antibody arises from specific IgG secreting lymphocytes called B cells. Although one cell clone can be expanded to generate a large antibody response, generally there are many B cells making different antibodies to the complexity of surface proteins and antigens of the invaders. The entire library of antibodies is called a polyclonal response. A polyclonal antibody response is good for fighting bacteria and viruses and a great insurance strategy for recurrent infections, but it is much less useful while using antibodies as exquisite binding tools. Kohler and Milstein developed a procedure from immunized mice generating a multitude of B cells making different antibodies in the spleen. Individual B cells were removed from isolated mice spleens, and they were fused with a class of cells called myelomas—cells that grow like tumor cells. When individual spleen cells making one antibody fused with the myeloma cell, the result was a cell called a hybridoma, a cell with two parents capable of making one antibody for many cell generations. Using special and selective media, hybrid cells could be isolated while individual spleen and myeloma cells were allowed to die. The successful hybrids were grown in mice in ascites fluid or in culture and represented a cell line capable of generating the specific monoclonal antibody for many cell generations.

Mouse hybridomas can be grown in culture flasks like bacteria, and these cultures produce and secrete an antibody with a single specificity. Now, monoclonal antibody cultures can be cultivated in special fermenters with synthetic media. The antibodies can be isolated, purified, and used as a specific protein drug, a reagent for immunoassays, or histochemistry, or as a diagnostic marker for a specific protein.

The Protein Chip

Although it took monoclonal antibodies more than 20 years to mature, they currently represent the greatest class of new biotechnology drugs that are in the pipeline. From cancer markers, to cytokines, to antireceptors, monoclonal antibodies are specific tools that have found many uses. One future use will be protein chips (28), also called protein microarray. Hundreds of specific monoclonal antibodies made, isolated, and characterized can be immobilized on chip substrates via their nonbinding end, so the working end, the antigen binding arms are above the chip free in solution and ready to interact with their antigens, complementary proteins in solution. To detect the presence of a particular protein in a given sample, the sample can be washed over a protein chip. If the sample contains proteins that the monoclonal antibodies on the chip can bind, those proteins will be bound, whereas others will be unattached and free in solution. After washing to remove unbound and nonspecifically bound contaminants, a reagent is added to detect antibody–antigen complexes. As in the gene chip procedure, the location of positives on the chip indicates what specific proteins are present or absent. This is done automatically, and data readouts report what specific proteins and at what concentration levels they are present in the sample.

Of course, not every protein will have a specific antibody and not every peptide or glycoprotein will be identifiable, but it is predicted that protein chips as powerful as gene chips will be available to confirm and even go beyond the information obtained with gene chips. In the future, the captured molecules need not be antibodies but can be allergens, nucleic acids, substrates, and carbohydrates. Robinson et al. (27) developed an array of more than 200 peptides and proteins to study antibodies to multiple sclerosis and its animal model. In the case of autoimmune diseases, specific antigens, drugs, or allergens might be immobilized on chips and the entire antibody repertoire in a person's serum can be probed and compared to a normal serum or an earlier or different sample from the same person. Thus a simple screening test would show if a person has antibodies to penicillin, is making antibodies to thyroid proteins, or has viral antibodies or an antibody to known cancer antigens. Clearly, the technology of protein chips has a more diverse and more quantitative use than gene chips and could replace gene chips for looking at specific protein problems, such as self-antigens, hormone deficiencies, or antibodies to viral and bacterial antigens. For example, in the case of Lupus, where a person makes antibodies to their own DNA, a protein or antigen chip could be used to detect and identify the problem, and therapeutic measures taken to alleviate it. In addition, protein chips with specific targets could permit a faster and cheaper analysis for patients undergoing hormone or other therapies with therapeutic drugs.

Mass Spectrometry

Another tool with great implications for biotechnology and proteomics in particular is the mass spectrometer (29). This machine permits the detection of small and medium size peptides/proteins and even permits their specific identification. There are several machine strategies, but all work by ionizing proteins and forcing them to move through an electric field in a way that permits selection and detection of different protein molecular weights. The best mass spectrometer (MS) machines not only detect proteins by their individual molecular weights but also are able to put selected proteins through a fragmentation process that in principle generates a series of amino acid sequences that are characterized by their molecular weights. Using the molecular weight data of fragmented peptides, and comparing this data with databases in libraries throughout the world with reference proteins, individual proteins in a complex mixture can be unambiguously identified. MS databases contain the amino acid sequences of thousands of mammalian, bacterial, and viral proteins. Very large proteins can be purified and fragmented with specific proteolytic enzymes to permit the ideal size to be analyzed by mass spectrometry. These machines can detect picomoles of proteins and peptides and offer a view into complex biological samples that simplifies protein detection. Quantitation of proteins is still difficult, as is the identification of proteins that are in less than 1% abundance levels. Nevertheless, coupled with typical high performance liquid chromatography and gel electrophoresis procedures, mass spectrometers are becoming the chosen method to identify proteins in the proteome. Especially important are the capabilities to identify modified proteins, such as glycoproteins, or phosphoproteins by molecular weights and then by using specific hydrolytic enzymes, to confirm their presence. Several labs are in the race and have rooms full of mass spectrometers working day and night to elucidate the entire human proteome, an accomplishment most experts don't expect to happen until the tools of proteomics improve.

A powerful strategy in proteomics development is the merging of the protein chip with the Matrix-assisted laser desorption ionization (MALDI) mass spectrometer (26). An unknown solution is reacted with a custom designed special surface to affinity capture a class of proteins, such as groups with acidic or basic components. After an incubation and binding step, the unbound proteins are washed away, leaving a surface with numerous target proteins. This surface is analyzed by a MALDI mass spectrometer, an instrument that knocks off bound proteins with a laser device and provides the molecular weight of the desorbed protein. This technique, called surface enhanced laser desorption/ionization (SELDI), is capable of rapid protein profiling, and can discriminate many protein classes based on different protein chips.

CURRENT AND FUTURE PRODUCTS FROM BIOTECHNOLOGY

Based on a listing of current products from biotechnology, we can gauge the depth and span of its application and make some estimation on how this technology would affect the personal care market. Table 2 shows a list of such products, which are all proteins but differ markedly as to their function. The first blockbusters were hormones, such as insulin, and such cell growth activators as Neupogen® and Epogen®. The newest set of products is monoclonal antibodies directed against a variety of cancer targets, such as breast cancer and non-Hodgkins cancer. Because there are so many monoclonal antibodies (more than 200!) in clinical development, they will dominate the list of new products

Table 2 Products of Biotechnology

Product examples	Function	2003 Estimate (in billion $)
Humulin®	Hormone	2
Interferons	Cytokines	16
Neupogen®/Epogen®	Growth stimulators	2
Targeted cancer antigens	Monoclonal antibodies	2
Therapeutic enzymes	Glycohydrolases	1
Detergent enzymes	Proteases, amylases, lipases	1

in the next five years. Another important protein class of products is enzymes, used both in commercial and therapeutic applications. In terms of volume and commercial value, protease enzymes, as used in detergents, represent the single largest use for recombinant products.

In personal care, the estimated market value for enzymes in lotions, contact lens, and dental products is $100 million. This is quite small compared to the market value of any product listed in Table 2. Now, a molecular understanding of skin disease is available. Because of this, a strategy to achieve more directed cosmetics is feasible. Skin care, for example, is an area in personal care where biotechnology could be used to develop targets and products. In this context, there are two general areas where biotechnology-derived products could make an impact: fixing such problems as psoriasis and inflamed skin and delivering products that will grant cosmetic wishes, such as elimination of age spots or the maintenance of baby-like skin.

For psoriasis, damaged tissue samples can be analyzed and compared with normal healthy tissue. Key genetic markers in the immune system and on such lymphocyte cell surfaces as HLA (human leukocyte antigen) molecules can be identified in the target population and compared with the total population. Both genomic and proteomic tools to compare tissues, individuals, and related reference samples can be used. With these tools, one could identify potential (genotypes) problems, such lack of an estrogen-synthesizing gene or presence of the gene but lack of estrogen-associated mRNA to make the hormones. After the genomic screens, a functional phenotypic screen to pinpoint and confirm the hypothesis could follow. Proteomic screens can be used to show real deficits in the target tissue for estrogen, estrogen receptors, or estrogen-synthesizing enzymes. Using other proteomic screens, one could look at specific immunological problems, such as self-antibodies to skin antigens or skin cell components, or increases or decreases in key skin biochemical molecules, including cytokines, normal degradative proteases, normal antibacterial peptides, and normal proteolytic inhibitors. Once the results of these screens are available, the best target for therapy that has minimal side effects could be chosen. The new data would help select a therapy to address structural, proliferative, or even nutritional and metabolic problems. Primary human keratinocytes are susceptible to gene transfer and have been genetically engineered (30) to contain foreign enzymes that act as bioreactors to detoxify excess metabolites.

The strategy to address cosmetic wishes is similar. Aging and wrinkled skin is caused by complex genomic, physiological, and environmental factors. In this case, the genetic and proteomic screens are focused on the target and the associated biochemistry. As cosmetic wishes have been pursued throughout history, there may be examples in the literature of successes based on evidence or anecdotal that may provide direction. The key to a strategy is the understanding of the underlying molecular and cellular processes and their interaction. The new products in this area will probably be cytokines that treat such skin problems as psoriasis, enzymes that remove old skin and make it smooth, and hair modifiers that remove, oxidize, or reduce hair. Skin coloration and skin spot reducers will be potential products, as will inflammation inhibitors and biochemical agents that maintain youthful skin. New biotechnology-based products will not be restricted to proteins but would also encompass such nonprotein products as polymers, hyaluronic acid, and its derivatives, as well as small molecules that will be useful in the cosmetics industry.

This was our introduction to biotechnology and the new tools and processes being used now and in the future. The following chapters will expand on these ideas in detail and explore research, applications, and therapies in personal care.

REFERENCES

1. Desrosier NW. Elements of Food Technology. Westport, CT: AVI Publishing Co. Inc., 1977.
2. Fishman HM. Cosmetics, past, present and future. In: Schlossman ML, ed. The Chemistry and Manufacture of Cosmetics. Carol Stream, IL: C.V. Mosby Co., 1988:1–10.
3. Barrett JT. Textbook of Immunology. Saint Louis, MO: CV Mosby Co., 1970.
4. Stanier RY, Doudoroff M, Adelberg EA. The Microbial World. 2d ed. Englewood Cliffs, NJ: Prentice-Hall, 1963.
5. Burnet FM, White DO. Natural History of Infectious Disease. 4th ed. New York, Cambridge University Press, 1972.
6. Avery OT, MacLeod CM, McCarty M. Studies on the chemical nature of the substance inducing transformation by a desoxyribonucleic acid fraction isolated from pneumococcus type III. J Exp Med 1944; 79:137–158.
7. Watson JD, Crick FH. Molecular structure of nucleic acids: a structure for deoxyribose nucleic acid. Nature 1953; 171:737–738.
8. Jackson DA, Symons RH, Berg P. Biochemical method for inserting new genetic information into DNA of Simian Virus 40: circular SV40 DNA molecules containing lambda phage genes and the galactose operon of Escherichia coli. Proc Natl Acad Sci USA 1972; 69:2904–2909.
9. Morrow JF, Cohen SN, Chang AC, Boyer HW, Goodman HM, Helling RB. Replication and transcription of eukaryotic DNA in Escherichia coli. Proc Natl Acad Sci USA 1974; 71:1743–1747.
10. Ying S-Y. Generation of cDNA Libraries. In: Ying SY, ed. Methods in Molecular Biology, Vol. 221. JM Walker, Series Editor. Towanda, NJ: Humana Press, Inc., 2003.
11. Stryer L. Biochemistry. 2d ed. San Francisco, CA: WH Freeman & Co, 1981.
12. Merrifield RB. Solid phase peptide synthesis. 1. The synthesis of tetrapeptide. J Am Chem Soc 1963; 85:49–54.
13. Smith LM, Sanders JZ, Kaiser RJ, Hughes P, Dodd C, Connell CR, Heiner C, Kent SB, Hood LE. Fluorescence detection in automated DNA sequence analysis. Nature 1986; 321:674–679.
14. Mullis KB, Faloona FA. Specific synthesis of DNA in vitro via a polymerase-catalyzed chain reaction. Methods Enzymol 1987; 155:335–350.
15. Cherry JR, Fidantsef AL. Directed evolution of industrial enzymes: an update. Curr Opin Biotechnol 2003; 14:438–443.

16. Gustafsson C, Govindarajan S, Minshull J. Putting engineering back into protein engineering: bioinformatic approaches to catalyst design. Curr Opin Biotechnol 2003; 14:366–370.
17. Sanford K, Valle F, Ghirnikar R. Pathway engineering through rational design. Gen Engg News 2004; 24:44–45.
18. Berry A, Dodge TC, Pepsin M, Weyler W. Application of metabolic engineering to improve both the production and use of biotech indigo. J Ind Microbiol Biotechnol 2002; 28:127–133.
19. Chong BF, Nielsen LK. Amplifying the cellular reduction potential of Streptococcus zooepidemicus. J Biotechnol 2003; 100:33–41.
20. International Human Genome Sequencing Consortium. Initial sequencing and analysis of the human genome. Nature 2001; 409:860–921.
21. Galas DJ, McCormack SJ. An historical perspective on genomic technologies. Curr Issues Mol Biol 2003; 5:123–127.
22. Rappuoli R, Covacci A. Reverse vaccinology and genomics. Science 2003; 302:602.
23. Roth CM, Yarmush ML. Nucleic acid biotechnology. Annu Rev Biomed Eng 1999; 1:265–297.
24. Mullner S. The impact of proteomics on products and processes. Adv Biochem Eng Biotechnol 2003; 83:1–25.
25. Greener M. Enzymology's new frontier. The Scientist 2004; 18:16–20.
26. Binz PA, Hochstrasser DF, Appel RD. Mass spectrometry-based proteomics: current status and potential use in clinical chemistry. Clin Chem Lab Med 2003; 41:1540–1551.
27. Robinson WH, Steinman L, Utz PJ. Protein arrays for autoantibody profiling and fine-specificity mapping. Proteomics 2003; 3:2077–2084.
28. Liotta LA, Espina V, Mehta AI, Calvert V, Rosenblatt K, Geho D, Munson PJ, Young L, Wulfkuhle J, Petricoin EF, 3rd. Protein microarrays: meeting analytical challenges for clinical applications. Cancer Cell 2003; 3:317–325.
29. Mann M, Hendrickson RC, Pandey A. Analysis of proteins and proteomes by mass spectrometry. Annu Rev Biochem 2001; 70:437–473.
30. Christensen R, Jensen UB, Jensen TG. Skin genetically engineered as a bioreactor or a metabolic sink. Cells Tissues Organs 2002; 172:96–104.

2

Personal Care Products via Fermentation and Biocatalysis Processes

Erick J. Vandamme and Wim Soetaert

Department of Biochemical and Microbial Technology,
Faculty of Bioscience Engineering, Ghent University, Ghent, Belgium

HISTORICAL

Ancient Egyptians, Greeks, and Romans, the Incas and Aztek cultures, all of them frequently used personal care products (cosmetics). Cleopatra's baths in asses' milk and the conspicuous makeup and malachite eye shadow of Nefertiti and of the pharaohs still appeal to our imagination. The embalmment of the deceased pharaohs and the makeup articles found in their tombs are evidence of their interest in and knowledge of cosmetics. They already tried to counteract the formation of wrinkles by means of an ointment based on the fenugreek plant. The Greeks and the Romans also applied massage oils on a large scale. The Greek Theophrastus (372 B.C.) and the Roman Galen (130–200 A.D.) wrote the first systematic books about the preparation of cosmetics through the introduction of distillation and extraction processes. Via the crusaders and the Portuguese and Spanish explorers, cosmetics gradually became known in Europe. During the Renaissance, cosmetics and perfumes were still mainly used at the royal courts. Not until 1900 did they come within reach of ordinary citizens.

Today, cosmetics and personal care products play an increasing role among primitive as well as so-called civilized societies. The level of cultural development of a society can usually be measured by the use of cosmetics and toiletries in general. Indeed, cosmetics are as old as the hills. Cosmetics are products with a complex composition, in very expensive packagings, and with high added value; in addition to a physiological function, they fulfill an important psychological role: looking good and feeling good.

After a brief explanation concerning cosmetics of chemical, vegetable, or animal origin, a general survey is presented here of personal care and cosmetic ingredients, which are made by or via microorganisms or their enzymes. More detailed aspects of cosmetic/personal care products of microbial origin and their bio-production processes have recently been published by the authors (1–4).

CHEMICAL SYNTHESIS OF COSMETIC INGREDIENTS

In a wider sense, the chemical "synthesis" of cosmetic ingredients also comprises the isolation of individual components from the essential oils, like rose oxide from Bulgarian oil of rose, which smells intensely of "green grass," such as citral from oil of lemon grass, eugenol from clove oil, geraniol from citronella, and terpinol from turpentine. These isolated base compounds are often chemically further derivatized. Moreover, a great many cosmetic ingredients that do not even occur in nature are now synthesized in the laboratory; this has led, among other things, to perfumes that are now available at prices the general public can afford. The famous civet and musk are so expensive that they have now been replaced by their synthetic equivalents, civetone and muscone. By simple synthesis from phenol, isobutene, and acetic acid anhydride, one obtains 4-tertiary butyl cyclohexyl acetate, a component with an intense smell of green/woods. Also most surfactants (detergents) that constitute the basis of many cosmetic products, such as shampoos, are produced by chemical means. The chemically prepared sugar alcohols sorbitol, glycerol, mannitol are widely used moisturizers (humectants). Chemical coloring agents (titanium dioxide), emulsifiers, coating agents, waxes, special fats, preservatives, metallic luster, and so on are employed especially in facial and eye makeup and in lipstick. Deodorants are mainly based on Al- and Zr-salts (aluminum chlorides, sodium zirconium lactate). Many sun protecting preparations contain cinnamates, p-aminobenzoic acid (PABA)-esters, and oils, which offer protection against ultraviolet (UV)-B radiation in particular. For further details concerning chemically prepared cosmetic ingredients, the reader is referred to the specialized literature.

So far, the majority of cosmetic ingredients are indeed synthesized chemically. The spirit of the times, the lifestyle, and growing environmental awareness have led to the "back-to-nature" phenomenon, resulting in an increasing (re)turn to natural raw materials, whether of vegetable, animal or, indeed, microbial origin. The term "cosmeceuticals" is coming to be used more and more, particularly when it concerns ingredients of a high degree of purity, which have a health effect, which are also biodegradable, and which have been "ethically" tested (i.e., in an animal friendly manner) (5).

PLANT- AND HERBAL-DERIVED PERSONAL CARE PRODUCTS

Components of plants, including perfumes derived from plants, have been used in cosmetics since time immemorial. Fatty acids and their alkaline salts, the basic ingredients of sol d and liquid soaps, are derived from coconut oil or palm oil, allantoin from the horse chestnut and azulenes, and α-bisabolol from camomile oil and yarrow oil (6). These ingredients occur in a large number of skin-care creams: cocoa butter and jojoba oil in lipstick and lip salve and avocado lipids, soybean sterols, and lecithins in various preparations. Selective plant extracts, which are specifically used in cosmetics, comprise among others:

> lichens (*Usrea barbata*), which are frequently used in deodorants because of their antibacterial properties
> liquorice (*Glycyrrhiza glabra*), which displays anti-irritant properties
> *Ginkgo biloba* leaves, used as radical scavenger and as antioxidant
> bearberry leaves (*Arctostaphylos uva-ursi*), containing high levels of arbutin and used for whitening the skin.
> green walnut shells (*Juglans regia*), rich in 6-juglon and which darkens the skin

Recently, α-hydroxy acids (AHA) and the polyunsaturated fatty acids (PUFAs), that is, γ-linolenic acid (GLA) and derivatives, extracted from plants and fruits, have become popular ingredients in many skin moisturizing and skin anti-aging cosmetic preparations. Volatile essential oils with a terpene character—such as lavender oil, jasmine oil, oil of rose, oil of citron, bergamot oil, patchouli oil, and others—are obtained from plants through steam distillation, extraction, or enfleurage and are used generally in perfumes. Pearlescent effects can be obtained by mixtures of fatty acids, glycerides, and derivatives, obtained from plant and animal sources (7).

ANIMAL-DERIVED PERSONAL CARE PRODUCTS

Certain very rare and now priceless components of animal origin are also used in cosmetics and perfume, such as civet (from the civet cat), ambergris (from the sperm whale), musk (from the musk deer), and castoreum (from the beaver). The well-known wool fat lanolin, collagen, elastin, and beeswax, which are widely used in skin-care creams, can also be mentioned (8). "Antiwrinkle" creams contain various animal proteins (bovine serum albumin, ovalbumin, pig placenta albumin) that subsequently dry into the skin and thus mechanically tighten it. There is a trend though to switch increasingly to plant-derived protein, that is, from wheat, oat, peas, *Acacia*, and so on. Mother-of-pearl glossy nail polish for the nails contains shiny substances that are derived from fish scales.

MICROBIAL PROCESSES AND PRODUCTS FOR COSMETIC USE: GENERAL ASPECTS

Today, many useful microorganisms are exploited as tiny but efficient factories: they are indeed capable of synthesizing a whole range of bulk and (chiral) fine chemicals, peptides, enzymes and so on via sophisticated fermentation processes, based upon renewable resources (starch, sugars, etc.) and performing very well under mild conditions of pH, temperature, and pressure in an aqueous medium (9,10).

Here we will focus on typical microbial processes and their products that find application in the cosmetic and personal care sector (Tables 1 and 2).

As is true for many other novel fermentation processes and products, Japanese companies have been in the frontline (i.e., Shiseido Co. since 1985; Tanabe Seiyaku Co.). In the meantime, several well-known "western" cosmetic and perfume companies have included such biocosmetics into their product range. Microbiological synthesis (fermentation) is generally accepted

Table 1 Microbial Products as Skin Moisturizers in Cosmetics

Product	Producing microorganism or enzyme	Applications in cosmetics
Hyaluronan	*Streptococcus zooepidemicus*	Water retention Gelling agent Diffusion of cosmetic ingredients
Poly-(1-4)β-D-glucuronan	*Rhizobium meliloti*	Gelling agent Water retention Emulsion stabilization
L-Fucose rich polysaccharide (Fucogel®)	*Klebsiella* sp., *Clavibacter* sp.	"Perfect touch" Water retention Decreasing allergic response
Chitosan	*Mucorales* fungi	Skin moisturizing Film forming on the skin Anti-*Candida* activity Bacteriostatical (skin, hair, and oral hygiene)
Xanthan	*Xanthomonas campestris*	Stabilization of emulsions and suspensions (toothpaste, etc.) Water retention (ointments, lotions, shampoos) Gelling agent (deodorant gels, etc.)
PUFAs (γ-linolenic acid, GLA)	*Mortierella* fungi	Water retention Anti-aging of the skin
Ceramide (sphingolipids)	*Pichia ciferri* en *Candida*—yeast fermentation, followed by chemical acylation	High water-retention capacity Against skin scaling Skin moisturizing (in gels, etc.)
Ectoines	*Halomonas* sp.; aerobic halophilic eubacteria	Skin moisturizing

Abbreviation: PUFAs, polyunsaturated fatty acids.

Table 2 Microbial Products for a Younger and/or Safer Tanned Skin

Product	Producing microorganism or enzyme	Applications in cosmetics
Dihydroxyacetone	*Gluconobacter oxydans*	Self-tanning products
Malyltyrosine,	*Micrococcus*	"Quick-tanning" molecule
tyrosineglucosinate	*caseolyticus* protease	Soluble melanin precursor
Urocanic acid	*Achromobacter liquidum* ammonialyase	Protecting agent against UV-B radiation
(Pro)vitamins (D-panthenol, niacine, vitamin E, vitamin C, β-carotene, PUFAs)	Various bacteria and fungi	Against skin aging Antioxidant
Ubiquinone (coenzyme Q_{10})	*Saccharomyces* yeast	Antiwrinkle effect
Amino acids (SER, ASP, GLU, OH-PRO) (+sorbitol, lactic acid)	*Corynebacterium glutamicum*	Moisturizing effect Cell growth stimulation Natural moisturizing factor (NMF)−effect
Yeast glucan derivatives (carboxymethyl-poly-β(1,3) glucan	*Saccharomyces cerevisiae*, other yeasts (*Tremella* sp., etc.)	Skin protecting Immunostimulant
Kojic acid	*Aspergillus* sp.	Skin lightening
α-Arbutin	Enzymatic glucosylation of hydroquinone (*Bacillus* sp., *Leuconostyoc* sp., *Xanthomonas* sp., etc.)	Treatment of age spots
Hydroxyguiacol	*Fungi, yeast (from ferulic acid)*	Antioxidant Suncare
Caffeic acid esters	Enzymatic hydrolysis of chlorogenic acid (in sunflower seed meal)	UV-A and UV-B absorbers Ethylhexylester is a liquid product, facilitating formulation
(Allo)Melanins	Enzymatic polymerization (polyphenoloxidase) of caffeic acid	UV-absorbers Antioxidant Skin pigmentation

Abbreviations ASP, aspartic acid; GLU, glutamic acid; CH-PRO, hydroxyproline: SER, serine; UV, ultraviolet.

as a natural process, in which simple sugars are converted via a controlled fermentation process into valuable molecules. Chemical synthesis of many of these "microbial" molecules is difficult or unknown, or the extraction from plants or animal tissue is too complex or even risky. The recent bovine

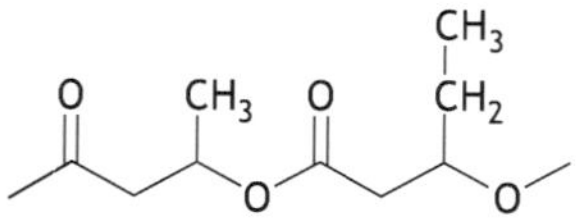

Figure 1   Structure of poly-β-hydroxybutyrate/valerate.

spongiform encephalopathy (BSE) scare and related prion diseases have forced industry to search for alternatives for animal (tissue) derived products (2,4).

It appears that the cosmetic industry is quite determined to give itself a sound environmentally friendly reputation, not only by increasing use of biologically produced ingredients but also by introducing recyclable packaging materials. A fine example here is the shampoo bottle marketed by Wella (Germany), moulded from poly-β-hydroxybutyrate/valerate (Biopol®) (Fig. 1). This biopolymer is an intracellularly stacked reserve material of among others the bacterium *Ralstonia eutrophus*. This polyester "bioplastic" has been produced on a large scale through fermentation, among others by Monsanto and formerly by Zeneca-ICI (U.K.). Another bioplastic material is a polylactide developed by Cargill Dow; it is based on lactic acid, produced by fermentation and then chemically polymerized into a biodegradable plastic.

MICROBIAL PRODUCTS FOR SKIN CARE

Hyaluronic Acid as a Second Skin

Hyaluronic acid (HA), a biological polymer, has long been known. HA is applied in ophthalmology, and new applications are found in surgery, drug delivery, orthopaedics and joint operations, cardiovascular medicine, and in cosmetics. It is a regular heteropolymer of the β-1,3 coupled dimer glucuronic acid and N-acetylglucosamine which is β-1,4 coupled to a following identical dimer (Fig. 2). HA is a highly viscoelastic glycosaminoglucan-polymer that forms part of the connective tissue in all vertebrates, where it lubricates the joints and acts as a "shock absorber"; this substance is also responsible for the maintenance of the semi-elliptical form of the human eye and the consistence of the aqueous humor. Highly pure HA, from whatever source, has an identical structure, although its molecular weight can vary depending on the source and the isolation procedure. The molecular weight is a critical factor depending on the application. Generally, the higher the molecular weight, the better (and more expensive) the product. Until recently, HA needed to be laboriously extracted and purified into a nonimmunogenic, noninflammatory fraction from cockscombs, shark skins, and umbilical cords! Estée Lauder was the first one in 1982 to apply animal HA in cosmetics. However, HA is also a component of the capsule occurring in certain *Streptococcus* bacteria (Lancefield group A or C).

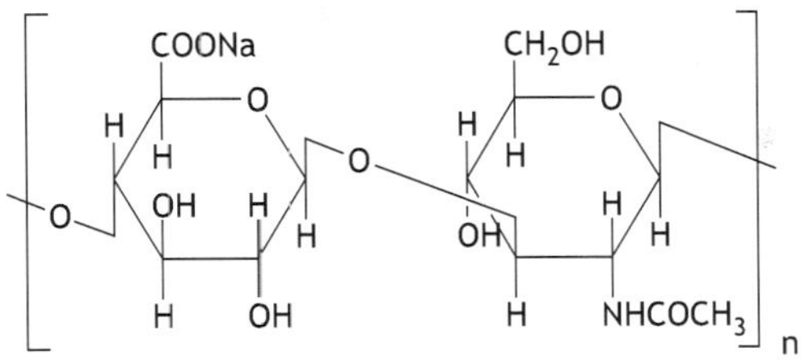

Figure 2 Structure of hyaluronic acid.

This has led to HA production through fermentation. Shiseido Co. has been producing HA since 1985 through fermentation with the capsule-forming bacterium *Streptococcus zooepidemicus*. Today HA is marketed by Biomatrix (U.S.A.), Bio-Technology General (Israel), Diagnostic Inc. (U.S.A.), Fermentech (U.K.), Genzyme (U.S.A.), Kibun Food Chemifar Co. (U.S.A.), Med. Chem. Products (U.S.A.), Pharmacia (Sweden), and Shiseido Co. (Japan) (11). Novozymes has recently announced the low-cost production of very pure high molecular weight HA that makes use of a *Bacillus* organism, a significant improvement over the use of the (pathogenic) *Streptococcus* organisms. In the cosmetics sector, the sodium salt of HA with a molecular weight of 1.1 to 1.6 million daltons is used as an ingredient of ointments, lotions, and makeup for skin care: it protects and lubricates the cells, helps in the transport of certain molecules, and controls moisture retention.

Fucogel® for a Perfect Touch

Recently, it has been demonstrated that the slimy capsular polysaccharide material, rich in the rare sugar L-fucose and produced by such bacteria as *Klebsiella* sp. and *Clavibacter* sp., can act as an efficient skin moisturizer. When applied as a film, it has a perfect psychosensorial touch and lowers the allergic response (12) (Fig. 3). Such a polysaccharide from *Klebsiella* sp. is marketed under the name of Fucogel and is also an excellent formulation agent.

Chitosan as Moisturizer and Biofilm

Chitosan is the deacetylated form of chitin (Fig. 4). Chitin is a β-1,4-polymer of N-acetylglucosamine, which is found in the cell wall of most fungi and the exoskeleton of crustaceans, krill, and insects. Chitosan occurs naturally only in the cell wall of the *Mucorales* fungi (*Mucor mucedo, Rhizomucor miehei, Absidia coerulea*), from which it must be extracted. It can be used as an encapsulating agent for biocides, seeds, fertilizer, and others in agriculture and as a flocculant in water purification. Oral ingestion has a cholesterol-lowering and fat-reducing effect. Mention has also been made of the use of chitosan as an agent in wound

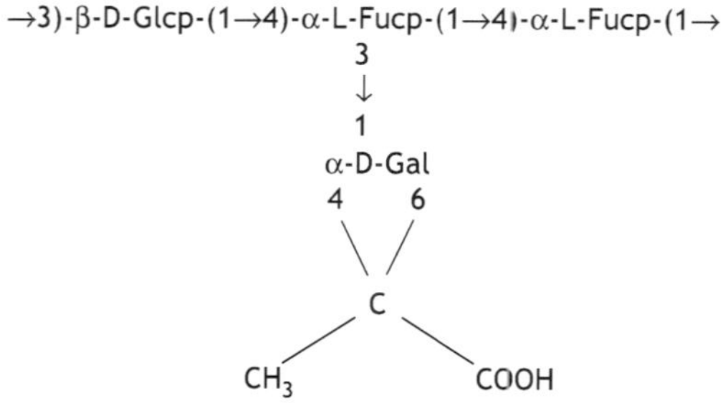

→3)-β-D-Glcp-(1→4)-α-L-Fucp-(1→4)-α-L-Fucp-(1→
                            3
                            ↓
                            1
                        α-D-Gal
                        4   6
                         \   /
                          \   /
                            C
                          /   \
                       CH₃   COOH

Figure 3 Structure of the repeating unit of *Clavibacter* sp. capsular polysaccharide.

healing and surgery, as an antitumor agent, and as an immunoadjuvant. It is also used in cosmetics, including in lotions for hair, skin, and oral hygiene. Producers are Cognis (Germany), Amerchol Corp (U.S.A.), Dainichiseika Color & Chem. Co. (Japan), American Cyanamid (U.S.A.), Protan (The Netherlands), Kyowa Oil & Fat Co. Ltd. (Japan), Novachem Ltd. (Canada), and others. The derivative N-carboxymethylchitosan also has several applications as a chelating substance, external protectant of seeds, skin moisturizer, transparent film former, stabilizer of emulsions. It is applied in cosmetic ointments for the sake of its permanent moisturizing capacity (e.g., Crema Idratante of Aleph, Italy) and film formation on the skin. It also contains bacteriostatic and *Candida*-cidal activity, a property that cannot be attributed to many other cosmetics ingredients!

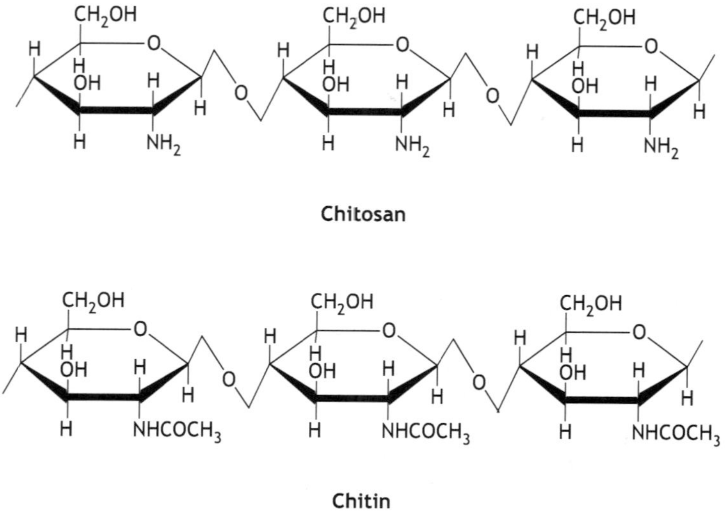

Chitosan

Chitin

Figure 4 Structure of chitosan and chitin.

Xanthan and Other Microbial Exopolysaccharides as Waterbinders

Xanthan is industrially produced through fermentation with the bacterium *Xanthomonas campestris* (20,000 ton/year). Xanthan is a biopolymer (which is formed extracellularly) with a β-1,4-glucan backbone. This chain has side chains consisting of mannose acetate, mannose, glucuronic acid, and pyruvate (Fig. 5). The combination of various unique physicochemical properties (pseudoplastic rheology, viscosity independent of pH, temperature, and salt concentration, etc.) renders this biopolymer extremely useful for numerous applications. By adding xanthan to paints, pesticides, detergents, fire-extinguishing agents, pharmaceutical preparations, explosives, printing inks for paper and fabrics, cosmetics, and so on, the viscosity, flocculation, jellifying, and rheological behavior can be controlled. Xanthan is marketed by Merck & SD-Kelco Inc. (Keltrol® and Kelzan®) (U.S.A.), Rhône-Poulenc (Rhodopol 23® and Rhodogel 1®) (France), Sanofi-Bioindustrie (Satiaxane) (France), Lohman Fermentations (Viskotan®) (Germany), Jungbunzlauer (Austria), Gist-Brocades (Maxaflo®) (The Netherlands), and others. In the cosmetics sector, it is applied in toothpaste and as an emulsion and suspension stabilizer and waterbinder in ointments, lotions and shampoos, and after-sun preparations. A mixture of xanthan gum and locust bean gum (St. John's bread) is also used in deodorant gels.

Another exopolysaccharide (EPS) with molecular weight ranging from 6.10^4 to 4.10^5 is produced by the bacterium *Rhizobium meliloti*. Chemical characterization has shown that the polymer is a (1-4)β-D-glucuronan, which is partially acetylated on the 2 and/or 3 position.

It forms a gel at low concentrations and does not precipitate in the presence of ethanol or polyethylene glycol and stabilizes emulsions that contain up to 50% oil. Its favorable moisturizing, jellifying, and thickening properties allow many applications in medicine, pharmacy, and cosmetics. Applications in cosmetics are primarily based on the special jellifying capacity, the water retention properties,

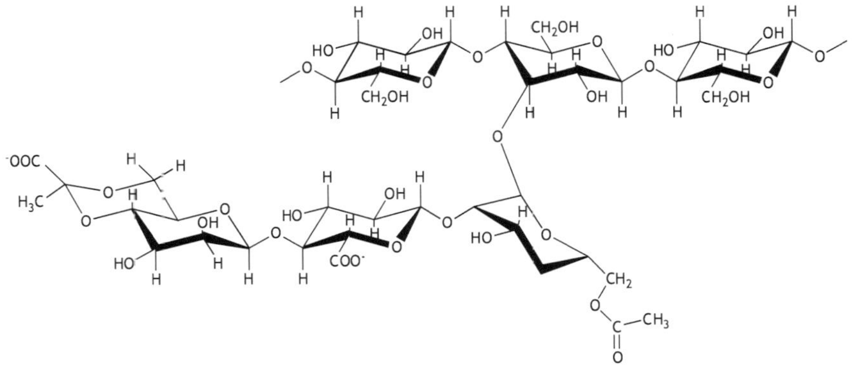

Figure 5 Structure of xanthan.

and stabilization of emulsions. It can compete with (microbial) products, such as xanthan and carboxymethylchitosan, which have been known longer.

Ceramide Against a Dry Skin

Ceramides are lipids with a high water retention capacity, which occur in the epidermis of the skin. They give the effect of a soft and shiny skin and prevent the formation of scales. Thus, it has been shown that the ceramide 1 content is too low in psoriasis patients. In a division of DSM, Cosmoferm BV (The Netherlands) and in the South Korean company Doosan-Serdary, a new process has been developed to produce specific ceramides (13).

Through fermentation, a ceramide precursor is synthesized by a yeast strain. This biosynthesis proceeds via desaturation of palmitoyl-coenzymeA and coupling with L-serine. This ceramide precursor is subsequently extracted from the fermentation medium and then converted into (phyto)sphingosine base (C-18 compound). This molecule is in turn converted into various (phyto)ceramides through acylation with various fatty acids, obtained via *Candida*-yeasts.

Two ceramides thus prepared with important cosmetic applications are ceramide 3 (Fig. 6), which contains phytosphingosine, acylated with stearic acid (C_{18}:0) and phytoceramide 1, a C_{18}-phyto-sphingosine base with a very low amide-coupled C_{27} α-hydroxy fatty acid, esterified with a C_{18} fatty acid (it is a so-called acyl-ceramide). Through this combined biotechnology and chemotechnology, it is possible to obtain ceramide derivatives with even better moisturizing properties. Such sphingolipids form highly stable liposomes (called "sphingosomes"), which can be used in moisturizing gels and slow-release systems. Certain (phyto)sphingosines also possess strong anti-inflammatory activity, and their glycosylated derivatives (the glycosphingolipids such as cerebrosides and gangliosides) play an essential role in brain cell and nerve cell membranes.

Amino Acid, Ectoines, and α-hydroxyacid (AHA) Mixtures as Natural Moisturizing Factor

Amino acids have been added to many cosmetic preparations with a moisturizing (fluid-regulating) effect. A mixture of the amino acids L-serine, L-aspartic acid,

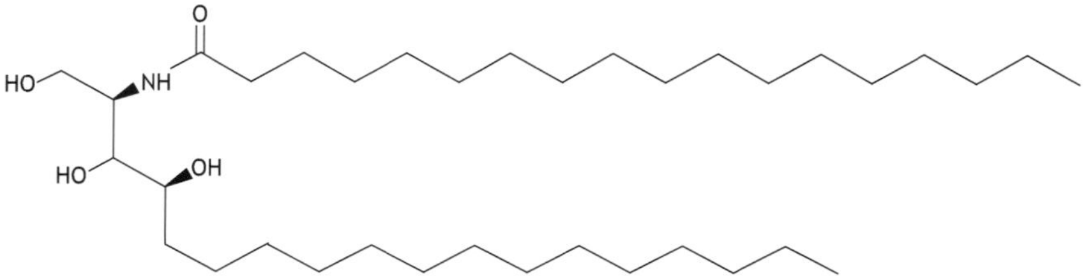

Figure 6   Structure of ceramide 3.

2-Methyl-3,4,5,6-tetrahydro-4-pyrimidine carboxylic acid (Ectoine)

2-Methyl-5-hydroxy-3,4,5,6-tetrahydro-4-pyrimidine carboxylic acid (S,S-β-Hydroxyectoine)

Figure 7 Structure of ectoine and hydroxyectoine.

L-glutamic acid, and L-hydroxyproline, in combination with sodium lactate and sorbitol, has a moisturizing effect comparable to the so-called natural moisturizing factor (NMF) of the skin. These L-amino acids and L-lactic acid and their salts are produced through industrial fermentation via *Corynebacterium* mutants and *Lactobacillus* strains, respectively.

Other skin moisturizing molecules related to amino acids are the ectoines. Natural ectoines protect the membranes of skin cells from destabilization and loss of water (Fig. 7). Ectoines are produced by extreme halophilic bacteria (*Halomonas elongate*, *Vibrio* sp., *Ectothiorhodospira*, *Marinococcus*, etc.) and by halotolerant aerobic bacteria (*Bacillus* sp., *Brevibacterium* sp., *Streptomyces parvulus*, etc.), when grown in the presence of high salt concentration (150 g/L). They are hygroscopic cyclic amino acid derivatives (ectoine and hydroxyectoine), which behave as an osmoprotectant (compatible solute) for the bacterial cells. They can be released from the bacterial cells by osmotic downshock. They aggregate large hydration shells and are therefore stabilizing natural polymers and membranes. As such, there is growing interest in producing these ectoines by fermentation for use as skin humectant in cosmetics or as a stabilizer of enzymes and cells during storage, (freeze) drying, and so on (14).

AHAs (α-hydroxyacids) are a class of compounds, which have unique effects on skin structure. Their application at a low concentration (below 5%) decreases intercorneocyte cohesion and induces skin peeling. Especially short chain AHAs, such as lactic acid and glycolic acids, exert very good exfoliating and moisturizing effects. At higher concentration, they become irritant and penetrate too quickly into the skin. To prevent such effects, AHAs can be grafted into lipophilic molecules or on carbohydrates. An example is the transesterification between α-butylglucoside and butyllactate into α-butylglucoside lactate with *Candida antarctica* lipase (Novozym 435) (15).

(Pro)Vitamins

Vitamins are eagerly used in various cosmetics and are sought after even more fervently as an item to be mentioned on cosmetic packagings. It is doubtful whether these added vitamins are really physiologically active upon topical application on the epidermis, the hair, and so on, unless it is possible, for instance, to enhance their skin migration through liposome or cyclodextrin inclusion. D-Panthenol, a vitamin B_5-analogue, niacin (vitamin B_3 or PP) and α-tocopherol (vitamin E) are used frequently in shampoos and in preparations against skin aging. Vitamin Q_{10} (ubiquinone) has a distinct antiwrinkle effect on the skin. A healthy diet and eventually oral vitamin supplementation usually have a more lasting effect.

Yet, they can also be extremely useful in cosmetics because of their additional properties, such as an antioxidant (β-carotene, vitamins C and E), acidulant (vitamin C), and biopigment (β-carotene, riboflavin) activity. For the production of almost all vitamins (both fat and watersoluble), fermentation processes have been developed on an industrial scale (16,17).

Sunless Tanning and Sunlight Protection Agents

Dihydroxyacetone (DHA) is the only nonchiral keto-triose sugar, and it has a strongly reactive keto group; it is a white, crystalline powder with a sweet, cool taste. It is highly soluble in water, alcohol, acetone, and ether. Thanks to its chemical structure, DHA is a product with many applications. Thus, it is a valuable intermediate in the synthesis of different organic chemicals. DHA is used in certain butadiene–styrene polymerization recipes and in the synthesis of certain fungicides. However, one of the most widely known commercial applications of DHA is in cosmetics, where it is used as an active component in self-tanning lotions. The keto group reacts with L-arginine, which is present in the proteins of the epidermis, so that a tanning effect is obtained. The speed and intensity of the reaction depends on the availability of free amino groups of epidermal proteins, the pH of the skin, the presence of inhibitors, and so on. The growing awareness of the dangers connected with excessive sunbathing is turning the market for self-tanning agents into one of the fastest growing markets within the cosmetics sector. Through esterification with fatty acids, such as palmitic acid, surface active agents are formed that have emulsifying properties, which is important for applications in food, detergents, cosmetics, and toiletries.

The formation of DHA through microorganisms from glycerol was already established in 1898 by Bertrand. Since then, a great deal of research into this microbial fermentation process has been conducted, which is nowadays carried out on a commercial basis. The bacterium *Gluconobacter oxydans* is used industrially today for the production of DHA from glycerol. Chemical synthesis copes with difficulties and with a lower yield.

Malyltyrosine is also a "fast-tanning agent." Its synthesis is carried out by a *Micrococcus caseolyticus* protease, which links malic acid and L-tyrosine (both also produced microbiologically) through a peptide bond (Fig. 8). This reversed protease-enzymatic reaction proceeds most smoothly in an organic solvent.

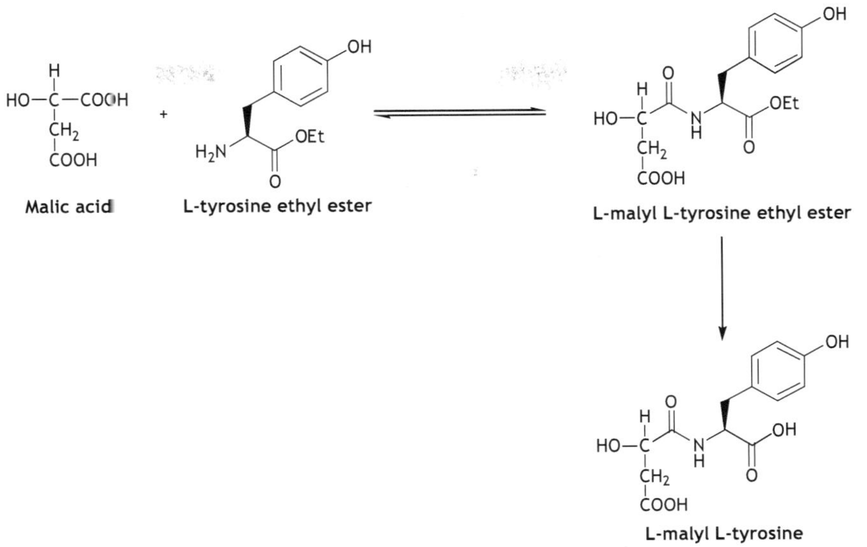

Figure 8 Enzymatic synthesis process of L-malyltyrosine.

Tyrosine glucosinate is also a natural tanning accelerator. Urocanic acid is a UV-B absorbing agent which is proper to the skin and is formed in the epidermal cells from L-histidine. Urocanic acid is now also produced microbiologically from the amino acid L-histidine, which is a fermentation product itself. This bioconversion is conducted commercially in Japan with the *Achromobacter liquidum* ammonialyase (7). It is used in suntan products that offer protection against UV-B.

Skin Depigmentation

Human skin pigmentation is the result of the synthesis and distribution of melanin pigments in the skin. The first steps in melanogenesis are catalyzed by tyrosinase (a copper containing polyphenol oxidase), catalyzing the oxidation of L-tyrosine via L-dihydroxyphenylalanine (L-DOPA) to dopaquinone. Pigmentation is principally determined genetically but can be stimulated by UV-irradiation, hormones peptides, chemicals, and so on. A healthy normal suntan appeals in Western society among young and old! Overexposure to UV and certain chemicals induces peroxidation of the skin, causing damage to epidermal cells, leading to local hyperpigmentation.

Skin color also plays a social role, in the sense that some black and Asian people tend to prefer a whiter skin pigmentation, whereas some westerners want to "hide" the dark spots on their skin, resulting from excessive sunning.

As a result, products are being developed to cause the desirable whitening effect, based on inhibition of tyrosinase: They include hydrochinon, arbutin, luteolin, kojic acid, and so on. Fermentations and biocatalytic processes have been developed to produce kojic acid and α-arbutin, respectively (18,19).

Others

The essential oil from the bud of *Eugenia aromatica*, which is generally called clove and known as a herb medicine, is widely used as a spice for cooking and as a balm. The main component, accounting for more than 90% of the clove essential oil is eugenol, which is used as a precursor for vanillin synthesis. Recently, it was found that eugenol shows an effect as a hair restorer. However, because eugenol is liable to sublimate and has a peculiar smell, its modification is needed for application as a component of hair restorers. Therefore, eugenyl-β-glucoside (β-EG) is being produced by organic synthesis and is now commercially used as an additive in hair restorers, since β-EG is gradually degraded into eugenol by the indigenous microorganisms of human skin and acts as a pro-drug of a hair restorer. Also eugenyl-α-glucoside is a useful derivative of eugenol; an efficient method for its selective production has been recently described, whereby eugenol was selectively α-glucosylated by α-glucosyltransferase from *Xanthomonas campestris*, with maltose as glucose donor (20). The ethylester of L-lysine can be "polymerized" with trypsin in a 2-propanol/H_2O mixture into oligolysine, a compound that limits rigidification of collagen skin fibers and counteracts wrinkle formation.

THE *CLOSTRIDIUM BOTULINUM* TOXIN FOR MEDICAL AND COSMETIC USE

The protein toxin produced and excreted by the anaerobic, endospore-forming soil bacteria *Clostridium botulinum* is probably the most poisonous molecule known on earth. It is known under the name of *botox*. This bacterial species was discovered and studied in 1895 by Prof. E. Van Ermengem, microbiologist at Ghent University, Belgium.

The *Clostridium botulinum* toxin complex consists of a neurotoxin and a stabilizing auxiliary protein. The heat-labile neurotoxin is itself a protein that contains about 1300 amino acids and consists of two protein chains linked through a cystein bridge. Seven antigenic serotypes (A to G) are known. A lethal dose (LD_{50}) consists of one nanogram per kilo body weight (21). The toxin can cause food poisoning, named botulism, through the eating of food that is contaminated with the bacteria or the toxin. The toxin migrates to the muscles and nerves, where it irreversibly blocks the release of the neurotransmitter acetylcholine (ACh), resulting in the weakening of muscles, dizziness, difficulty in breathing, paralysis, and ultimately death. In the 1930s, botulism was a much feared phenomenon, for instance in the production and introduction of canned food that was not always optimally prepared.

The toxin is heat-labile (inactivated at 85°C after 15 minutes), but *Clostridium* endospores can survive this heat treatment and subsequently turn quickly—anaerobically—into actively growing cells that excrete the toxin. Humans can also be contaminated through wound infections or through *in vivo* intestinal growth of the toxin-producing bacteria. Animals as well die of botulism, for example, water birds, especially when the water becomes oxygen-deprived, for instance because of the growth of other aerobic (oxygen-consuming) microorganisms (bacteria, algae, etc.). Several *Clostridium botulinum* types are known: A and B in humans, C and D in cattle, and so on. As recently as 2002, 164 cows were contaminated on a dairy farm in England: one hundred and forty-one of them died within two weeks. All symptoms pointed toward botulism as the cause, but the source of contamination (drinking water, feed, silage, etc.) and the *Clostridium*-neurotoxin could not be established unambiguously! This has led to increasing cautiousness (and uncertainty) concerning our "great" knowledge of botulism. This "botox" toxin can however be used medically, when applied in very low doses, as a "medicine" in the treatment of dystonia—these are involuntary and undesired muscle contractions in humans and animals. This principle was already tested in 1973 by Dr. E.J. Schantz (University of Wisconsin, Madison, U.S.A.), in collaboration with Dr. A.B. Scott (an ophthalmologist from San Francisco, California, U.S.A.), in order to treat, among other things, strabismus (squint, lazy eye, etc.), blepharospasm (closed eyelid) and other hemifacial spasms (22). In 1989, National Institutes of Health (NIH) experts and the U.S. Food and Drug Administration (FDA) gave permission to the therapeutic use, in nanogram doses, of a bacterial toxin! Nowadays it is used medically to cure focal dystonia around the neck, jawbone, vocal cords, (tennis) elbow, and so on, or to stop stuttering and migraine. It has made many operations and other medications redundant. However, repeated topical injections of the toxins remain necessary. Unfortunately, some patients develop antibodies to the toxin, which makes the desired effect disappear. Other (potential) medical applications are a.o. the weakening of muscles that control the activities of the stomach and the intestines or that cause clumbfoot, or to remedy the paralyses that are the consequence of a stroke, and so on. For a few years now, neurotoxin A is also being used in the cosmetic sector "to make disappear" wrinkles (crow's feet, etc.) in the skin (by relaxing skin muscles) or to counter excessive sweating and hyperhydrosis, and so on.

Also here there are very recent medical indications that long-term use of botox can lead to headaches, nausea, and heart disorders, and that after a cosmetic facial treatment with botox injections, new wrinkles ("face lines") can come into being. The botox toxin is produced through industrial fermentation processes with the appropriate *Clostridium botulinum* strains (especially type A, produced by the "Hall" strain, is clinically used). One either aims at the production of the toxin itself, or this toxin is subsequently transformed into a vaccine (23). As *Clostridium botulinum* produces endospores and is strictly anaerobic, special culture conditions need to be observed. The best growth is obtained at

35°C on glucose, protein hydrolysates, and yeast extract under nitrogen atmosphere. Contained fermentors with incinerators for exhaust gas and with control of pH, stirring speed, temperature, gas, and foam are necessary to obtain high exotoxin titers. The toxin is excreted by the cells in the culture fluid. After separation of the bacterial cells the toxin is again purified and eventually crystallized. This preparation is then applied in therapy and cosmetics. Already 50 years ago the principle of production and purification was laid down in the microbiological labs of the U.S. Army, in Fort Detrick, Maryland, U.S.A. At the moment several firms produce the toxin: Oculinum, Berkeley, California, U.S.A.; Oculinum®; Allergan Inc., Irvine, California, U.S.A. (Toxin A); Botox®; Elan Pharmaceuticals, U.S.A. (Toxin B); Myobloc®; Ipsen, U.K. (Toxin A); Dysport®; CAMR, Porton Down, U.K.

MICROBIOLOGICAL PRESERVATIVES AND "SKIN" PREBIOTICS

Many cosmetics contain preservatives, including various ones of microbiological origin. The fermentation products L(+)-lactic acid, propionic acid, citric acid, L-tartaric acid, L-malic acid are generally used as acidulants in this connection. Tests are under way to make it possible to use bacteriocins, bacterial oligopeptides with a narrow antimicrobial spectrum, as biological preservatives (e.g., nisin, pediocin) or as an agent to counteract acne (epidermin, gallidermin). It has also recently been demonstrated that certain short sugarchain molecules (gluco-oligosaccharides, GOS), prepared with *Leuconostoc mesenteroides* lactic bacteria from sucrose and maltose, have a beneficial effect on the healthy microbial skinflora; they promote the growth (and skin colonization) of useful skin bacteria such as *Lactobacillus pentosus*, *Micrococous kristinae*, etc.). This GOS preparation acts as a prebiotic, by favoring the growth of (lactic) bacteria, having a role in preventing undesirable microbial growth, leading to irritation, odor, acne, and so on. Such GOS compounds were recently incorporated in dermocosmetic formulations (such as Liphaderm®, Merck) with beneficial results.

MICROBIAL ENZYMES FOR PERSONAL CARE

Certain microbial enzymes are more and more added directly to cosmetics and toiletries. Some examples are:

Dextranase and/or glucose oxidase in toothpaste (to remove dextran in dental plaque).

Gluco-amylase/glucose oxidase, added to toothpaste and mouthwash, generate H_2O_2, which, together with thiocyanate (SCN) compounds, is converted into oxidised-SCN-compounds due to the lactoperoxidase in saliva; these oxidised-SCN-compounds subsequently inhibit the cariogenic bacterial flora.

Catalase which after perming the hair converts an excess of H_2O_2 and thus prevents discoloration of the hair; during the perming of the hair, thioglycolate is used to reduce the cystine bonds (—S—S—) in hair keratin to cysteine residues (—SH HS—) that—after application of the desired hairdo—are oxidized again by means of H_2O_2 upon which new cysteine and cysteine–lysine bonds are formed, fixing the new hairdo.

Superoxide dismutase allegedly protects the skin against radicals.

Keratinase is said to dehair more efficiently; lipoxygenase is claimed to slow down the regrowth of hair after depilation.

Serineprotease (Erase®) can be applied to remove old skin.

Tyrosinase stimulates the formation of the melanin pigment, thereby protecting against sunburn.

Photolyase (from cyanobacteria *Anacystis nidulans*) reverses DNA damage due to UV-B radiation.

CYCLODEXTRINS: JACK-OF-ALL-TRADES

α, β, or γ-Cyclodextrins (CDs) are cyclic α-1,4-D-glucose oligomers, which contain 6, 7, or 8 glucose units, respectively (Fig. 9). They are only produced

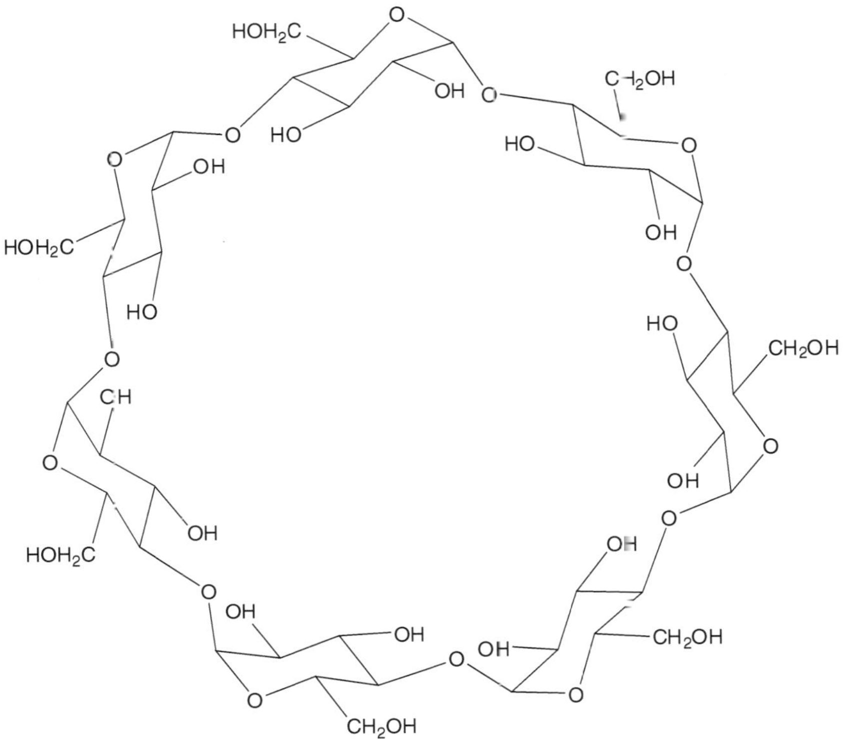

Figure 9 Structure of β-cyclodextrin.

from starch through the enzyme GGT-ase (cyclodextrin glucosyl transferase), which occurs exclusively in several bacteria (certain *Bacillus*, *Klebsiella*, *Micrococcus*, and *Thermoanaerobacter* strains). These torus-shaped molecules are hydrophilic on the outside and lipophilic in the central cavity. CDs form reversible molecular inclusion complexes with many "guest molecules" inasmuch as they are lipophilic and fit sterically in the CD cavity: This "micro-encapsulation" results in stabilization/protection (against light, oxidation, volatility, temperature) and/or alteration of the reactivity and physicochemical properties of the "guest molecule" (better water solubility, detoxification, masking of scent/taste, slow-release, conversion of liquids into powders, etc.). They are also suited as chiral selectors for the chromatographic separation of enantiomers. Countless applications already exist in the food industry, pharmacy, agrochemistry, and cosmetics, while new ones present themselves. Industrial producers are Akzo-Avebe (The Netherlands), Roquette (France), Rhône-Poulenc (France), Sanraku Inc. (Japan), Toyo Jozo (Japan), Nihon Shokukin Co. (Japan), Meito Sangyo Co. (Japan), Bioestron (Estonia), and Cerestar-American Maize (U.S.A.). The annual production now amounts to more than 20,000 tons; CDs were first produced commercially in Japan in 1976 (24). In cosmetics, CDs (particularly β and γ-CD) and their derivatives (e.g., methyl-CD) are used to solubilize lipid ingredients (e.g., essential oils, fat-soluble vitamins, steroids, etc.), in order to reduce irritation, to stabilize perfumes in soap and detergents, to absorb excess fat of the skin (in Matité® crème, Yves Rocher), or otherwise to promote the migration of molecules (e.g., L-carnitine) through the skin. "Empty" CDs are used as tablets or in chewing gum against halitosis and in deodorant sticks to complex lipophilic skin components and odors. Recently they are being marketed as textile deodorizers (Febreze®, Procter & Gamble) and as perfume–CD complex (Bounce®, Procter & Gamble) to obtain a slow release effect.

BIOSURFACTANTS

D-Glucose is industrially prepared through enzymatic (amylase, amyloglucosidase, pullulanase) hydrolysis of starch. The enzymes used are all of a microbial origin. Glucose can be derivatized in various ways—chemically or enzymatically—to surfactants with cosmetic applications, among others (25). Via the linking of the hydrophilic glucose molecule to a hydrophobic (fatty acid) molecule, amphiphilic compounds are formed, which possess surfactant-like properties (26).

Alkylglycosides, obtained through a chemical reaction of glucose with fatty alcohols, are efficient and mild surfactants: particularly well known are the alkylpolyglucosides (APG). APGs with a C10–C12 residue show good water solubility and foam stabilization and react synergetically with anionic and amphoteric surfactants, so that they are suited best as cosurfactants in shampoos and liquid soaps. Glycolipids with longer fatty acid chains are hardly soluble but display excellent emulsification properties. Particularly sugar (saccharose) esters have been developed for this purpose and are an excellent formulation aid in many cosmetics. Although these surfactants are mainly produced chemically, enzymatic esterification can also be performed with the *Candida (Pseudozyma) antarctica* lipase (27,28).

Surfactants are expected to be increasingly produced by fermentative processes. These biosurfactants have several advantages over the chemical surfactants, such as lower toxicity, higher biodegradibility, better environmental compability, high selectivity and specific acitivity at extreme temperatures, pH, and salinity, and the ability to be synthesized from renewable feedstocks.

A number of fermentation processes have been developed for the production of sophorolipids, rhamnolipids, and other glycolipids (29,30). High yields and concentrations of more than 100 g/L are generally obtained in these fermentations. For instance, the yeast *Candida bombicola* is able to convert a mixed carbon source of glucose and vegetable oil into sophorose lipids in a scale of 300 to 400 g/L with product yields up to 90% based on substrate weight (31).

BIOPIGMENTS FOR PERSONAL CARE PRODUCTS

Indigo: From the Plant over Chemical to Microbiological Synthesis

There is a trend toward substituting chemical/synthetic dyes by natural colors of (micro)biological origin (32–34). Indigo (E312) is one of the oldest natural blue colors. Mummies were wrapped since about 1500 BC in garbs dyed with indigo. In Western Europe, indigo was obtained indirectly from the woad (*Isatis tinctoria*) and from the 16th century onward from the tropical indigo plant *Indigofera tinctoria*. These plants contain in their green leaves the uncolored indigo precursors isatan B and indican, respectively. *Murex brandaris* (a kind of mussel) also yields a purple dye, called Tyrian purple. All these indogoid colors are derived from indigotine (Fig. 10). Fermentation of the leaves by the natural microbial flora yields from these precursors the yellowish water-soluble "indigo white." Through oxidation with air this transforms to the water-soluble indigo blue. Chemical or microbial reduction of indigo blue again forms indigo white. In such an indigo white solution, blue jeans cloth (jeans cotton) gets soaked and colored. When the cloth is taken out of the dye bath, it colors, through oxidation with the air, slowly from yellow to green to "jeans blue."

In 1870, the chemical formula of indigo became known and attempts for the chemical synthesis started. Success followed in 1896. From the 1920s

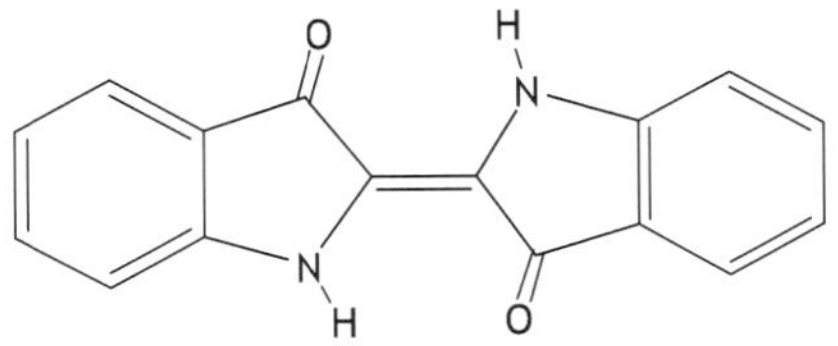

Figure 10 Structure of indigotine.

onward indigo blue was chemically synthetized on a large scale on the basis of aniline, formaldehyde, and natriumcyanide—which was not exactly a "green process." The synthetic indigo has nevertheless supplanted the natural indigo almost completely.

Indigo can now also be produced biotechnologically through bacteria from glucose. Several bacteria (*E. coli*, *Serratia* sp.) can produce the amino acid L-tryptophan from glucose through well-known pathways of fermentation; L-tryptophan is subsequently split into indol by the enzyme tryptophanase. After the genetic transfer of a *Pseudomonas* gene, which codes for naphthalene dioxygenase, these recombinant *E. coli* strains were able to convert the L-trypto-phan via indol into an intermediary, which then spontaneously oxidizes into indigo (35,36). The current yield of bacterial indigo from glucose does not yet permit to make this bioprocess economically attractive.

Other Blue and Purple Biopigments

Phycocyanin is a blue color that chemically consists of a protein that is coupled to chromophore tetrapyrrol groups. It is a component of the photosynthetic pigment of cyanobacteria. It is, among other methods, produced with the cyanobacteria *Arthrospira platensis* and is used in human food in Japan. The salt-loving red micro-alga *Porphyridium cruentum* is a source of the red-violet phycoerythrin that is structurally similar to phycocyanin. Such biocolors from micro-algae are produced in Israel for cosmetic applications, among others (17,37).

Microbial Synthesis of Yellow Flavin Pigments

Vitamin B_2 or riboflavin is an intensely yellow colored compound (Fig. 11). Next to its function as vitamin, riboflavin is increasingly used as a yellow biocolor. Through fermentation with *Ashbya gossypii* fungi riboflavin is produced on a

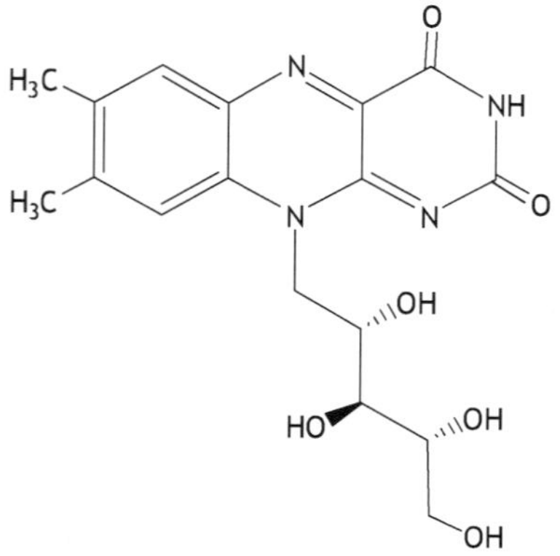

Figure 11   Structure of riboflavin (vitamin B_2).

large scale (4000 t/yr) by various companies, BASF (Germany), Coors Biotech Inc. (U.S.A.), E. Merck (Germany), Hoffmann-Laroche (Switzerland), Merck Sharp & Dohme (U.S.A.), Pfizer (U.S.A.), and so on (17).

Another commercial bioprocess (Takeda Chem. Ind., Japan) is based on the microbial synthesis of D-ribose from sugars with *Bacillus subtilis* transketolase-negative mutants. D-Ribose then is chemically converted into riboflavin (38).

Microbiological Synthesis of β-Carotene, Astaxanthin, and Other Orange–Red Carotenoids

Pure β-carotene is used not only as a vitamin A precursor and an antioxidant but also as orange-red pigment in the food industry, pharmacy, and cosmetics (Fig. 12). It also possesses antitumor/anticancer characteristics. In the 1980s, a commercial bioprocess has been developed on the basis of the controlled cultivation of salt-loving green micro-algae (*Dunaliella salina, D. bardawil*) in basins, salt lakes, and lagoons. This happens in areas with favorable climatological conditions (a lot of sunlight, high temperatures, and a high salt content: 20–30% NaCl), in Australia, Chile, China, Israel, Mexico, Spain, the Russian Federation, the United States, and South Africa. The harvested algal cells contain up to 14% β-carotene in the dry mass, with glycerol and protein-rich alga powder as rest products.

Another microbial process is based on the culture of the *Blakeslea trispora* fungus in large fermentors, a.o. by DSM (The Netherlands). Mixed cultures of the two sexual forms of this fungus produce up to 10 times more β-carotene as a consequence of the induction of trisporic acid, a "hormone" that stimulates the β-carotene biosynthesis. This process is industrially applied for the production of purified β-carotene as well as of β-carotene rich fungus mycelium, which is then used in animal feed (17,39).

Astaxanthin (3,3'-dihydroxy-4,4'-diketo-β-carotene) is the pigment that, through the natural food chain, turns salmon, trout, certain crustaceans, and the feathers of fowl pink. When those fishes, crustaceans, and birds are reared, one has to add astaxanthin for instance to the feed in order to turn them into pink color. Synthetic astaxanthin and cantaxanthin (4,4'-diketo-β-carotene) are also used. Related colors, lutein and zeaxanthin (from maize), are also employed in the feed of fish and poultry. There is, however, a strong trend to produce these colors through microbiological processes (40,41).

In this respect, DSM (The Netherlands) has devised a fermentation process in which the yeast *Xanthophyllomyces dendrorhous* (previously *Phaffia rhodozyma*) produces relatively large amounts of (3R, 3R')-astaxanthin. A similar process has been developed by Sensient Technologies Corp. and by Igene in the United States, companies that market an astaxanthin-rich yeast preparation. Astaxanthin has recently also been found in salt-loving bacteria, for example, *Halobacterium salinarum*. Also micro-algae, such as *Haematococcus* sp., produce carotenoids and are now cultured on a large scale.

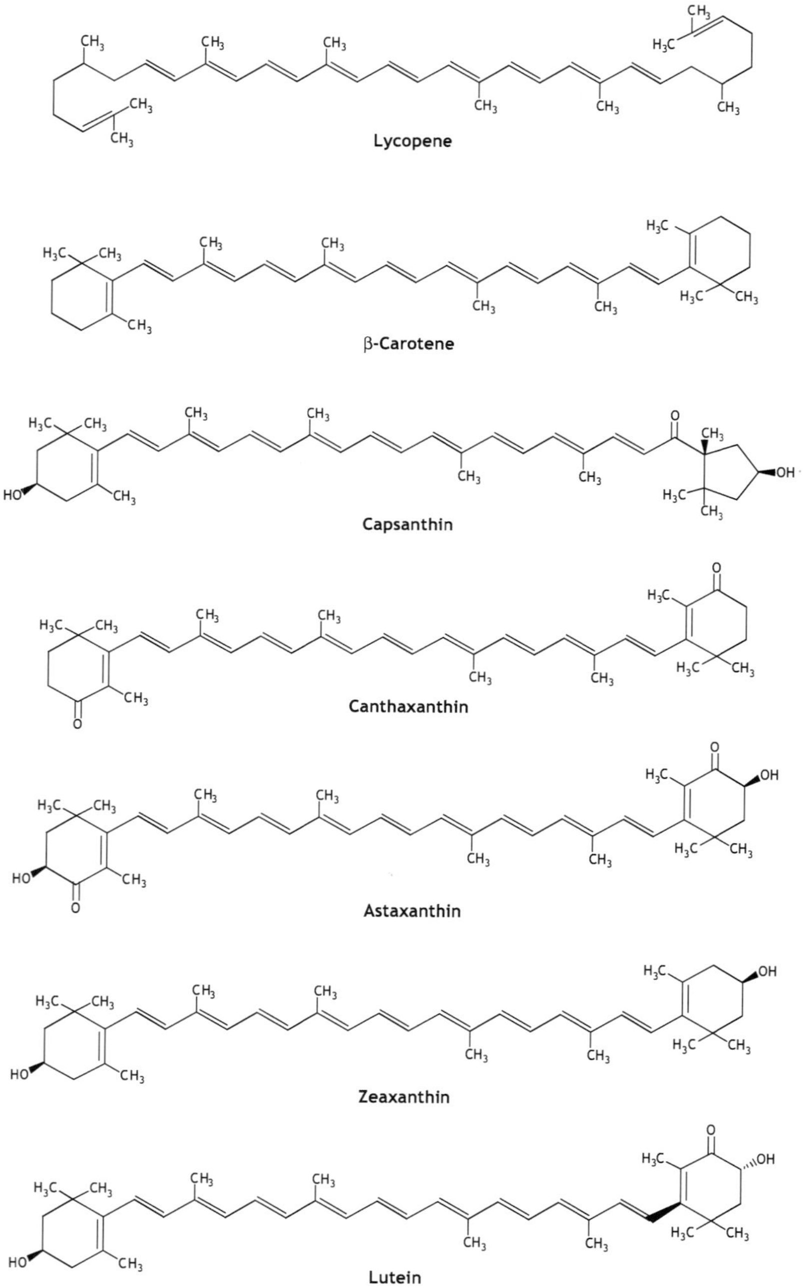

Figure 12 Structure of carotenoid pigments.

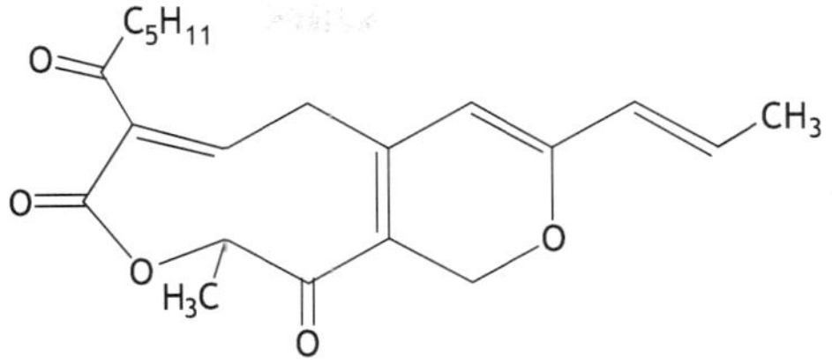

Figure 13 Structure of the fungal monascin M pigment.

Some years ago, in 1995, all the genes that code for asthaxanthin biosynthesis had been identified and cloned in the host cell bacterium *E. coli* (42). Also, several carotenoids can now be produced via genetic modification of the food yeast *Candida utilis* (43). Whether this "spectacular" intervention will lead to an industrial fermentation process remains an open question, in view of the distrust of the consumer toward genetically modified organisms (GMOs). The bacterium *Flavobacterium* on the other hand is able to form high amounts of the yellow "maize"-pigment zeaxanthin (3,3'-dihydroxy-β-carotene).

Other Microbial Red Pigments

In the Far East (Japan, China, etc.) the red color monascin is used in fermented "red-rice" (ang-kak) and in surimi, fish paste, and pink saké wine (Fig. 13). This color is produced by the fungi *Monascus purpureus*, *M. ruber*, and *M. anka*, especially through "solid-state" fermentation processes on moist rice. Monascin consists of six closely related polyketide structures that vary in color from bright yellow to deep red. It is a natural color that could replace the synthetic erythrosin (E127) or insect derived cochineal. It could also be used for cosmetics (lipstick) and textiles (silk, linen), where it also displays antimicrobial action (44).

The Japanese textile and cosmetics manufacturer Kanebo Co. markets lipstick containing the vegetable pigment "shikonin" (Fig. 14). Formerly this red naftochinon pigment was laboriously extracted from the roots of *Lithospermum erythrorhizon*. Recently it has become possible to produce this pigment through plant cell cultures in bioreactors (45). Besides being employed in "bio-lipstick," it also has medical applications as an inflammation inhibitor.

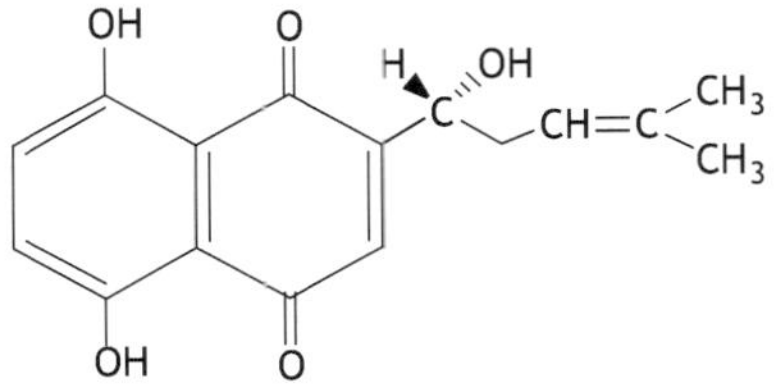

Figure 14 Structure of the plant pigment shikonin.

Other pigments derived from plant tissue culture concern safflower pigment, arbutin (which counteracts the tanning of the skin), and melanin.

Synthetic Pigments vs. Biopigments

Nowadays synthetic colors are increasingly replaced in diverse applications by their biological or microbiological counterparts. As has been mentioned earlier, some microbial colors are already employed. Many other microorganisms (bacteria, yeasts, fungi, and micro-algae) are known to be able to produce various other colors (phenazin, prodigiosin, violacein, porfyrine, chrysogenin, pulcherrimin, melanin, etc.), but they have not yet been further examined for possibilities of production and application. The fact, however, that they are of biological origin is clearly to their benefit—now that producers as well as consumers are increasingly more aware of health and environment. However, natural colors still display technical deficiencies: A higher concentration (2 to 50 times) is often needed to arrive at the same color effect as that of an equivalent chemical color; they are often more dispersive in water rather than soluble; and they are more sensitive to light. Toxicity tests of chemical as well as natural biocolors are performed on laboratory animals for nutritive, cosmetic, and pharmaceutic purposes. Whether the results of those tests are also valid for humans mostly remains a moot point. Depending on the application, sensitivity to temperature and pH, and the influence of other ingredients or additives also plays an important role in the desired color effect.

PERFUME/FRAGRANCE SYNTHESIS THROUGH MICROORGANISMS AND THEIR ENZYMES

Biosynthesis of 2-phenylethanol

2-Phenylethanol is an important flavor/fragrance component (threshold: 125 ppm) of not only certain fruit and beverage flavors, but also of rose fragrances. It can be produced chemically, or via extraction from roses; the naturally obtained product is extremely expensive (4,46–48). During conventional yeast fermentations (*Saccharomyces cerevisiae*, *Kluyveromyces marxianus*), low levels of 2-phenylethanol can be recovered from the fermentation gases or broth using specific resins. To improve the process, *S. cerevisiae* mutants and *Aspergillus niger* strains have been selected (49–51), which convert added L-phenylalanine via deamination, decarboxylation, and subsequent reduction into 2-phenylethanol, without very little further metabolization; high yields (>2 g/L) are now obtained by solvent extraction of the fermentation broth.

Fatty Acids as Substrate for Bioflavor Synthesis

Many valuable flavors and fragrances can be produced by microorganisms from fatty acids, added as precursors, including compounds that provide "green notes,"

Table 3 Sources of Precursor Fatty Acids

Precursor fatty acids (chain length: unsaturation)	Typical commercial source
Saturated fatty acids	
C_4 to C_{12}	Milk fat
C_8 to C_{12}	Coconut oil fractions
C_{10} to C_{18}	Butter fat
(Poly)unsaturated fatty acids (PuFAs)	
C_{18}:1 oleic acid	Plant oils, animal fats
C_{18}:2 linoleic acid	Most plant oils
C_{18}:3 α-linolenic acid	Linseed oil
C_{18}:4 arachidonic acid	Animal fats, fungi
C_{20}:5 EPA	Fish oil, fungi
C_{22}:6 DHA	Fish oil, fungi
Hydroxylated fatty acids	
C_{16}: 0—OH 11-hydroxypalmitic acid	Jalap root (sweet potato)
C_{18}: 1—OH ricinoleic acid	Castor oil (seeds of *Ricinus communis*)

Abbreviations: EPA, eicosapentaenoic acid; DHA, docosahexaenoic acid.

mushroom flavors, specific lactones, and methylketones (52,53). Commercial sources of such precursor fatty acids are given in Table 3 (54).

Starting from α-linolenic acid (C_{18}:3; found in linseed oil), the fungal plant pathogen *Botryodiplodia theobromae* can form jasmonic acid. This can then be esterified, using commercial lipases to obtain the final flavor product, methyl (+)-7-isojasmonic acid, which displays a sweet floral, jasmine-like odor. A complex pathway—which occurs normally in plants—involves lipoxygenase (a dioxygenase that acts on cis–cis-pentadiene units of PUFAs), allene oxide synthase, cyclase enzymes, followed by β-oxidation steps, and double bond reduction (55).

As mentioned before, musk and civet components evaporate very slowly and fix other odors. In this respect, musks are important components of many fragrances; most are of a polycyclic aromatic nature and are produced via petrochemical synthesis. Naturally occurring macrocyclic lactone musks are found in some plants (ambrette seed oil, galbanum), whereas keto-musks are produced by musk deer and civet cats, now very expensive and unethical sources.

Mutants of the yeasts *Candida bombicola* and *Pseudozyma antarctica* have been obtained, which are able to convert palmitic acid into juniperic acid (16-OH-hexadecenoic acid), which can then be cyclized into hexadecanolide lactone musk (46).

Another process, based on the yeast *Candida tropicalis*, converts C10–C18 alkanes, into α, ω-dicarboxylic acids, which can then be polymerized and cyclized into macrocyclic musks: For example, brassylic acid is prepared from tridecane

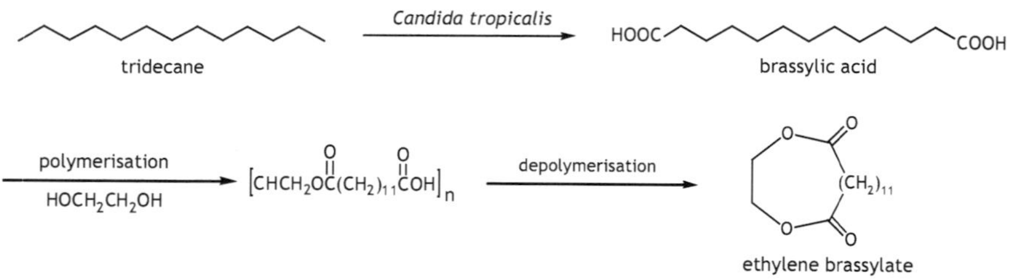

Figure 15   Conversion of alkanes into macrocyclic musk fragrance.

and then converted into ethylene brassylate (54) (Fig. 15). Another bioprocess has been described to produce the fragrance ingredient called Ambrox®, a terpene furan. It is one of the important components of ambergris, an excretion product of sperm whales. It is, just like musk, a fixative for other fragrances. A chemical process starts from the terpene sclareol, extracted from the *Salvia sclarea* plant, which is converted via sclareolide into ambrox. Also here, fungal and yeast strains (*Hyphozyma roseoniger, Cryptococcus* sp.) that have been screened are able to use sclareol as sole carbon source and to accumulate sclareolide, which is then chemically converted via its diol into Ambrox (46,47,56).

CONCLUSIONS

This survey shows that many biotechnological/microbial products, more than could be expected at first sight, are already being applied in cosmetics. Plant-derived cosmetic ingredients are not only more difficult to produce but also their composition changes in function of the harvest, origin, extraction procedure, and so on. Animal derived cosmetic ingredients are now under pressure: Not only are certain exotic compounds almost "extinct" (if not prohibitively expensive), but also others are now considered a suspicious source of viral or prion diseases. Chemical syntheses also have lost their gloss; enforced environmental regulations and the consumer demand for natural products (biodegradable/compostable/safe, etc.) have contributed largely to this attitude.

Animal/skin cell culture techniques, for example, epidermal cells (keratinocystes), neurons, and so on, are being developed to test cosmetics as to their toxic, allergic, and other effects so as to make animal testing superfluous.

Also plant or algal protein or lipid cosmetic extracts still contain variable amounts of chlorophyll and pheophytins, which are difficult to remove by conventional bleaching techniques. This can be achieved by treatment with chlorophyllase (from algae) or by switching toward microbial synthesis.

A novel idea to be further studied deals with the anti-skin-aging effect of heat shock proteins (HSPs), which act normally in all cells as molecular chaperones to stabilize cell metabolism; HSP can be induced in human cells by extracts from *Artemia* or be added as HSP-rich yeast extract. The extracellular matrix (ECM), protein molecules, collagen, fibronectin, laminin are very important for skin integrity, appearance, regeneration, wound healing, anti-aging, and so on. Synthetic ECM-like peptides are now being developed and could be very useful in the future to promote dermal repair.

Already several microbially prepared cosmetic ingredients have been introduced, without the above mentioned disadvantages or risks. Only recently is the astonishing versatility of the synthetic capabilities of beneficial microorganisms beginning to be valued by the layman—so far mainly informed and alarmed about the disease-causing microbes! Indeed, a wide range of microbial compounds has already found application in medicine, pharmacy, food and agriculture, and bulk and fine chemistry. This is now completed with quite a number of known and novel microbially derived molecules with specific cosmetic application.

Today, not only chemical and pharmaceutical companies (and of course the personal care and cosmetic sector) but also food companies develop and produce such biocosmetics! The fact that microbial products are "natural," that they show the desired chirality, are biodegradable, are formed from renewable agrosubstrates, and that fermentation and bioconversion processes proceed under mild reaction conditions, all have contributed to an increasing implementation of such "green processes" and their "bioproducts" in a sector that must—by nature—have an eye for health, freshness, and natural well-being.

REFERENCES

1. Vandamme EJ. Bacteria in front of the mirror: biocosmetics via microbial synthesis. Agro-Food-Industry Hi-Tech 1996; 7(4):3–8.
2. Vandamme EJ. Biocosmetics produced via microbial and enzymatic synthesis. Agro-Food-Industry Hi-Tech 2001; 12(1):11–18.
3. Vandamme EJ. (Micro)biological colours. Agro-Food-Industry Hi-Tech 2002; 13(2):11–16.
4. Vandamme EJ, Soetaert W. Bioflavours and fragrances via fermentation and biocatalysis. J Chem Technol Biotechnol 2002; 77:1323–1332.
5. Dutton G. Cosmetic companies move forward in adopting biotechnology techniques. Gen Eng News 1994; 15:11–12.
6. Marks A. Herbal extracts in cosmetics. Agro-Food-Industry Hi-Tech 1997; 8(2):28–31.
7. Ansmann A, Kawa R. Pearlescent concentrates, modern technology and formulations. Agro-Food-Industry Hi-Tech 1996; 7(3):16–18.
8. Thewlis J. Lanolin for cosmetics application. Agro-Food-Industry-Hi-Tech 1997; 8(4):10–15.
9. Vandamme EJ. The search for novel microbial fine chemicals, agrochemicals and biopharmaceuticals. J Biotechnol 1994; 37:89–108.
10. Demain AL. Small bugs, big business: the economic power of the microbe. Biotechnol Adv 2000; 18:499–514.

11. Hagesawa S, Nagatsuru M, Shibutani M, Yamamoto S, Hasebe S. Productivity of concentrated hyaluronic acid using a Maxblend® fermentor. J Biosci Bioeng 1999; 88:68–71.
12. Vanhooren P, Vandamme EJ. L-Fucose: occurrence, biological role, chemical and microbial synthesis. J Chem Technol Biotechnol 1999; 74:479–497.
13. Keuning W, Lambers JWJ, van der Winden W, Farin F. Ceramides, an update. The Gist 1994; 94(58):14–16.
14. Bunger J. Ectoin, added protection and care for the skin. Euro Cosmetics 1999; 3:22–24.
15. Bousquet MP, Willemot RM, Monsan P, Boures E. Enzymatic synthesis of AHA derivatives for cosmetic application. J Mol Catal B 1998; Enzymatic, 5:49–53.
16. De Baets S, Vandedrinck S, Vandamme EJ. Vitamins and related biofactors: microbial production. In: Lederberg J, ed. Encyclopedia of Microbiology. 2nd ed. New York: Academic Press, 2000:837–853.
17. Vandamme EJ, ed. Biotechnology of Vitamins, Pigments and Growth Factors. London: Elsevier Applied Science, 1989.
18. Blume G, Teichmuller E, Orndorff S. Tyrosinase inhibitors and their role in skin whitening. Agro-Food-Industry Hi-Tech 2001; 12(3):9–12.
19. Kurosu J, Sato T, Yoshida K, Tsugane T, Shimura S, Kirimura K, Kino K, Usami S. Enzymatic synthesis of α-arbutis by α-anomer-selective glucosylation of hydroquinone using lyophilized cells of *Xanthomonas campestris* WU-9701 J Biosci Bioeng 2002; 93:328–330.
20. Sato T, Takeucmi H, Takamashi K, Kurosu J, Yoshida K, Tsugane T, Shimura S, Kino K, Kirimura K. Selective α-glucosylation of eugenol by α-glucosyl transfer enzyme of *Xanthomonas campestris* WU-9701. J Biosci Bioeng 2003; 96:199–202.
21. Morin RS, Kozlovac JP. Biological Toxins. In: Fleming DO, Hunt DL, eds. Biological Safety: Principles and Practices. 3rd ed. Washington, D.C.: ASM-Press, 2000:261–272.
22. Johnson EA. Clostridial toxins as therapeutic agents: benefits of nature's most toxic proteins. Ann Rev Microbiol 1999; 53:551–575.
23. Vandamme EJ. Biotoxins: a poison as well as a medicine? Chem Today (Chimica Oggi) 2003; 21:55–58.
24. Allegre M, Deratini A. Cyclodextrin uses: from concept to industrial reality. Agro-Food-Industry Hi-Tech 1994; 5(1):9–17.
25. Vandamme EJ, Soetaert W. Biotechnical modification of carbohydrates. FEMS Microbiol Rev 1995; 16:163–186.
26. Beck R, Röper M. Starch derived cosmetic and toiletry ingredients. Agro-Food-Industry Hi-Tech 1994; 5(3):24–25.
27. De Goede ATJW, Woudenberg-Van Oosterom M, Van Rantwijk F. Selective lipase-catalyzed esterification of carbohydrates. Carbohydrates in Europe 1994; 10:18–20.
28. Sarney DB, Vulfson EN. Enzymatic synthesis of surfactants. Communications in Agricultural and Applied Biological Sciences, University Ghent (Proc. 8th FAB Symposium), 1994; 59(4b):2321–2330.
29. Hommel RK, Weber L, Weiss A, Himmelreich U, Rilke O, Kleber HP. Production of sophorose lipid by *Candida* (*Torulopsis*) *apicola* grown on glucose. J Biotechnol 1994; 33:147–155.
30. Lang S, Wullbrandt D. Rhamnose lipids—biosynthesis, microbial production and application potential. Appl Microbiol Biotechnol 1999; 51:22–32.

31. Rau U, Hammen S, Heckmann R, Wray V, Lang S. Sophorolipids: a source for novel compounds. Industrial Crops and Products 2001; 13:85–92.
32. Dean K. Biotech pigments poised to challenge synthetic colors. Industrial Bioprocessing 1992; 14(5):4–6.
33. Artz R. Natural food colours. Food Tech Europe 1994; 2:204–208.
34. Piccaglia R, Venturi G. Dye plants: a renewable source of natural colors. Agro-Food-Industry Hi-Tech 1998; 9(4):27–34.
35. Murdock D, Ensley BD, Serdar C, Thalen M. Construction of metabolic operons catalyzing the de novo biosynthesis of indigo in *Escherichia coli*. Biotechnol 1993; 11:381–386.
36. Wick CB. Blue dye. Gen Eng News 1995; 1(5):22–23.
37. Borowitzka LJ, Borowitzka MA. β-Carotene (provitamin A) production with algae. In: Vandamme EJ, ed. Biotechnology of Vitamins, Pigments and Growth Factors. London: Elsevier Applied Science, 1988:15–26.
38. De Wulf P, Vandamme EJ. Production of D-Ribose by fermentation. Appl Microbiol Biotechnol 1997; 141–148.
39. Nelis HJ, De Leenheer AP. Microbial sources of carotenoid pigments used in foods and feeds. J Appl Bacteriol 1991; 181–191.
40. Nagodawithana T. Production of colors. In: Nagodawithana TW, Reed, G, eds. Nutritional Requirements of Commercially Important Microorganisms. Milwaukee: Esteekay Associates, 1998:513–533.
41. Parajo JC, Santos V, Vazquez M. Optimization of carotenoid production by *Phaffia rhodozyma* cells grown on xylose. Process Biochem 1998; 33:181–187.
42. Kajiwara S, Kakizono T, Saito T, Kondo K, Ohtani T, Nishio N, Nagai SS, Misawa, N. Isolation and functional identification of a novel cDNA for astaxanthin biosynthesis from *Haematococcus pluvialis* and astaxanthin synthesis in *Escherichia coli*. Plant Mol Biol 1995; 29:343–352.
43. Miura Y, Kondo K, Saito T, Shimada H, Fraser PD, Misawa N. Production of the carotenoids lycopene, β-carotene and astaxanthin in the food yeast *Candida utilis*. Appl Environ Microbiol 1998; 64:1226–1229.
44. Juzlova P, Martinkova L, Kren V. Secondary metabolites of the fungus *Monascus*: a review. J Ind Microbiol 1996; 16:163–170.
45. Fugita Y, Takanashi S, Yamada Y. Selection of cell lines with high productivity of shikonin derivatives by protoplast culture of *Lithospermum erythrorhizon* cells. Agri Biol Chem 1985; 49:1755–1759.
46. Cheetham PSJ. The use of biotransformation for the production of flavours and fragrances. Trends Biotechnol 1993; 11:478–488.
47. Cheetham PSJ. Combining the technical push and the business pull for natural flavours. Adv Biochem Eng/Biotechnol 1997; 55:1–49.
48. Schrader J, Etschmann MMW, Sell D, Hilmer JM, Rabenhorst J. Applied biocatalysis for the synthesis of natural flavour compounds current industrial processes and future prospects. Biotechnol Lett 2004; 26:463–472.
49. Atika O, Ida T, Obata T, Hara S. Mutants of *Saccharomyces cerevisiae* producing a large quantity of β-phenetyl alcohol and β-phenetyl acetate. J Ferment Bioeng 1990; 69:125–128.
50. Lomascolo A, Lesagee-Meesen L, Haon M, Navarro D, Antona C, Faulds C, Marcel A. Evaluation of the potential of *Aspergillus niger* species for the bioconversion of L-phenylalanine into 2-phenylethanol. World J Microbiol Biotechnol 2001; 17:99–102.

51. Etschmann MMW, Sell D, Schrader J. Screening of yeasts for the production of the aroma compounds 2-phenylethanol in a molasses-based medicin. Biotechnol Lett 2003; 25:531–536.
52. Janssens L, De Pooter HL, Schamp NM, Vandamme EJ. Production of flavours by microorganisms. Process Biochem 1992; 27:195–215.
53. Hagedorn S, Kaphammer B. Microbial biocatalysis in the generation of flavour and fragrance chemicals. Annu Rev Microbiol 1994; 48:773–800.
54. Häusler A, Munch T. Microbial production of natural flavours. ASM-News 1997; 63:551–559.
55. Liu S, Li C, Xie L, Cao Z. Intracellular pH and metabolic activitiy of long chain dicarboxylic acid producing yeast *Candida tropicalis*. J Biosci Bioeng 2003; 96:349–353.
56. Cheetham PSJ. Use of enzyme and microbial technologies for the production of cosmetic ingredients and aroma chemicals. Proc. 13th FAB Symposium, Communications in Agricultural and Applied Biological Sciences, Belgium University Ghent, 1999; 64(5a):239–245.

3

Proteins and Peptides in Personal Care

Manoj Kumar and Roopa Ghirnikar

Genencor International, a Danisco Company, Palo Alto, California, U.S.A.

OVERVIEW

The success of the multibillion dollar cosmetic and personal care industry has been in large part due to constant innovation. This has resulted in bringing many value-added products to the market. Whether it is use of naturally derived ingredients for gentler effects or, more recently, the use of therapeutic high-tech ingredients, changes in the cosmetic industry have been driven by competitive challenges as well as "baby boomer" consumer needs. Advances in genomics and proteomics have led to a deeper understanding of how the human body functions and have changed the way the personal care industry today identifies and develops new products. The industry trend is to now use bioactive ingredients that naturally play a role in growth, maintenance, and repair of our body to enhance natural processes. This approach has brought proteins and peptides onto the list of performance bioactive agents that could be used, either in the form of purified ingredients or as protein extracts. Advances in recombinant DNA technology have enabled a variety of modifications to be made in proteins and peptides, either to increase their performance or production or improve their compatibility with other ingredients, making them more suitable for cosmetic formulations. This chapter briefly summarizes the nature and properties of proteins and peptides, discusses their current use in personal care products, and highlights additional potential applications for their use. The impact of recombinant DNA technology on identification and production of proteins and peptides as well as its role in designing knowledge-based performance proteins is reviewed.

The future trends for applications of proteins and peptides in personal care products are also discussed.

PROTEINS

Proteins are a primary constituent of all living things and one of the chief classes of macromolecules. They occur as natural polymers—polypeptide chains constructed from the building blocks of 20 different amino acids. A condensation reaction in which the carbon of the carboxyl group of the first amino acid forms a chemical bond with nitrogen of the amino group of a second amino acid with the elimination of water across the bond results in the formation of peptide bonds. The amino acids are generally classified as acidic, basic, hydrophilic (polar), or hydrophobic (nonpolar) based on the properties of their side chains. The sequence and properties of these side chains determine the unique characteristic of a particular protein, including its biological function and its specific three-dimensional structure. To be biologically active, proteins must adopt specific folded three-dimensional, tertiary structures. Changing amino acids in the polypeptide chain changes the structure of the protein, which in turn changes function. Modification of a single amino acid in a key location, such as the active site on a protein, can lead to significant changes in the protein's properties. A typical protein contains 200 to 500 amino acids (Fig. 1).

The primary structure of a segment of a polypeptide chain or a protein is determined by the amino acid sequence of the chain(s). The polypeptide chain starts with a free amino group called the "N-terminal" end of the protein, whereas the end with the free carboxyl group is termed the "C-terminus." The local spatial arrangement of the main-chain atoms without regard to the conformation of the amino acid side chains gives rise to the secondary structure of the protein. There are three common secondary structures in proteins, namely alpha helices, beta sheets, and turns. Those structures that cannot be classified as one of these three standard classes are usually grouped into a category called "random coil."

The alpha helix and beta-structure conformations of proteins are generally the most thermodynamically stable secondary structures. The tertiary structure of

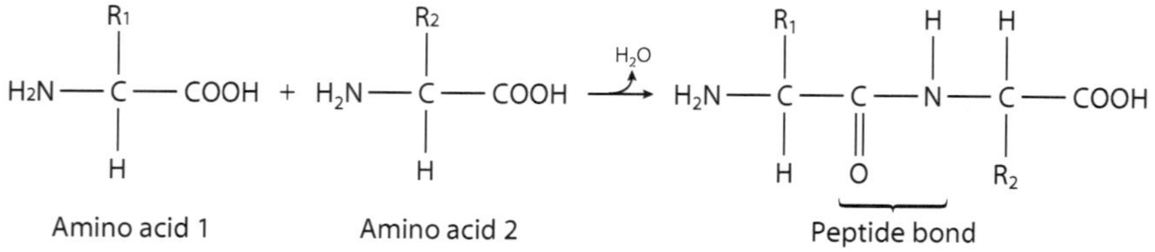

Figure 1 Peptide bonds are formed when the carbon of the carboxyl group of the first amino acid forms a chemical bond with nitrogen of the amino group of a second amino acid, with the elimination of water across the bond.

a protein molecule comprises the arrangement of all its atoms in space, without regard to relationship with neighboring molecules. Several proteins, for example, hemoglobin, ion channels, and microtubules, function as part of the larger assembly or protein complex (i.e., as multiple subunits of the same or different polypeptide chains). The quaternary structure of a protein is reflected by the arrangement of these subunits in space and the grouping of intersubunit contacts and interactions, without regard to the internal geometry of the subunits. The subunits in a quaternary structure are usually in noncovalent association. Proteins with covalently linked carbohydrate groups, such as collagen or bromelin, are called "glycoproteins." Proteins modified at their N-terminal with lipid modifications are termed "lipoproteins" (Fig. 2).

Proteins are either globular or fibrous in nature. Globular proteins are compact spheroids whose active surface represents about 25% of the total protein. The globular conformation is formed when the polar amino acid side

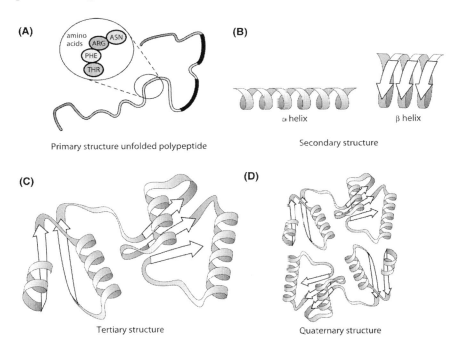

(A) Primary structure unfolded polypeptide

(B) α helix β helix
Secondary structure

(C) Tertiary structure

(D) Quaternary structure

Figure 2 Protein structure: (**A**) The primary structure of a protein is the specific sequence of amino acids in the polypeptide chain, held together by peptide bonds. (**B**) The secondary structure is the occurrence of regular repetitive patterns over short regions of the polypeptide, held together by hydrogen bonds. (**C**) The tertiary structure is the overall folding of the polypeptide chain, formed by bonds between side chains of amino acids. (**D**) The quaternary structure is the result of linking, often by purely noncovalent interactions, of several protein molecules to form a larger unit with distinct properties. *Abbreviations*: ASN, asparagine; ARG, arginine; PHE, phenylalanine; THR, threonine.

chains tend to gather on the outside of the protein, where they can interact with water, and the nonpolar amino acid side chains are buried on the inside to form a hydrophobic core that is "hidden" from water. For fibrous proteins, much or most of the polypeptide chain is organized approximately parallel to a single axis. Fibrous proteins are often mechanically strong, usually insoluble, and play a structural role in nature (1) (Fig. 3).

Proteins provide most of the molecular machinery of cells and are involved in practically every function performed by the cells. Chemical reactions within cells are catalyzed by specialized proteins called "enzymes." In these specialized proteins, residues widely dispersed in the primary sequence are folded into proximity to create a catalytic center in the tertiary structure. Depending on the type of

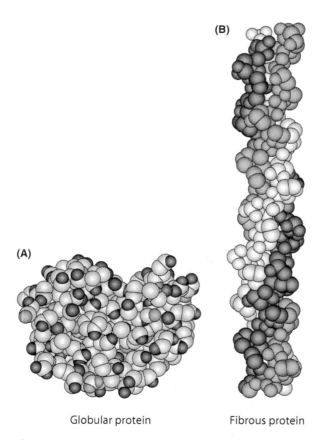

Globular protein   Fibrous protein

Figure 3   (**A**) Globular proteins are relatively spherical in shape and highly soluble. They usually play a dynamic role in body metabolism. (**B**) Fibrous proteins are those in which the polypeptide chain is organized approximately parallel to a single axis. Such proteins are often mechanically strong and generally play structural roles in organisms.

reaction they catalyze, enzymes are classified into such groups as oxidoreductases, transferases, hydrolases, lyases, isomerases, and ligases (see chap. 4 for more information on enzymes). Storage of various small molecules and other metabolites is achieved through complex formation (e.g., storage of iron by ferratin). Proteins have various functions. For example, hemoglobin transports oxygen to various body tissues, whereas hormones, transporter permeases, and cytokines play a role in cellular regulation through transmission of nerve impulses or other messages, or substrates, across cell membranes. Antibodies bind to specific foreign particles and provide protection via the immune system. Some proteins, like collagen and keratin have a structural role, as they provide mechanical support to the body. Muscle movement occurs through the coordinated action of proteins, such as actin and myosin.

The remarkable effects of proteins in the care of skin and hair were only speculative in early days. But through years of research, it is now firmly established that these bioactive molecules, through their structure and function, can provide beneficial effects (2,3). Thus, proteins from natural sources have been realized as building blocks for today's modern skin- and hair-care products. Proteins have been incorporated in personal care products in two ways: proteins that have structural and functional similarities to those naturally present in hair, skin, and cortex and proteins that have been derived from other sources and used as specialized ingredients because of their unique properties. Isolated from a variety of sources of animal, vegetable, and microbial origin, proteins possess properties essential for the care and protection of skin and hair that have been scientifically recognized (4–6). Today, there are several proteins and protein derivatives that provide raw ingredients that can be formulated in cosmetic products. A list of suppliers and their web sites is given in the reference (7).

Proteins have been part of a variety of cosmetic bases, including oil in water emulsions, liquid detergents, lotions, aqueous gels, and simple aqueous systems from both "in-house" and customer formulations. Studies using analytical instrumentation, such as a cutometer and chromometer in protein-based personal care formulations, have confirmed the functional benefits of the protein and have illustrated a relationship between functionality and the molecular weight of the protein under evaluation (8). Some of the products currently on the market include proteins derived from many sources, such as almond, collagen, elastin, keratin, lupine, milk, silk, wheat, soy, rice, and vegetable/plant. Proteins of marine origin have also found applications in cosmetics. Most protein molecules are too large to penetrate the hair shaft in their original state as they usually have molecular weights in the range of tens of thousands. Hydrolyzed (i.e., broken down into fragments with lower molecular weights) proteins, however, can penetrate the hair shaft. The optimum molecular weight of the protein fragments for maximum reconstructive effect is reported to be between 200 and 2200 daltons molecular weight (9). In addition, proteins modified with silicone or quarternary ammonium salts have found numerous applications in hair and skin care formulations (10–12).

The next section will discuss the properties of proteins that have enabled their use in cosmetic formulations and how they have been used in products for skin and hair care applications.

Collagen, Elastin, and Keratin

Collagen and elastin are produced in the skin dermis by fibroblasts, the major cells of the dermis. In conjunction with other proteins they form a framework called the extracellular matrix (ECM), and contribute structure, strength, elasticity, and durability. Collagen is the most abundant protein of the skin, accounting for 70% of the total protein content and is responsible for maintaining skin tone and elasticity. Interlacing of the elastin fibers with the collagen fibers is what gives the skin its elasticity. As humans grow older, collagen synthesis slows down and loses its flexibility and capacity for absorption so that the elastin fibers become thick and brittle. The skin becomes thinner, and the protein fibers decrease in diameter. The external effects of this process are the appearance of wrinkles and dry skin.

Because of its high potential to bind water, collagen helps to promote skin hydration and accelerates skin soothing. It has both film-forming and skin-moisturizing properties (13). Its excellent smoothing and hydrating qualities have resulted in its use in both hair- and skin-care applications. Hydrolyzed collagen from different animal/fish sources is incorporated in skin regenerating products designed to counteract skin dryness and help mature skin, as well as prevent damage to the skin caused by environmental influences, especially UV exposure (14,15). Modified collagen is also used in shampoos and conditioners to provide an overall conditioning effect without buildup. Collagen, in combination with quarternary ammonium salts, has demonstrated enhanced substantivity (16). Injections of natural human collagen similar to that found in skin are also used to correct facial wrinkles, frown lines, nasolabial folds, or vermilion borders (17). Hydrolyzed elastin with high affinity to skin and hair has also been shown to provide a natural protein layer of protection against environmental factors. It has been added to skin-care formulations and shown to firm/tighten mature skin and activate regeneration of new elastic fibers (18).

The sea is a huge store of natural ingredients for application in cosmetics. In addition to such proteins as collagen and elastin that have been isolated from fish, specialized proteins of marine origin have also been used. Hydrolyzed conchiolin marine protein, found in the pearl oyster, has been shown to restore hair to a healthy condition. Studies at Seiwa Kasei (or Silab (Rita)) have shown that the protein gently coats the hair cuticle, thereby leaving hair looking shiny and smooth (19,20).

Keratin is the major protein in hair. Hair contains a high amount of sulfur because the amino acid cysteine is a key component of the keratin proteins in hair fiber. Sulfur in the cysteine molecules from adjacent keratin proteins links together and forms disulfide chemical bonds, which are very strong and difficult to break apart. These bonds linking the keratins together are the key factor in the durability and resistance of hair fiber to degradation under environmental stress. Hair perming processes, which use alkaline solutions and reducing agents, result in breaking the disulfide bonds in the keratin protein. Thus, repeated perming results in hair damage due to constant breaking down of keratin. Hydrolyzed keratin is thought to penetrate the hair shaft to rebuild damaged hair and give it increased body. Cationic keratin containing cystine has been used in shampoos and conditioners and has been shown to increase the smoothness of hair and add body and shine (21,22).

Silk

Silk is another naturally occurring protein whose composition has facilitated its use in hair- and skin-care applications (23). Natural organic silk is rich in those amino acids that are the main constituents of skin and hair proteins. Silk protein is compatible with most cosmetic ingredients, including anionic, cationic, and nonionic substances. A high molecular weight, natural, soluble protein constituent of silk has been shown to bind to the keratin of skin and hair, forming a protective film. Because of its soothing, film-forming, and hydrating properties, it has been used in a broad range of scalp- skin- and hair-care products (24). When used in hair care products, it has been shown to increase gloss and improve manageability/texture of hair.

The application of highly functional hybrid polymers composed of hydrolyzed silk protein, alkyl chain, and silicone chain, as moisturizers, skin and hair protectors, and antidiscoloring agents for hair has also been demonstrated (25,26). Pure sericin—silk gum—has been shown in Japanese studies to protect from ultraviolet (UV radiation) damage. This product gives strength and body to fine hair making it more manageable. It has also been shown to prevent and reverse damage from sunlight, chlorine, seawater, and chemical treatments (27,28).

Whole globular silk protein is able to make up a protective film on the skin that produces a feeling of elasticity and keeps the skin properly hydrated. Silkall^{TM} 100 (Ikeda Corp.) is a highly purified grade of natural silk, carefully processed to retain its original physical structure and chemical composition. A unique property of Silkall^{TM} 100 silk powder is its ability to hold and release moisture depending on the temperature and humidity of the ambient environment. For many years, Silkall^{TM} 100 has been used by a number of leading cosmetic manufacturers in the United States, Europe, and Japan in many mosturizing and antiwrinkle cosmetic products. SilkPRO^{TM} (Ikeda Corp.) is another hydrolyzed form of pure silk protein that has found cosmetic applications. Being readily soluble in water, it is compatible with most cosmetic ingredients, including anionic, cationic, and nonionic surfactants and has been used in formulating many hair-care, skin-care, and cosmetic products (29). Fibro-Silk^{TM} (film-forming, moisturizing silk protein fibers in powder form) from Arch

Personal Care Products, L.P., has been shown to retain moisture and entrap oil and is recommended for use in shampoos to enhance hair shine (30).

Milk Proteins

Milk is one of nature's oldest and best-known skin softeners, and its benefits in the world of beauty care have been known for a long time (31). Milk proteins have been incorporated into aqueous and aqueous-alcoholic hair care formulas, designed for preventive care of scalp and hair. Follicusan™ (bioactive signaling milk proteins, CLR) has been shown to vitalize the cells of the scalp, including those in hair follicles and counteract premature, accelerated hair loss (alopecia), and normalize excess sebum secretion, thus counteracting formation of dandruff (32). Milk bio-proteins have been shown to reinforce moisturization of the outer layers of the skin, providing suppleness and comfort. Lactokine™ fluid with milk proteins in a dose range of 2.0% to 5.0% has been shown to minimize reactions caused by skin irritation, such as release of inflammatory mediators or reduced cell vitality, resulting in accelerated recovery of the skin. Lactokine™ fluid was also shown to reduce the melanin production of melanocytes in vitro and in vivo, leading to even skin pigmentation (33).

Milk peptide complex (MPC), containing functionally valuable milk components as carrier and stabilizers, has been used in emulsified and gel-type skin-regenerating products that are designed to rejuvenate mature skin and to smooth wrinkles. These products have been shown to prevent environmentally induced, accelerated aging of skin (biological and environmental skin aging) by increasing thickness of epidermis and stimulating cell–cell communication between epidermis and dermis (34,35). Studies at Estée Lauder have shown that whey protein in combination with vitamins protects the skin from free radical damage. The effect was shown to occur through increased natural collagen production that led to refirming the skin. Whey proteins have also found applications in cosmetics for infants and children (36).

Vegetable/Plant

Hydrolyzed vegetable/plant proteins have gained importance in cosmetic applications since the trend of avoiding animal products in food and cosmetics has gathered momentum. The use of proteins extracted from plants has become important to give formulations a "green" aspect by providing the consumer recognizable, environmentally safe ingredients (37). Hydrolyzed vegetable protein is moisture-retentive and can be used as a protective film-former. Studies have shown its application for skin-moisturizing and hair-conditioning products (38). Some products containing vegetable protein have been shown to stimulate growth of new hair, delay the hair-loss process, and improve hair and scalp condition. Plant-based protein products offer hydration protection to hair and better moisturization to skin. Studies with a copolymer of hydrolyzed vegetable protein and silicone (Keravis™) have shown that the low molecular weight components penetrate the cortex and moisturize from within, and the high molecular weight components form a film on the hair shaft and lubricate and reinforce the cuticle. In combination, these properties strengthen the hair and help it withstand the stresses of chemical treatment, environmental insults, and styling practices. In these studies, flexabrasion, a technique that examines tensile strength, bending modulus and fiber–fiber friction of hair fibers was used to measure hair strength. These studies showed that the addition of Keravis™ provides a conditioner with three times the strengthening performance as compared to conditioners without Keravis™ (39).

The increasing use of products that contain no polyoxyethylene has led to the creation of new classes of basic materials that are of vegetable origin and free of polyoxyethylene but at the same time are versatile with pleasing cosmetic qualities. In this category, vegetable lipoproteins are receiving considerable attention (40). Surfactants and emulsifiers based on coconut oil or fatty acids and vegetable proteins are routinely used in several formulations. A soluble form of the protein extensin, derived from carrots has an amino acid distribution similar to that of soluble collagen, including a high hydroxyproline content, and has been shown to possess moisturizing, smoothing, and firming properties (41,42).

Oats are an amazing and powerful seed that seem to be as helpful for skin treatment as they are for nutrition (43). Hydrolyzed oat protein, which has a well-balanced amino acid profile, is a very rich emollient. Its effect has been most dramatic for hair conditioning. Some studies have claimed that oat protein actually penetrates the hair shaft, protects damaged hair, and maintains its structure without buildup over time. Oat protein (along with oat beta glucan) has been shown to possess anti-inflammatory and anti-itch properties. These agents together have been shown to reduce irritation and inflammation and protect against damaging free radicals as they lubricate and moisturize skin (44). Other studies have shown that hydrolyzed oats retain significantly more moisture and gain up to 50% more moisture at relative low humidity when extra moisture is most needed (45).

Proteins and glycoproteins isolated from soybean seeds have been widely used in cosmetics (46–48). Products containing high concentrations of extensive glycoprotein and polysaccharides from hydrolyzed soy flour, such as Raffermine® (Silab/Rita), have been used in skin care products where skin firming and elastin protection is desirable. Raffermine® also has proven anti-elastase activity (49). Hydrolyzed soybean extract has served as an alternative to mammal derived protein extracts in products designed to counteract the signs of biological and UV-induced premature skin aging. As a "biological sun protection factor" it is claimed to reduce UV-induced DNA damage when applied as a pretreatment and prevent release of ECM-decomposing proteases. Soy protein has also been shown to stimulate skin regenerative functions and improve skin firmness. Products containing soy protein have been shown to inhibit skin enzymes (elastase and tryptase) and reduce damage to skin and promote soothing.

For example, Elhibin® (Pentapharm) has been shown to improve skin firmness with regular use. When used in skin care products it has been shown to increase the ability of skin to hold moisture and provide a smoothing effect for minimizing roughness and wrinkles. In hair-care products, Elhibin® claims to improve gloss and texture, increase moisture retention, and improve manageability and body (50,51).

Hydrolyzed sweet almond protein extract is used for its soothing and insulating properties and has been an active ingredient in applications where anti-irritation properties are desired (52). It has hydrating and protective properties and is recommended for dry and delicate skin. Studies at Silab (Rita) have demonstrated that a high molecular weight biopolymer of sweet almond proteins spreads at the skin surface to form a tensor film that allows an immediate, visual and perceptible decrease of wrinkles and fine lines. Almond extract is also a natural restructuring and conditioning agent for hair because of the high affinity of the keratin peptides of hair to the hydrolyzed proteins in the extract. Amandu-laine™ SG, (Silab, France) has been shown to have a high substantivity for hair as a result of negative charge of the damaged hair. Because the material consists of branch-chained glucosides and peptides, the film formed on the hair improves its structural integrity and is said to add volume and shine to hair fibers (53). Shampoo and conditioners containing protein extracts of lupine plant, a legume that produces seeds high in protein, claim to increase hair microcirculation, facilitate penetration of nutrients, renew hair cycle, and stimulate hair growth. Lupine extract has also been recommended for application to scabby blemishes and additive to facial steams and masks to reduce oiliness and invigorate skin (54). Hydrolyzed sesame extract, Cohesine (Silab, France), is composed of purified glycoproteins obtained from sesame. Cohesine increases the number of intercorneocyte junctions ensuring cellular cohesion of skin, thereby enhancing flexibility and skin softness.

Research carried out at Laboratoires Serobiologiques has shown the potential benefits in cosmetic applications of protein fractions derived from the tree *Moringa oleifera*. Puricare® LS, containing protein fractions of relatively low molecular weight has been developed and shown by scanning electron microscopy and traction tests to have very good hair-conditioning as well as strengthening effects (55).

The beneficial actions of natural wheat protein, hydrolyzed wheat protein, hydrolyzed wheat protein polysiloxane copolymer, and hydrolyzed wheat protein polyvinylpyrrolidone copolymer have also been recognized. Hydrolyzed wheat protein has remarkable substantivant, conditioning, and antistatic properties for hair and skin and has been extensively used in the formulation of conditioners, shampoos, cleansers, and various skin-care products (56–59). Heat activated wheat protein/silicone copolymer has been shown to polymerize on drying and cross-link to provide thermal protection from styling damage (60). It has also been shown to reconstitute the lipid membranes in the intercellular spaces of the horny layer of skin and reduce trans epithelial water loss. Its anti-irritant, sebum-replenishing, and moisturizing properties have led to its use in aftershave lotions (61). Native wheat protein fraction, because of its low ionic strength and lower negative net charge, has been shown to possess enhanced binding to human hair and thereby reduce hair roughness and improve hair shine (62). Recently, low molecular weight fractions from wheat proteins (Gluadin®, Cognis Deutschland Gmbh & Co. KG) have been shown to provide deep penetration into hair cortex, leading to anti–hair-breakage efficacy and anti-inflammatory effects on keratinocyte cell cultures (63).

Microbial Extracts

Microbial extracts have found applications in skin-care formulations as well as in hair care for hair smoothing, styling, and conditioning effects (64–66). Melawhite® (microbial extract) from Pentapharm has been recommended for use in whitening gel and tan-preventing day cream applications and is claimed to be an effective skin whitener in combination with alphahydroxy acids. The extract minimizes formation of skin tanning, freckles, liver spots, and aging pigmentation (67).

In particular, Biofactor® HSP [Yeast extract rich in heat shock proteins (HSP) and heat shock factors (HSF)] has been shown to protect the skin from such everyday stresses as heat. The inclusion of heat shock factors along with other proteins allows collagen, elastin, keratin, and enzymes from the skin to function to their full extent without any damage and is included in sun cosmetics, antipollution care, and antiaging care products. In in vitro experiments, 86.7% of fibroblasts kept at a temperature of 47°C in the presence of 3% Biofactor® HSP survived as opposed to only 33% of the cells without it, showing a 57% increase in survival rate (68).

Extracts of special strains of *Saccharomyces cervisiae* have been shown to activate tissue regeneration through significant stimulation of cell respiration. Their revitalizing capacity strengthens the skin's natural ability to protect itself against damaging environmental influences (69,70). Studies with Revitalin®-BT (Pentapharm) have shown a boost in skin's oxygen content and consumption in skin with concomitant increases in cellular respiration. Such extracts have been recommended for use in night repair creams, soothing night creams, and body-firming lotions (71). Antarcticine™ (*Pseudoalteromonas* Ferment Extract; Lipotec, SA) a high molecular weight glycoprotein has shown cryoprotective effects providing stability to proteins and lipid membranes exposed to extremes of cold or dryness. Formulations containing such extracts have shown to reduce the dryness and roughness of skin.

The preceding section has described many different proteins that are in use today for hair- and skin-care applications. These have been derived from animal, plant, and microbial origins. Over the years, there has been a gradual shift from including proteins from animal sources to those derived from plant sources, driven partly by the consumer desire for "naturally derived ingredients." Based on their inherent properties, these proteins have been claimed to impart several beneficial effects, including improving body and shine to hair and smooth supple feel to the skin. Although such claims at first were highly subjective, recently, formulators and manufacturers have used a combination of clinical observations, bioinstrumentation, photography, and other technologies for claim substantiation. Moreover, continued research in this area has shown that modified proteins exhibit properties that are much different than their parent protein. For example, the use of quarternary salts or silicone in combination with various proteins has been shown to enhance the product's substantivity and give it greater conditioning effects. Today, increasing demand for performance-driven personal care products has resulted in the need to understand the mechanism of action of individual components. This has led to a trend of using "purified" components as opposed to the use of hydrolyzed protein extracts in products. Such extracts, however, will remain an important active ingredient for use in personal care products and constitute a primary means to test protein fractions from new sources.

PEPTIDES

Peptides are generally defined as short sequences of amino acids ranging from 2 to 30 amino acid residues. Hormones were the first group of biologically active agents that were characterized as peptides. Several peptide hormones—such as insulin, oxytocin, corticotropin, angiotensin, bradykynin, ankephaline, and so on—were soon found to play key roles in human physiology. In the last 50 years, vast progress in the area of both natural and synthetic peptide research has been made with applications in human health and pharmaceuticals. Recently peptides have started to show their potential in personal care and cosmetics applications.

Biologically active peptides are universal and have very diversified functions. One of the most commonly known groups of peptides other than hormones includes antimicrobial peptides. More than 650 natural antimicrobial peptides have been documented (72). Many of these are present on the skin surface, as well as in the oral cavity, and constitute a first line of defense against pathogens (73).

Personal care applications of peptides thus seem a natural fit for hair, skin, and oral cosmetic purposes. Some of the concerns regarding use of peptides in cosmetic products have been related to their penetration and subcutaneous delivery, long-term stability, and long-term effects. Although some of the solutions to diffusion and penetration of peptides have been documented (74), they have only recently been applied in development of commercial products (75,76). Concerns regarding long-term stability on application are being circumvented using clever chemical/biological modifications of peptides (77).

Studies on methods and applications of naturally derived, bio-inspired, and/or synthetic peptides for cosmetic purposes have seen an exponential growth in the last decade. These studies demonstrate the rapid progress in this research area and serve as an indicator of the realized opportunity for commercialization of peptide-based cosmetic products. The availability of such products may thus fulfill the "hope in a bottle" desired by millions of young and aging individuals globally.

Current use of peptides in personal care is mostly confined to either the use of natural proteins that are hydrolyzed to generate peptides or to their derivatized versions, which make them more accessible to the target. In the last few years, however, several synthetic peptides have appeared in the marketplace to address many key cosmetic applications. The following section will cover current applications of peptides in the cosmetic framework based on both natural and synthetic materials and their application area. Examples of recently identified peptides with potential for use in personal care applications have also been included.

Skin Care

The skin (*integumentum commune*), the largest organ of the body, plays an important role in many body functions, including regulation of body temperature, protection, and immunity. The dermis contains fibroblasts necessary for skin material synthesis (collagen and elastin) and immune cells, which combat foreign bodies (i.e., pathogens) that have permeated through epidermis.

Just as proteins derived from natural sources have found numerous applications in skin care, peptides from natural sources are being discovered and added to the formulators' basket (78). Peptides derived from collagen, elastin, and keratin continue to dominate this pool for use in skin care. A highly functional collagen tripeptide from fish has recently been reported to efficiently permeate the stratum corneum, epidermis, and dermal layers and improve collagen synthesis in human fibroblasts. This has led to the development of a skin lotion formulation with excellent moisture retention and improved effects on skin elasticity (79). Polyaspartate peptide and collagen peptides have been used to prepare gel cosmetics that give a "good feeling" with moisturization and are compatible with skin and hair (80). Furthermore, oral ingestion of marine collagen peptides has been reported to reduce dryness and roughness of the human skin (81). Silk peptides are also a common theme in many skin-care creams and lotions and are being reported as nourishment agents (82,83). Silk fibroin peptides having excellent film-forming, moisture-holding, and foaming ability, as well as luster, gloss, and long-term stability have become key ingredients in both skin- and hair-care formulations. In addition, soy peptides have also become a choice for cosmetic applications, in particular in skin-lightening applications (84). Cosmetics containing fish and shellfish peptides are being explored for control of skin discoloration (85), whereas whey peptides have been shown to have antioxidant properties (86). Recently, a new laminin peptide has been shown to stimulate ECM biosynthesis and cell adhesion and may have potential as a cosmetic ingredient in anti-aging creams (87).

Pepsyn, a United Kingdom-based company, is pursuing milk peptides for nutraceutical and cosmetic applications (88). Vegetable based peptides, such as Vegeseryl®, developed from fractionation of soy peptides seem to improve skin elasticity, while a water soluble peptide isolated from pea (Proteasyl® TPLS8657) shows anti-elastase activity. Purisoft™, a complex of two peptides from *Moringa* seeds has been shown to be effective as a skin cleanser. In vitro, it has shown protective abilities against heavy metals and cigarette smoke by decreasing the level of heat shock protein 27. In vivo results have shown reduced binding of particulates to skin. These three vegetable based peptide products were developed by Laboratorie Serobiologiques. Silab has recently launched rice based di and tri peptides. Neutriskin™, for example, stimulates fibroblast proliferation, increases cell recovery and collagen production following a UV challenge. In an in vivo study, this product was shown to be effective in reducing crow's feet wrinkles. Vincience, another ingredient supplier with a focus on peptide research, has developed a significant peptide-based cosmeceutical portfolio. This portfolio includes anti-irritant peptides, elastase inhibitors, anti-aging peptides, and peptides (Lys-Leu-Asp, Ala-Pro-Thr) to stimulate collagen, laminin, and fibronectin synthesis (89). Modulene (immunomodulator and anti-irritant biopeptide), an acetyl-hexapeptide has biomimetic cytokine modulator/regulator properties, with applications in anti-aging, regeneration, and repair of sensitive skin, and after-sun treatment. MAP (Photo-protector and immunomodulator) is another acetyl-hexapeptide that shows melanin regulating activity with application in day care (UV-protection), acne cosmetics, aftershave, and preventive sun cosmetics. Melanostatine-DM (pigmentation modulator), a hexapeptide, showing inhibition of melanin synthesis during UV-induction, is useful in skin-brightening products. ETF (natural anti-aging biopeptide) is mimetic to thymulin, a natural thymus messenger that stimulates keratinocytes and immune cells, and may have applications in sensitive skin, anti-aging, and skin regeneration. Collaxyl (collagen peptide) is a hexapeptide that is mimetic to collagen IV and XVII proteins, which play an important role in dermo-epidermic connection and thus may have application in anti-aging and healing. Kollaren CPP (collagen potentiating tripeptide) is shown to increase collagen I and III synthesis, and is thus marketed for anticellulite, anti-aging, and reduction of stretch marks applications. IEL (Leucocytar Elastase Inhibitor), a biomimetic peptide of the physiological inhibitor of cutaneous elastase has been shown to preserve skin elasticity and firmness. Pentapeptides Vinci 01 and Vinci 02 derived from laminin and fibronectin respectively, have shown anti-aging and skin-regenerating properties. Laminin-5 is a key molecule of the cell membrane and is involved in the aging process. Fibronectin is a key component of the ECM.

The ionic and hydrophilic nature of several peptides results in their poor penetration of the stratum corneum of the skin. In order to make them penetrate and reach the viable epidermis and dermis, scientists have resorted to derivatizing them. Such modified peptides have been extensively researched for cosmetic applications. For example, polyethylene glycol (PEG) peptide conjugates such as methoxy-PEG-FGAL tetra peptide with an RCHO group, have been shown to inhibit one or more protease enzymes present on skin. This PEG conjugated peptide once incorporated in a body wash, lotion, or cream application, is anticipated to aid in the reduction of protease associated damage of aging skin (90). Peptides derived from keratin and milk casein linked to palmitic acid as a carrier have been shown to have hygienic benefits and are used in cleaning, shaving, lipsticks, and cosmetic aerosols (90,91). Similarly skin cosmetics, containing peptides with antibacterial properties bound to quaternary ammonium compounds, have made it to the marketplace (92). Cosmetics containing phosphorylated peptides or salts derived from natural sources are reported to hold moisture in the skin and have buffering actions in a wide range of pH spectrum (93).

Neutrogena Inc. has introduced peptide copper complexes in the market, which were initially discovered by Procyte Corporation (94). GHK–Cu complex in a moisturizing lotion has shown efficacy in preserving, improving, and regenerating skin tissue, as well as hair follicles, mucosa, bone, and intestinal linings. The naturally occurring GHK peptide is generated by proteolysis during skin turnover and has been suggested to be involved in wound healing. This peptide appears to stimulate ECM production and evidence indicates that it has better antioxidant properties than vitamin C or retinol. Tripeptide copper complexes are being used in cosmetic skin renewal procedures and laser resurfacing to improve post-treatment skin recovery (95). Furthermore, complexing of two to five amino acid peptides containing glycine, hydroxyproline, proline, arginine, lysine, or histidine with metals and nonmetals has been shown to improve their beneficial effects on skin (96). A hand cream containing GHK–Mg complex has been shown to have skin beneficial properties. Skin Biology Inc. has now developed the next generation of peptides by isolating peptides from soy proteins that have the correct characteristics to chelate copper (97).

Sederma Corp. (74) has introduced a number of peptides to the market that have found many applications in skin care. Many of these peptides have been derivatized by acylation of the N terminal end or esterified at the C terminal end. For example, Senicalmine[TM] as N-acetyl-Tyr-Arg or as cetyl esters, when present in a skin cream at 300 ppm was shown to be effective in reducing negative sensation and thermal stimulus (98). Palmitated GHK peptide (Maxilip[TM]) has been shown to redensify connective tissue for voluminous lips. Two other peptides, valyl-Tryptophan (valyl-Trp) and palmitoyl-GQPR peptides are active ingredients in Eyeliss[TM], an eye gel formula designed for reduction of puffiness around the eyes. Valyl-tryptophan is described to be an effective angiotensin converting enzyme inhibitor, thus helping in drainage of excess fluid. Palmitoyl-GQPR peptide is said to be anti-inflammatory in nature. These two peptides, along with hesperidin methyl chalcone, have demonstrated reduction in eye-bag thickness in clinical studies (99). Sederma's biopeptide series are based upon palmitated GHK and VGVAPG peptides and have been shown to be effective in multiple ways: stimulating collagen synthesis, glucosaminoglycan synthesis in vitro, increasing skin thickness in vivo, reducing wrinkle depth in vivo, stimulating fibroblast mobility in vitro, and inducing cutaneous firmness in vivo (100).

Palmitoyl-G-gln-P-Arg (Rigin™) is another peptide that has been reported to be useful in maintaining cytokine balance. It has been shown to induce IL-6 levels in vitro and improve skin firmness and elasticity together with smoothness and hydration in vivo (101). Yet another product, which consists of palmitoyl-GHK and palmitoyl-VGVAPG, is targeted for improved skin firmness possibly by stimulating fibroblast proliferation (102). In addition to these, Lipotec Inc. has developed acetyl-EEMQRR peptide (Argireline™) for muscle relaxation in a manner similar to Botox®. This peptide is shown to be a neurotransmitter release inhibitor that acts by inhibiting the synthesis of SNARE vascular fusion complex. In vivo studies have shown that it possesses antiwrinkle properties.

Pentapeptides identified by Sederma that are released during wound healing have been used in skin-care compositions (103). Pentapeptide KTTKS, a breakdown product of procollagen-1, stimulates ECM synthesis and in vivo testing has led to claims that it is as effective as retinol products (104). KTTKS when formulated in a skin care lotion or cream shows efficacy in reduction of fine lines and wrinkles.

Binary polymer mixtures of albumin and glycosaminoglycan have been reported as being useful for treatment of skin wrinkles or other skin irregularities. Aqueous compositions of the ternary mixtures have been shown to have pH dependent phase change properties and form skin activated films (105). Cosmetic skin-care compositions containing peptide thymolysin-b4 have been claimed to improve the appearance of skin (106).

Cosmetic preparations using peptides to improve radical protection factor (RPF) have also been investigated (107). Peptide cecropin, when included in cosmetic preparations, has been shown to improve RPF between 40 and 400, depending on the amount used in the formulation. Another repeat peptide of proline-arginine, with one to three repeats in number, has been shown to have efficacy in cosmeceutical applications for skin care (108). By reducing IL-6 and IL-8 tissue concentrations to achieve rates similar to those in young tissues, this peptide has been shown to prevent cutaneous inflammation and immunological dysfunctions caused by physiological aging and normal exposure to UV radiation. Furthermore, esterification or acylation of C-terminal end of the dipeptide multimer has been shown further to enhance its efficacy.

In recent years, hundreds of peptides showing antimicrobial properties have been isolated, designed de novo, or synthesized. (109). These peptides serve as a nonspecific defense system that complements the highly specific cell-mediated immune response. They act rapidly to neutralize a broad range of microbes (110). Such peptides have been used for skin-care applications where control of microbial growth is targeted. For example, researchers from Hercules Inc. (111,112) have demonstrated the use of hexapeptides and their chemical modifications for inhibiting and controlling the growth of microbes,

especially *Burkholderia cepacia*. Antimicrobial skin creams using cyclic peptides, such as iturin (0.2 wt%), and 0.5-wt% surfactin, have been shown to be
efficacious against fungal growth (113).

Hair Care

Peptides derived from digested or denatured keratin, the major structural protein
in hair, are used extensively in the hair-care industry. The peptide fragments are
small enough that they can actually enter the hair shaft through defects in the
cuticle from weathering, permanent waving, or permanent dyeing and temporarily strengthen the hair shaft. The peptides can also act as humectants for the
hair shafts, increasing manageability and hair shine (114). Thus, various formulations containing peptides derived from keratin have been explored for promoting hair growth, luster, and elasticity (115). Use of thioredoxin-derived, or
thioredoxin-like dithiol peptides have also been the subject of innovative research
for various hair-care applications, such as waving, straightening, softening, or
removing hair. Thioredoxin peptides decrease the amount of sulfite or bisulfite
needed for breaking disulphide bonds of hair keratin. These peptides also
allow the hair to be treated at a lower pH to minimize hair damage when
waving, straightening, or softening the hair. When used in hair removing
formulations, they aid in minimizing or eliminating objectionable odors of
thioglycolate-based depilatories (116,117). Modified calycins (calycins comprise
a binding domain and a targeting domain) are used for targeting hair fibers for
various applications, such as color cosmetics (118). Development of milk whey
peptides and their derivatives for hair-care applications has been reviewed (119).

Peptides modified using an esterification reaction to yield acylated or
palmitated peptides have been used to deliver active agents for hair care. Acylated peptides have been reported to show good moisturizing, softening, hair protecting, and gloss giving properties to the hair (120). Another common
derivatization approach seen in peptide products targeted to hair care is silylation.
Polypeptides and peptide-polysiloxane copolymers prepared by thermal copoly-
merization of amino acids with organofunctional polysiloxanes are known for
their use in hair care as interface-active substances (121–125). For example,
hydrolyzed wheat protein peptides were reacted with y-glycidoxypropylmethyl-
dichlorosilane to give a silated peptide, which was formulated into a shampoo.
The shampoo provided better manageability, gloss, moisture, and combability
to hair (126). Several companies, such as Croda, L'Oreal, Phoenix Chemicals,
Siltech, Biosil, Noveon, Shiseido, and Seiwa Kasei, have peptide–silicone
copolymer products for hair applications on the market. To improve substantivity
of collagen peptides to hair, cysteine conjugated peptides have been made that
show better adhesion to hair (127).

Peptides developed for hair care have not only been restricted to applications for hair but have also been used to improve the appearance of eyelashes.
For example, cosmetic bases containing peptide–rosin condensates have been

created for improved luster and film-forming effects for mascara applications (128). These peptides are derived from partial hydrolysis of proteins originated from animal, plant, or microorganisms. Likewise, an emulsion-based mascara using water-soluble silk fibroin peptides (129) with fine eyelash curling properties has been developed. Similarly, an eye shadow formulation using collagen-based peptides PA-100 and PA-300 has been described in literature (130).

Oral Care

Antimicrobial properties of certain peptides have also been exploited for use in oral care. Several peptides that prevent bacterial adherence to teeth have been identified. Cationic amphiphilic peptides derived from bovine and human lactoferrins with antimicrobial activity against oral pathogens have been documented (131). Dimers and cyclomonomers of antimicrobial peptides are preferred because they have enhanced stability in the acidic conditions of mouth. These peptides (e.g., YWFWYN; Tyr-Trp-Phe-Trp-Tyr-Gln) may be used in various oral hygiene formulations, such as mouthwash, chewing gum, and toothpaste to inhibit the growth of dental plaque (132). Recently, two antibacterial peptides produced by *Lactobacillus lactis*, 35 and 39 amino acids in length, have been shown to control endocarditis and thus have potential for use in oral care (133). Furthermore, the use of metal binding peptides, peptide derivatives, and dimers that reduce tissue inflammation in the mouth and thus reduce damage done by reactive oxygen species to oral tissues, has been documented (134). Peptides containing phosphoryl residues have been shown to stabilize amorphous calcium phosphate and have been implicated in the regulation of biomineralization process. Casein-derived phosphorylated tetra peptide SSEE (S = Ser, E = Glu) has been shown to reduce dental caries and also help in repairing early stages of tooth decay (135). These phosphorylated peptides thus can be added to the existing list of oral-care products for the control of dental caries.

USE OF RECOMBINANT DNA TECHNOLOGY FOR IDENTIFICATION AND PRODUCTION OF PROTEINS AND PEPTIDES

"Designer Proteins" are needed as active ingredients to perform a variety of functions and to impart desired characteristics to personal care product formulations. Advances in genetic engineering offer unique opportunities to design proteins with specific, targeted properties, as well as produce consistent fermentation-based protein polymers that can impart specific benefits. Additionally, engineering of multiple protein motifs to provide useful characteristics for a given personal care formulation is also possible. Thus novel proteins with well-defined modular structures and properties for desired applications in personal care formulations are currently in demand.

Repeat sequence protein polymers (RSPP), produced through molecular biological design and fermentation, and targeted to incorporate the characteristics needed in personal care formulation are currently being investigated at Genencor International, a Danisco Company. For example, a case study of an RSPP product called SELP47K for possible personal care applications has been reviewed recently (136). This protein polymer illustrates a new concept of hybrid proteins that can deliver multifunctionality in personal care formulations using genetic and protein engineering techniques.

Although proteins have been widely used as ingredients to perform a variety of functions and to impart desired characteristics to product formulations, they may not provide all of the desired characteristics when used in personal care products. For example, natural silk proteins may impart durability but may also form tight, hard fibers that are not suitable for film formation. Also, the low isoelectric point of many natural proteins may result in a reduction in their affinity for the negatively charged skin and hair. Additionally, when more than one protein is needed to impart all of the desired characteristics to a given formulation, the cost and production time for a given personal care product may be increased.

Furthermore, proteins generally have poor solubility due to their high molecular weight and hydrophobicity. Commercially available proteins, including structural proteins, such as silk and collagen, are typically chemically degraded, giving a diverse mixture of molecular weight fragments with variable properties. As such, these proteins are often modified chemically to enhance solubility for inclusion in personal care products. However, even chemically modified proteins may not have all desired characteristics. Thus, there remains a need in the industry for personal care compositions that have desired characteristics without chemical modification of the proteins.

Natural protein polymers, such as silk fibroins, have found use in personal care products. Currently, synthetic protein-based biopolymers (137) are made using recombinant DNA technology and fermentation methods (138). Recombinant biopolymers offer the ability to screen for desired properties based on the tremendous potential diversity of amino acid combinations. Furthermore, the existing fermentation technology allows for large-scale manufacturing. Using recombinant DNA methods, one can precisely control the molecular weight, size, monodispersity, stereochemistry, and distribution of the biopolymer (139) to create composite biopolymers that simulate natural protein polymers (140). Thus, using the 20 natural amino acids, one can create a protein polymer designed for a specific function.

Representative examples of natural small peptide-based RSPPs and their block copolymers (repeated amino acid sequences, using the one letter code, in parentheses), include elastin (GVGVP, VPGG, APGVGV), silk fibroin (GAGAGS), byssus (GPGGG), flagelliform silk (GPGGx), dragline silk (GPGQQ), GPGGY, GGYGPGS), collagen (GAPGAPGSQGAPGLQ, GAPGTPGPQGLPGSP), and keratin (AKLKLAEAKLELA). The relative environmental stability of these families of structural proteins, in combination with their biocompatibility, unique mechanical properties, and leverage for genetic control of sequence, provide the foundation on which one may exploit naturally derived RSPPs for personal care.

The presence of regularly repeated sequences also implies a propensity to adopt a regular structure and to self-assemble. Such new generation RSPP biomaterials will, by design, harness the power of surfaces and self-assembly to direct specific orientations desirable for skin, hair, and oral care. Surfaces of these newly designed materials are precisely defined at equilibrium and are resistant to contamination. This is in contrast to present naturally derived materials (141), which are amorphous or polycrystalline, drift in structure and composition with time and suffer from uncontrolled contamination. The key elements in molecular self-assembly, a phenomenon ubiquitous in nature, are chemical and structural compatibility through noncovalent interactions. Silk-elastin protein polymers, are simple, versatile, easy to produce, and self-assemble.

Producing a silk-elastin protein polymer requires an understanding of the protein structure, the ability to manipulate protein polymer structure through control of amino acid sequences, and an efficient method to synthesize sequences in a reproducible and precise fashion. Genencor International has developed technology that allows production and stable maintenance of repetitive genes and gene products in microorganisms by specifically designing the genes to avoid recombinational deletion. This process has included exploiting the degeneracy of the genetic code such that adjacent, identical oligopeptide blocks can be encoded by nonidentical DNA sequences. Additionally, by properly choosing and engineering microbial production strains, high expression of SELP47K has been achieved from these genes. By using microorganisms deficient in the deletion mechanisms of homologous recombination (i.e., DNA-modifying functions) and using precise sequence design and gene construction, recombinant genes of more than 5000 base pairs have been stably maintained in *E. coli*. Thus, RSPPs are the result of knowledge-based polymer design that relies on the knowledge that repeated sequences adopt specific structural motifs that provide the basis for polymer formation.

RSPPs are similar to a chemically polymerized block of copolymers but do not exhibit heterogeneity. They are unique, defined, monodispersed, and have molecular weights generally between 30 kD and 250 kD. For example, in SELP47K (Unit block structure: Fig. 4), individual units are composed of silk fibroin (S = GAGAGS), and elastin (E = GVGVP). In this nomenclature,

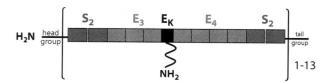

Figure 4   Schematic block representation of the protein polymer SELP47K. Individual units are composed of silk fibroin (S = GAGAGS), and elastin (E = GVGVP). SELP47K (silk-elastin-like protein) consists of four silk repeat peptides, seven elastin repeat peptides, and one lysine modified elastin repeat peptide.

SELP47K (silk elastin like protein) consists of four silk repeat peptides, seven elastin repeat peptides, and one lysine modified elastin repeat peptide. Cross-linking functionality is provided to the SELP47K by substitution of one of the amino acids, valine, for a lysine in one individual unit of elastin. This modification also increases the water solubility of the polymer.

Results from physico-chemical studies indicate that the silk-elastin protein polymer offers unique properties that are desirable for possible hair- and skin-care applications. These tailor-made protein polymers have been designed using molecular biology, gene-expression methods, and modern fermentation engineering. Specifically, SELP47K, has shown ease in manufacturing and possesses key structural and mechanical properties relevant to personal care. Moreover, personal care application data demonstrate the potential for repeat sequence protein polymers to become key active ingredients in upcoming cosmetic products (142). Thus repeat sequence protein polymers, genetically designed based on the combined benefits of natural proteins, potentially can offer biotechnological solutions in personal care.

CURRENT STATUS OF PROTEINS/PEPTIDES IN THE COSMETIC INDUSTRY

The cosmetic industry has successfully used proteins and peptides for the following applications and functionalities: exfoliation, skin firming/anti-aging, skin whitening, sun/photo-oxidation protection, antioxidants/free radical scavengers, moisturizer or protecting moisture barrier, anti-inflammation, anti-irritating or enhancing skin immune power/system, hair, skin, or oral stimulants, hair growth inhibitors, and potential angiogenic agents. In summary, here are a few examples to illustrate such products already on the market: (*i*) Pentapharm's Colhibin™ and Elhibin®, collagenase and elastase inhibitors respectively, derived from rice grains, (*ii*) Croda and Sederma's Rigin™, a lipopeptide with DHEA-like activity, (*iii*) IMPAG Cosmetic's IEL, a tetrapeptide with leucocyte elastase inhibitor activity, (*iv*) Codif's Dermochlorell™, a protein extract from *Chlorella* microalgae showing elastase and collagenase inhibition and supporting collagen synthesis, (*v*) Epernon's Actimp™ 1.9.3, low molecular weight peptides derived from white *Lupin* inhibiting elastase, which protects DNA and has anti-lipoperoxidising properties, (*vi*) Lipotec's Argireln®, a hexapeptide that inhibits SNARE complex on chromofin cells and inhibits catecholamine release, thereby claiming to prevent aging induced by repeated facial movements mediated by catecholamine release.

New active ingredients in the form of proteins and peptides designed for preventive and restorative cosmetics have gained acceptance and importance in both the younger and baby-boomer generation, as evidenced by the number of peptide- and protein-based products in the cosmetic industry. It is estimated that suppliers offering biological materials make up about 10% of the ingredient suppliers to the cosmetic industry. Today, this number is growing. Proteins and peptides as active ingredients form a group that makes up a substantial portion of the biological materials used in the industry. Their share is also growing very rapidly due to the substantive benefits already demonstrated both in clinical trials and consumer satisfaction.

FUTURE FOR PROTEINS/PEPTIDES IN PERSONAL CARE PRODUCTS

In recent years, many proteins that can deliver a "perceptible benefit" have been identified. Their use in personal care products, however, has been primarily as hydrolyzed extracts of animal, plant, or microbial origin. Being highly specific and environmentally friendly, proteins offer a favorable solution to the use of chemicals. In particular, the use of protein extracts from such plants as soy and wheat has flourished as a result of consumers associating "safe and wholesome" with "naturally derived." The immense biodiversity of plants makes them a valuable source for additional protein-based ingredients. Similarly, marine organisms offer a variety of readily available resources for the development of new, innovative, and high value-added protein products for use in cosmetics. The immense reservoir of proteins derived from these life forms will offer new sources for proteins.

Although proteins have provided the personal care industry with a variety of functional constituents, it has been difficult to include them in very high concentrations because of their use as extracts. Using them in purified form may offer a solution to obtain larger and more diverse desired benefits. Advances in genetic and protein engineering can enable a variety of modifications to be made in proteins to increase their activity and improve their pH and temperature stability as well as their compatibility with other ingredients, making them more suitable for cosmetic formulations.

Modifying the behavior of proteins by conjugating them with other chemicals to produce products with novel behavior is being exploited. For example, protein-silicone copolymers represent a family of functional proteins for use in cosmetic preparations. Being chemically linked as opposed to a simple combination of the two components, these polymers possess unique behavioral characteristics that may find applications in skin and hair care formulations. In addition, naturally derived glycoproteins (e.g., Revitalin®-BT) and lipoproteins are being used in cosmetic products that claim to impart an excellent soothing and restoring effect on the skin (40,143).

Research efforts in the area of screening of peptides for delivery, binding, or acting against specific targets will be at the forefront of discovery activities to create efficacious cosmetic formulations. These peptides may come from direct screening of relevant environments. Various technologies have been used successfully to screen for skin and hair binder peptides. Genencor is exploring these peptides for various applications including personal care (144).

Supramolecular networks, such as aggregates, polymers, and networks made by beta-sheet self-assembly of rationally designed peptides, offer a structural and functional scaffold for both targeting and delivery of active ingredients to the desired site. These networks are thus expected to be a hot topic of research for use in personal care applications. This research work will use the power of rDNA technology to create functional peptide libraries based on first principles and engineering (145), making engineered peptides increasingly available for use in personal care applications. For example, in hair- and skin-conditioning applications, peptides will be designed taking into consideration the percentage of cysteines and prolines needed for respective applications (146). The antimicrobial efficacy of peptides also will be explored in developing new cosmetic formulations that not only nourish the skin and hair but also provide protective benefits against spread of microbes.

An increase in research and development activities for use of peptides in oral care hygiene "cosmeceuticals" is resulting in the generation of a healthy pipeline of potential ingredients. More efficacious oral care compositions specifically in the area of peptide-based antiplaque agents are expected in the future. For example, peptide structures in polymers could be designed to specifically recognize bacterial adhesins or plaque bacterial antigens. Such peptide coated colloidal antiplaque agents (such as colloidal ZnO) can then be specifically targeted in the oral cavity, where an external stimulus, such as acidic pH, will cause the active agent to be released (147).

Finally, protein and peptide-based active ingredients for personal care applications are now on a solid performance base and will gain increasing importance in the personal care products formulary. Conducting appropriate safety assessments on the products to assure that the planned application will be safe for the consumer will further enhance the utility of these ingredients. It is both anticipated and desirable that the cosmetic industry will offer more preventive, restorative, and preservative active ingredients that are biotechnology driven and clinically proven. A desirable course of action for ingredient suppliers to the industry would be to respond quickly to biotechnological developments taking place in understanding the physiology, biochemistry, and metabolism of skin, hair, and oral cavity so that they can then be translated into valuable cosmetic products.

REFERENCES

1. Stryer L. Biochemistry. 4th ed. New York: W H Freeman & Co., 1995.
2. Griesbach U, Klingels M, Horner V. Proteins: classic additives and actives for skin and hair care. Review and new findings. Cosmet and Toilet 1998; 113(11): 69–73.
3. Kushida T. Multifunctional hydrolyzed-protein derivatives for hair care products. Fragrance J 1998;26(5):71–78.
4. Abrusci C, Corrales T, Catalina F, Bosch P. Proteins in cosmetics. Revista de Plasticos Modernos 2003; 86:451–459.
5. Sikora M. Animal and vegetable proteins in cosmetics. Tluszcze, Srodki Piorace, Kosmetyki 1997; 41:488–495.

6. Challoner NI, Chahal SP, Jones RT. Cosmetic proteins for skin care. Cosmet and Toilet 1997; 112:51–56, 58, 62–63.
7. Web sites for suppliers of proteins and protein derivatives: Arch Personal Care (http://archpersonalcare.com/); Ceterchem (www.centerchem.com/Cosmetics. html); CLR (www.clr-berlin.de/index-shockneeded.html); Croda (www.croda. com/europe/pc); Induchem (www.induchem.ch/); Javenech (www.javenech.com); Maybrook (Tri-K) (www.tri-k.com/); Pentapharm (www.pentapharm.ch/ sw152.asp); Provital (www.provital.org); Sederma (www.sederma.fr/); Silab (Rita) (www.ritacorp.com/); Sinerga (www.sinerga.it/eng/azienda.htm); Vincience (www.vincience.com/); Ikeda (www.ikedabussan.com/english/index.html); Kalichem Italia SRL; and Lipotech, kelli@kalichem.it, and www.lipotec.com.
8. Packman E, Gans E. The panel study as a scientifically studied investigation: moisturizers and superficial facial lines. J Soc Cosmet Chem 1978; 29:91–98.
9. www.lancerlabs.com/conditioners-reconstructors.htm (Accessed May 2004).
10. Humphries M. Protein-silicone copolymers. Cosmet News 1993; 16:313–318.
11. Chester J, Dixon M. Quarternised proteins in modern hair care. Seifen, Oele, Fette, Wachse 1987, 113(17):617–622.
12. Koester J. Properties and application of cation additives for hair-care preparations. Parfuem Kosmet 1991; 72(4):218–225.
13. Shirai T, Shirai K, Hattori S. Collagen for cosmetic use. Kagaku Kogyo 1996; 47:451–457.
14. Kushida T. Multifunctional hydrolyzed-protein derivatives for hair care products. Fragrance J 1998; 26:71–78.
15. www.skin-healthcare.de/en/skincare/matricol_main.html (Accessed May 2004).
16. Cade PH. Collagen derived proteins. HAPPI, Household Pers Prod Ind. 1984; 21:50, 53, 54.
17. www.lookingyourbest.com/articles/cosmoderm_physician.php. (Accessed May 2004).
18. Sato H, Yajima I. Cosmetics containing moisturizers and polymer emulsifying agents. 2000; JP 98-250419.
19. Nakane T. Development of marine materials for cosmetic in recent year. Fragrance J 1999; 27:58–68.
20. Yoshioka M, Adachi T, Omi S. Cosmetic compositions containing sponge protein hydrolyzate N-quaternary ammonium derivatives 2002; JP 2002179520.
21. Yoshioka M, Shintani H, Matsukawa Y, Adachi T. Hair preparations containing protease digests of keratin oxidative degradation products 2003; JP 2003040727.
22. Gesslein BW, Jones RT. Kerasol, a new keratin protein. Cosmet and Toilet 1987; 102:52, 56.
23. Philippe M, Garson JC, Arraudeau JP. Cosmetic or dermatological composition containing at least a natural, recombinant, or analogous spider silk protein. 1999; FR 2774588.
24. http://smiss.cn/smissEnglish/silk derivatives/silk powder.asp (Accessed May 2004).
25. Ikeda N, Goto N, Yoshioko M. Evaluation of novel hydrolyzed silk protein and alkyl-silicon hybrid polymer. Fragrance J 2003; 31:113–118.
26. Daikai S, Nagao S, Uchida S. Application of polypeptides and their derivatives in shampoo and rinse. Fragrance J 2000; 28:65–71.
27. Kushida T. Multifunctional hydrolyzed-protein derivatives for hair care products. Fragrance J 1998; 26:71–78.

28. http://158081.pub.diysite.com/sc.deliver/main/0-4-5/4/0-pr-1-314655.html?siteid = 158081 (Accessed May 2004).

29. Zhang Y. Use of silk sericins in cosmetics and nutrition. Fangzhi Xuebao 2002; 23:70–72.

30. http://archpersonalcare.com/Products/Category.asp?CatID = 53 (Accessed May 2004).

31. Tamura Y, Fukuwatari Y. Application of milk protein hydrolyzate to cosmetics. Fragrance J 1991; 19:119–121.

32. www.clr-berlin.de/(Accessed May 2004).

33. www.cscm-net.com/images/CLR%20Product%20Summary.pdf (Accessed May 2004).

34. Itoh H. Effects of milk peptide complex (MPC) on anti-aging and anti-cellulite. Fragrance J 1998; 26:92–97.

35. Chigarina KM. Gel for skin care around the eyes 2003; RU 2204984.

36. Negishi H, Otomo H, Gotou T, Ueda T, Kuwata T. Cosmetic properties of whey minerals and their application to skin care products for babies. International Dairy Federation [Special Issue] S.I. 1998; 9804:337–350.

37. Komaki Y. The recent trend of utilization of hydrolyzed natural protein as cosmetic ingredient. Fragrance J 1994; 22:80–88.

38. Kowata Y. Application of vegetable protein hydrolyzates to cosmetics. BioIndustry 1993; 10:344–350.

39. www.crodausa.com/product_list.lasso?product_section=pc&new_product_search=1 &Product2=Keravis&Ctfaname=&CommonName=&PCApps=&PCCats=&- Nothing=Start+Search (Accessed May 2004).

40. www.keminova.com/e_materie.htm (Accessed September 2004).

41. Benaiges A. Extensin functionality tests. Applications of plant protein cosmetics. Cosmet News 1995; 18:252–255.

42. Itoh H, Matsuzaki Y, Ohyoshihara T. The function and application of plant extracellular matrix. Extensins, arabinogalactan proteins. Fragrance J 1996; 24:69–74.

43. Potter R, Castro JM, Moffatt LC. Oat oil compositions with useful dermatological properties 1995; WO 9517162.

44. www.pennyisland.com/healing_oats.html (Accessed May 2004).

45. www.theherbarie.com/botanicalex.html#hydrolyzedOats (Accessed May 2004).

46. Wu W, Hettiarachchy NS. Foaming and emulsifying properties of soy protein isolate and hydrolyzates in skin and hair care products. J of Surfactants and Detergents 1998; 1(2):241–246.

47. Chen H, Hua Y. Functionality of soybean protein products and their application in cosmetics. Riyong Huaxue Gongye 2000; 30:62–64.

48. Voegeli R, Stocker K, Mueller C. Protein fraction for cosmetic and dermatology care of the skin (5,322,839) 1994.

49. www.chembuyersguide.com/partners/ritacorp.html (Accessed May 2004).

50. www.theherbarie.com/botanicalex.html#soyProtien (Accessed May 2004).

51. Yoshioka M, Kamimura Y. Manufacture of shampoos containing plant proteins 1992; JP 04139115.

52. Nawaz Z. Cosmetic compositions comprising a proteinaceous material and a polyol ester 1998; WO 9855089.

53. www.creative-developments.co.uk/papers/Hair Care 2002.htm (Accessed May 2004).

54. Sasaki I, Takemoto Y. Regulation of skin moisture: keeping and enhancing the Natural Moisturing Factor. In: Suzuki M, ed. Roka Boshi-Bihaku-Hoshitsu Keshohin no Kaihatsu. Tokyo, Japan: Shi Emu Shi, 2001:114–120.
55. Armand-Stussi I, Basocak V, Pauly G and McCaulley J. Moringa *oleifera*: an interesting source of active ingredients for skin and hair care. SÖFW-Journal 2003; 129:45–52.
56. ESPERIS S.p.A. Wheat proteins in cosmetics. Use of proteins in cosmetics: animal and plant proteins. Cosmet News 1995; 18:248–251.
57. Nosaka K. Possibility of cereal proteins as cosmetics ingredients. Fragrance J 1998; 26:19–24.
58. Phillips JE, Resch BS. Topical skin and/or hair compositions containing an hydrolyzed protein 2003; WO 2003063816.
59. http://www.deltatecnic.com/Kelisen.htm (Accessed May 2004).
60. Croda Italiana S.p.A. Effects of a new wheat protein isolate on the mechanical properties of hair. Cosmet News 1994; 17:36–39.
61. Okamoto M, Noda I, Yoden E. The functions and applications of hydrolyzed wheat protein and its derivatives. Fragrance J 1998; 26:25–32.
62. Vollhardt J. Native hydrophobic wheat proteins with intelligent hari care properties. SÖFW-J 1999; 125:2–9.
63. Hütter I. Hair care with depth effect by low molecular proteins. SÖFW-J 2003; 129:12–16.
64. Brooks GJ, Burmeister F, Parish D. Pseudocollagenous proteins from yeast. Drug & Cosmet Industry 1992; 150:42, 44, 86, 88, 91.
65. Ohmura T, Nanba T. Hair-smoothing and -styling preparations containing cationic polymers and silyl peptides 2000; JP 98-280547 19980916.
66. Westphal G. Transdermal skin-conditioning compositions containing hyaluronic acid and proteins or peptides 1997; DE 19533038.
67. www.advancedskintherapy.co.uk/newbies.htm (Accessed May 2004).
68. www.impag.de/english/kosmetik/z11stres.htm (Accessed May 2004).
69. www.twaian.com/privatelabelproducts-littlemiracles.htm (Accessed May 2004).
70. Paufique JJ. Process for the extraction of an active principle from yeast for the treatment of wrinkles and cosmetic compositions thereof 6,531,132, 2003.
71. http://www.pentapharm.ch/sw193.asp (Accessed May 2004).
72. Holz CM, Stahl U. Ribosomally synthesized antimicrobial peptides in prokaryotic and eukaryotic organisms. Food Biotechnol 1995; 9:85–117.
73. Hancock REW. Cationic peptides: effectors in innate immunity and novel antimicrobials. Lancet Infect Dis 2001; 1:156–164.
74. Morelle, J.F., Palmitoyl peptides from keratin for cosmetic and hygienic skin care, FR, 1967, FR 1491262; Acylated Protein Hydrolyzates, MORELLE JEAN VALENTIN, GB1153408, 1969.
75. www.sederma.fr/(Accessed September 2004).
76. Lintner K, Peschard O. Biologically active peptides: From a laboratory bench curiosity to a functional skin care product. Int J Cosmet Sci 2000; 22(3):207–218.
77. Ueda Y, Segawa A, Yoshida M. Poster # 216 22nd IFSCC Congress Edinburgh, 2002.
78. Tomatis I, et al. Biopeptides and immunity. In: Actifs et Additifs en Cosmetologies (2nd edition). Martini, Marie-Claude, Seiller Monique. Lavoisier: Tech. & Doc., 1999:245–250.

79. Kikuta T, et al. The development of highly functional collagen tripeptide, Fragrance J 2003; 31:61–67.
80. Hatsutori T, Gel cosmetics containing poly (amino acids), peptides, and inorganic salts 1997; JP 09020614.
81. Kikuchi K, Matahira Y. Efficacy of orally-ingested marine collagen peptide on dryness and roughness of the human skin. Fragrance J 2003; 31:97–102.
82. Zhou X, et al. Preparation of quick-dissolving health care perfumed film soap containing water soluble polymer, surfactant, sterilizing agent, skin nourishing agent, filler and colorant 1996; CN 1134450.
83. Zhang Y, et al. Skin-care creams containing silk peptide, marten oil and other substances 1994; CN 1096669.
84. Tamura H. Properties and applications of soy peptides. Fragrance J 1994; 22:32–37.
85. Nochi R. Cosmetics containing fish or shellfish peptides 1994; JP06157233.
86. Yakult Honsha. Cosmetics containing whey peptides as antioxidants 1983; JP 58198409.
87. Bauza, et al. New laminin peptide for innovative skin care cosmetics. Cosmet and Toilet 2003; 118:43–46, 48, 50, 52.
88. www.pepsyn.co.uk/ (Accessed September 2004).
89. www.impag.de/english/company/index.htm (Accessed September 2004).
90. Underiner TL, et al. PEG-peptide conjugates as protease enzyme inhibitors for cosmetics 2003; US2003143186.
91. Morelle JV. Nouvelle composition biologique a base de keratine, destine aux soins esthetiques de la peau humaine, 1967, FR1491262.
92. Morelle JV. Nouvelle biologique destinee aux soins hygieniques et esthetiques de la peau humaine, 1966, FR1461423.
93. Yoshioka M, Kamimura Y. Skin cosmetics containing peptides bound to quaternary ammonium compounds 1992; JP 04082822.
94. Yoshioka K, Kamimura Y. Cosmetics containing phosphorylated peptides derived from natural proteins 1989; JP 01019013.
95. Patt LM. Skin care compositions containing peptide copper complexes and retinol or its derivatives 2003; US2003134780.
96. Pickart L. Copper peptides for tissue regeneration. Specialty Chem Magazine 2002; 22:29–31.
97. Wank A. Cosmetics comprising peptides and peptide-metal complexes 1993; DE 4127790.
98. Lintner K. Antiaging cosmetic and dermopharmaceutical composition containing hesperidin, dipeptides, and oligopeptides, WO2003068141, 2003.
99. Malnou A, Martinez F. Cosmetic composition for nails, free of phthalates, camphor, and aromatic solvent. WO02100322, 2002.
100. Lintner K. Biologically active peptides: New perspectives in topical applications. SOFW Journal 2000; 6:8–10.
101. Lintner K. Compositions containing mixtures of tetrapeptides and tripeptides. 2004; US 2004132667 A1.
102. Mas-Chamberlin C, Mondon P, Peschard O, Lintner K. Collagen deficit and wrinkles: a new method to reverse cutaneous ageing. Eurocosmetics 2000; 8:3, 43.
103. Robinson LR, et al. Skin care compositions containing pentapeptides 2000; US6284802.

104. Thorel JN, Redziniak C. Cosmetic compositions comprising a peptide or a protein and a nucleotide, polynucleotide or nucleic acid 2004; Fr. Demande, FR 2849376 A1.
105. Band, et al. Polymer mixtures useful in skin care 1991; US5153174.
106. Marini J. Cosmetic skin care compostions containing thymosin-b4 2003; US2003228266.
107. Karin ZL. Cosmetic preparation of active substances with a synergestically increased radiation protection factor, 2001.
108. Lintner K. Peptides as cosmetics or pharmaceuticals for the regulation of immunological dysfunctions and cutaneous inflammation 2000; WO 2000043417.
109. www.bbcm.univ.trieste.it/∼tossi/pag1.htm (Accessed September 2004).
110. Hancock REW. The Lancet (Infectious Diseases) 2001; 1:156–164.
111. Kuhner CH, Romesser JA. Chemically modified peptides, compositions and methods of production for antimicrobial use 2000; WO2001098362.
112. Kuhner CH, Romesser JA. Peptides, compositions, and methods for the treatment of Burkholderia cepacia 2001; WO2001098364.
113. Kitakuni E, et al. Antimicrobial compositions containing cyclic peptides, and cosmetics containing them 2003; JP2003128512.
114. http://www.dermatologytimes.com/dermatologytimes/article/articleDetail.jsp?id= 65551 (Accessed September 2004).
115. Vissarionov VA, et al. Development and utilization of milk whey peptide derivatives. Hair care balsam 2003; RU 2210355.
116. Pigiet VP. Use of thioredoxin, thioredoxin-derived or thioredoxin-like dithiol peptides in hair care preparations 1990; US 4804223, WO 8906122.
117. Pigiet VP. Use of thioredoxin and other dithiol peptides in hair care 1986; EP 183506.
118. Findlay J. Modified calycins for targeting hair fibers or skin surface 2000; WO 0048558 A1.
119. Suzuki A. Fragrance J. 1999; 27, 79–84.
120. Hattori N, Okumura M. Acylated peptides and cosmetics containing them 1998; JP 10298196.
121. Dietz, et al. Polypetide-polysiloxane copolymers 2002; US Patent 6,358501.
122. Jones RT, Humphreys MA. Silicone modified proteins, 1995, US Patent 5,412,074.
123. Humphries MA, Jones RT. Protein-silicone copolymers and compositions containing them. EP0540357, 1993.
124. O'Lenick, Jr., Anthony J. Silicone protein polymers, US Patent 5,243,028, 1993.
125. Yoshioka M, Shintani H, Segawa A, Yoshihara T. Silane copolymer and a method for producing the same, US Patent 6,228,968, 2001.
126. Masato Y, et al. Silated peptides for cosmetics 1996; EP699431.
127. Yoshioka M, et al, Preparation of peptides by introducing cysteine into protein hydrolyzates via amide linkage 1999; JP 11124395.
128. Masato, et al. Cosmetic bases containing peptide-rosin condensates for improved luster and film-forming effects 1998; JP 10095726.
129. Takatsu A, Kanayama H. Emulsion type mascara containing water soluble fibroin peptides 1992; JP 04305515.
130. Takagishi I, Watabe H. Pen-type liquid cosmetics 1985; JP 60116622.

131. Groenink J, et al. Cationic amphipathic peptides, derived from bovine and human lactoferrins, with antimicrobial activity against oral pathogens. FEMS Microbiol Letts 1999; 179: 217–222.

132. Charbonneau DL, et al. Oral care compositions containing peptides with anti-adherence activity 1997; GB 2307476.

133. Sonomoto K, et al. Lactobacillus lactis producing antibacterial peptide for food preservation 2004; JP 2004105118.

134. Bar-Or D. Methods and products for oral care 2003; US 2003158111.

135. Reynolds R. Anticarcinogenic casein phosphopeptides. Proteins and Peptides 1999; 6:295–303.

136. Kumar M. Biotechnology for Personal Care: A Case Study of Silk-Elastin Protein Polymer, 23rd IFSCC Meeting, Orlando USA, Poster #99, 2004.

137. Langer R, Tirrell DA. Designing materials for biology and medicine. Nature, 428, 487–492, 2004.

138. Alper J. Protein structure: stretching the limits. Science 297, 329–331, 2002.

139. Ferrari F, Cappello J. Protein-Based Materials, chapter 2. Boston: Birkhauser, 1997.

140. Tirrell DA, Fournierb MJ, Masonb TL. Current Opinion in Structural Biology 1991; 1:638–641.

141. Roy I, Gupta MN. Smart polymeric materials emerging biochemical applications. Chem & Biol 2003; 10:1161–1171.

142. Kumar M, Cuevas WA. Use of repeat sequence protein polymers in personal care compositions. U.S. Pat. Appl. Publ. 2004; US 20040180027 A1.

143. http://www.stimulife-ind-dist.com/hydrating-eye-therapy-yv.htm.

144. Murry C, et al. Peptides binding to phenolic compuncs found in tea and wine stains and their biological and industrial uses 2004; WO 2004033482.

145. Naville B, Agelli A, Ingham Eileen, Kirkham J. Networks 2004; WO 2004007532.

146. Buffa CW, O'Lenick AJ, Genjale M. Engineered polypeptides in personal care applications 2003; US 6551997.

147. Carr SW, Pickup KM, Smith PM, Schilling KM. Antiplauqe oral care compositions US Patent 5,824,292, 1998.

4

Introduction to Enzymes and Their Applications in Personal Care

James T. Kellis, Jr. and Raj Lad

Genencor International, a Danisco Company, Palo Alto, California, U.S.A.

BASIC PRINCIPLES

Introduction

Enzymes are biological catalysts. They are found both inside and outside of cells, and these fascinating molecules dramatically accelerate chemical reactions, often by many orders of magnitude compared to the uncatalyzed reaction. Enzymes are protein molecules and are very complex. A protein consists of a linear chain of hundreds of amino acid building blocks, which are produced in the cell, like beads on a string. Each chain of amino acids folds up into a very specific compact form, dictated by its linear amino acid sequence. Proteins are composed of 20 different types of amino acids, and it is the chemical properties of these amino acids and the interactions between them that dictate the particular compact form the amino acid sequence will adopt. In this manner, the linear sequence of the amino acid chain dictates the three-dimensional shape of a protein and consequently its function. The three-dimensional structure of a protein determines the location of crucial amino acids and puts them in position to carry out the function of the protein, such as catalysis of a chemical reaction or recognition and binding to such molecules as DNA, proteins, hormones, metabolites, or drugs. Some enzymes are composed of multiple protein molecules that are associated noncovalently in a specific arrangement.

The linear sequence of amino acids in a given protein is determined by the linear DNA sequence of the gene representing the protein. Protein synthesis

87

occurs through an intermediary molecule, messenger RNA, which is "transcribed" from the DNA sequence. At the ribosome, the messenger RNA sequence is "translated" into the corresponding amino acid sequence. Thus results the central dogma of molecular biology: DNA → RNA → Protein (see chap. 1 for details.)

The specific three-dimensional fold of an enzyme molecule places its amino acid side chains in a spatial arrangement, which dictates that the functional groups on crucial side chains are in precise position to carry out the chemistry of the reaction. Sometimes enzymes contain nonprotein species, such as metal ions, cofactors (e.g., NADH), or prosthetic groups (e.g., heme), that participate in the chemistry of the reaction. Figure 1 shows four structural representations of

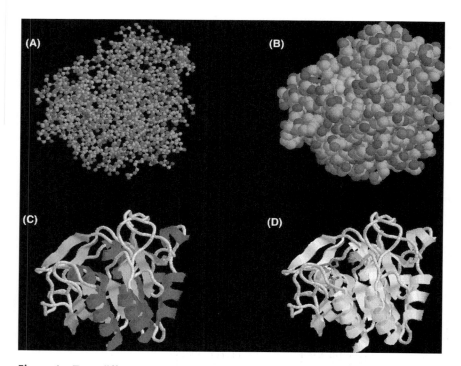

Figure 1   Four different structural representations of an enzyme, subtilisin. All four panels depict the enzyme in the same orientation. (**A**) Ball-and-stick model showing the very complex atomic structure. (**B**) Space-filling model depicting the actual atomic volumes. Color code: carbon, lightest gray; nitrogen, medium gray; oxygen, darkest gray. (**C**) Schematic structure showing the path of the amino-acid chain and the elements of regular secondary structure. Color code: α-helix, dark gray; β-strands, light gray; irregular structure and loops, white. (**D**) Schematic structure as in **1C**, the three amino-acid residues involved in the catalytic mechanism are in the upper portion of the structure, left of center.

subtilisin, a well-characterized enzyme that had its three-dimensional structure determined by X-ray crystallography at very high resolution (1). Subtilisin is a protease, an enzyme that catalyzes the breakdown of proteins via the hydrolysis of peptide bonds linking the amino acids. Three amino acid residues in subtilisin are crucial in the catalytic mechanism of this enzyme. Their location is highlighted in Figure 1. It should also be noted that these amino acid side chains reside in a cleft in the surface of the enzyme, a very common general feature of enzymes.

Historical Background

The term "enzyme" means "in yeast" and was coined in 1877. Much earlier, however, it was suspected that biological catalysts are involved in the fermentation of sugar to produce alcohol. J. J. Berzelius published the first general theory of chemical catalysis in 1835 and included a description of the hydrolysis of starch by the enzymes contained in malt extracts. In 1897, E. Buchner extracted the enzymes that catalyze alcoholic fermentation from yeast cells. This demonstrated that enzyme action is independent of intact cell structure. The first enzyme isolated in pure crystalline form was urease from jack bean. This was accomplished by J. B. Sumner in 1926. He determined that the crystals consisted of protein and concluded that enzymes are proteins. Today thousands of different enzymes are known, and hundreds have been isolated in pure crystalline form (2).

The Lock-and-Key Model and Mechanisms of Catalysis

The molecular structure of many enzymes has been elucidated by X-ray crystallography. Nuclear magnetic resonance (NMR) spectroscopy has been used for precise structural studies on a number of enzymes, as well. Each enzyme's unique three-dimensional structure usually includes a pocket or cleft presenting an array of functional groups deriving from amino acid side chains positioned to bond to complementary groups on the substrate molecule. The three-dimensional fold of the protein chain provides the scaffold to create the substrate-binding pocket and endows the enzyme with its remarkable specificity of action. In 1894, Emil Fischer made the classic postulation that the substrate molecule fits the active site of its enzyme in a "lock-and-key" relationship. This model has been confirmed many times over by structural studies of enzymes carried out in molecular detail. Depending on their structure and biological function, enzymes vary widely in the precision of their substrate specificity (3).

Enzymes are thought to accelerate reactions in a number of ways, and understanding the fundamental basis of their diverse mechanisms is an area of active research. *General acid-base catalysis* occurs when a proton is transferred to or abstracted from the substrate by an acidic or basic amino acid side chain of the enzyme. Positive and negative charges developing in the substrate during the course of a reaction can be stabilized by complementary charges in the enzyme during *electrostatic catalysis*. Nucleophilic catalysis is an example of *covalent catalysis*, where the enzyme provides a nucleophilic group that attacks the substrate to form an enzyme-bound intermediate, which then undergoes, for example, hydrolysis by water to form the products of the reaction. Some enzymes contain metal ions that function in *electrophilic catalysis*, in some cases, for example, stabilizing negative charges that form in the transistion states of some reactions.

Enzymes also accelerate reactions by binding reactants, bringing them into close proximity to one another, and positioning them optimally for the reaction to occur. This considerably decreases the activation entropy of the reaction, leading to dramatic rate accelerations compared to the analogous nonenzymatic reaction. This lowering of the entropy barrier is "paid for" by the highly organized nature of the three-dimensional fold of the enzyme.

TYPES OF ENZYMES

Enzymes catalyze a wide range of reactions. The specific reactions of interest in personal care applications will be discussed in more detail later in this chapter. Table 1 lists the official enzyme classes, some of the major reactions that fall under these classes, and the code numbers used to identify them. Particular enzymes, which are not listed in this general table, have additional code numbers to further delineate them within these categories.

ENZYME KINETICS

Enzyme-Substrate Interaction

Consider the simplest enzyme-catalyzed reaction:

$$\text{Substrate} \xrightarrow[\text{Enzyme}]{} \text{Product} \tag{1}$$

One of the hallmarks of enzyme catalysis is the dependence of the *initial reaction rate* on *substrate concentration*. (The initial rate is the rate of product formation with respect to time before the substrate has been appreciably depleted by conversion to product.) A plot of rate versus substrate flattens out at high substrate concentration (Fig. 2A), indicating that there is a limited number of sites at which the reaction is catalyzed. This theory of enzyme-catalyzed reactions was proposed by Michaelis and Menten (4) and is based on the assumption that the enzyme (the catalyst, E) and the substrate (the reactant, S) form a complex (ES) by a reversible reaction. The complex is then converted into the product (P) with the reaction rate constant k_2.

$$E + S \underset{k_{-1}}{\overset{k_1}{\rightleftharpoons}} ES \xrightarrow{k_2} E + P \tag{2}$$

Table 1   Classification of Enzymes as Recommended by the International Union of Biochemistry and Molecular Biology

1. Oxidoreductases (oxidation–reduction reactions)
    1.1 Acting on the CH–OH group of donors
    1.2 Acting on the aldehyde or oxo group of donors
    1.3 Acting on the CH–CH group of donors
    1.4 Acting on the CH–NH_2 group of donors
    1.5 Acting on the CH–NH group of donors
    1.6 Acting on NADH or NADPH
    1.7 Acting on other nitrogenous groups as donors
    1.8 Acting on the sulfur group of donors
2. Transferases (transfer of functional groups)
    2.1 Transferring one-carbon groups
    2.2 Transferring aldehydic or ketonic groups
    2.3 Acyltransferases
    2.4 Glycosyltransferases
    2.5 Transferring aryl or alkyl groups other than methyl groups
    2.6 Transferring nitrogenous groups
    2.7 Transferring phosphorous-containing groups
    2.8 Transferring sulfur-containing groups
3. Hydrolases (hydrolysis reactions)
    3.1 Acting on ester bonds
    3.2 Acting on glycosidic bonds
    3.3 Acting on ether bonds
    3.4 Acting on peptide bonds
    3.5 Acting on C–N bonds other than peptide bonds
    3.6 Acting on acid anhydrides
4. Lyases (addition to double bonds)
    4.1 Carbon–carbon lyases
    4.2 Carbon–oxygne lyases
    4.3 Carbon–nitrogen lyases
    4.4 Carbon–sulfur lyases
    4.5 Carbon–halide lyases
    4.6 Phosphorous-oxygen lyases
5. Isomerases (isomerization reactions)
    5.1 Racemases and epimerases
    5.2 *cis–trans* isomerases
    5.3 Intramolecular oxidoreductases
    5.4 Intramolecular transferases (mutases)
    5.5 Intramolecular lyases
6. Ligases (formation of bonds with concomitant ATP cleavage)
    6.1 Forming carbon–oxygen bonds
    6.2 Forming carbon–sulfur bonds
    6.3 Forming carbon–nitrogen bonds
    6.4 Forming carbon–carbon bonds
    6.5 Forming phosphoric ester bonds

Source: From Ref. 101.

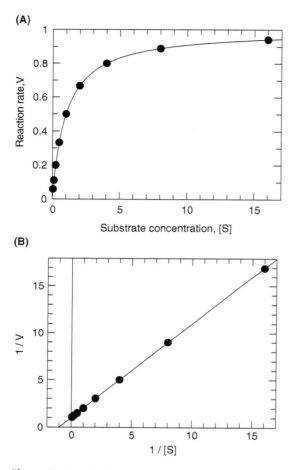

Figure 2 (A) Typical dependence of enzyme reaction velocity, V, on substrate concentration, [S]. Note that the velocity levels out at high [S]. V, when extrapolated to infinite [S], is known as V_{max}, the maximal velocity. K_M is [S], which gives $\frac{1}{2}$ V_{max}. (B) Lineweaver–Burk double-reciprocal plot of the data from **2A**. $1/V$ is plotted against $1/[S]$. The y-intercept is $1/V_{max}$, and the x-intercept is $-1/K_M$.

Using these assumptions, we can derive the mathematical relationship between reaction rate and substrate concentration. This relationship is of extreme fundamental importance, because it allows one to experimentally characterize an enzyme's binding affinity for its substrate and its maximal catalytic rate, two of the most important properties of an enzyme.

The rate of product formation, also termed the reaction velocity, is $d[P]/dt$. It can be seen from the reaction scheme that

$$d[P]/dt = k_2[ES] \tag{3}$$

It is convenient to convert $[ES]$ to the experimentally controlled parameters $[E]_{total}$ and $[S]$. Under commonly used conditions of enzyme activity measurement, $[ES]$ can be considered to be constant during the observed reaction period, thus the sum of its synthesis and breakdown are zero:

$$d[ES]/dt = k_1[E][S] - k_{-1}[ES] - k_2[ES] = 0 \tag{4}$$

Rearranging gives

$$k_1[E][S] = (k_{-1} + k_2)[ES] \tag{5}$$

Now we introduce $[E]_{total}$, which is $[E] + [ES]$, and substitute:

$$k_1([E]_{total} - [ES])[S] = (k_{-1} + k_2)[ES] \tag{6}$$

Solve for $[ES]$:

$$[ES] = k_1[E]_{total}[S]/(k_{-1} + k_2 + k_1[S]) \tag{7}$$

Thus:

$$dP/dt = k_2[ES] \tag{8}$$
$$= k_1 k_2 [E]_{total}[S]/(k_{-1} + k_2 + k_1[S]) \tag{9}$$
$$= k_2[E]_{total}[S]/(((k_{-1} + k_2)/k_1) + [S]) \tag{10}$$

Let $(k_{-1} + k_2)/k_1 = K_M$, the Michaelis constant, and let $k_2 = k_{cat}$, the catalytic constant. Thus:

$$dP/dt = k_{cat}[E]_{total}[S]/(K_M + [S]) \tag{11}$$

Now we have defined the reaction rate in terms of enzyme and substrate concentration.

Please refer to Figure 2A. $d[P]/dt$ is termed V, the reaction velocity, and $k_{cat}[E]_{total}$ is termed V_{max}, the reaction rate extrapolated to infinite substrate concentration. K_M is equal to the substrate concentration that yields a reaction velocity of $\frac{1}{2}V_{max}$. Note from the final equations above that when $k_{-1} \gg k_2$, $K_M = k_{-1}/k_1$, which is the dissociation constant for the E–S complex. The kinetics of more complex reaction schemes can be found in works such as that of Segel (5).

Historically, the determination of K_M and V_{max} was accomplished using algebraic linear transformations of the Michaelis–Menten equation, such as that of Lineweaver and Burk (6), using reciprocals:

$$1/V = K_M/V[S] + 1/V_{max} \tag{12}$$

Please refer to the plot shown in Figure 2B. The intersections with abscissa and ordinate allow the determination of the values for K_M and V_{max}. This type of plot is useful for conceptualizing different types of enzyme inhibition (see below), but with the ubiquity of powerful computer software, direct fitting of untransformed experimental data by nonlinear regression is now preferable for determination of K_M and V_{max}. To illustrate the inadequacy of Lineweaver-Burk plots, the same data points are plotted in Figures 2A and 2B. Note how Figure 2B magnifies the data at low [S] (i.e., high 1/[S]). Therefore, this type of analysis gives undue weight to data obtained at low [S], where there is the lowest amount of product formed. This is often the most unreliable data in an enzyme kinetics experiment.

Michaelis constants for enzymes usually range from 10^{-2} to 10^{-5} mol/L; a low K_M value indicates a high affinity between enzyme and substrate, and a high K_M value indicates low affinity. The catalytic efficiency of an enzyme is indicated by its turnover number, which is the moles of product molecules formed per mole of enzyme molecules per unit time. Average turnover numbers range from 10^3 to 10^4/min; peak values have been measured for acetylcholinesterase at 1×10^6/min and for catalase at 5×10^6/min. The specific activity of an enzyme is the moles of product molecules formed per unit mass of enzyme per unit time. Turnover number and specific activity can be interconverted if the molecular mass of the enzyme is known.

Enzyme Inhibition

Enzyme inhibition is a decrease in the rate of an enzyme-catalyzed reaction caused by a chemical agent. Enzyme inhibitors are of enormous importance. Many drugs are enzyme inhibitors, enzyme inhibition plays a major role in modulation of enzyme activity in vivo (such as the regulation of flux through metabolic pathways), and studies of in vitro enzyme inhibition have contributed greatly to our understanding mechanisms of enzyme function. Enzyme inhibition can be either reversible or irreversible. The following mechanisms of enzyme inhibition may be distinguished (5):

Irreversible Inhibition. An irreversible inhibitor frequently forms a stable adduct with the enzyme by covalent bonding with a crucial amino acid residue at the active site. For example, diisopropyl fluorophosphate (DIFP) reacts with a serine residue at the active site of acetylcholinesterase to form an inactive diisopropylphosphoryl enzyme. Alkylating reagents, such as iodoacetamide, inactivate enzymes that have thiol groups at their active sites, by reacting with the amino acid cysteine.

Reversible Inhibition. Reversible inhibition, in contrast, is characterized by an equilibrium between enzyme and inhibitor. Inhibition can be relieved by diluting the enzyme-inhibitor complex into a solution lacking inhibitor. Several main groups of reversible inhibitory mechanisms can be differentiated: competitive inhibition, noncompetitive inhibition, and uncompetitive inhibition. These are described below.

Competitive Inhibition. The inhibitor competes with the substrate or coenzyme for a common binding site, forming an enzyme-inhibitor complex EI. In many cases, the chemical structure of the inhibitor resembles that of the substrate. The inhibitor can be displaced by excess substrate. Figure 3 shows that V_{max} is unchanged whereas K_M is increased by the presence of inhibitor.

Noncompetitive Inhibition. The inhibitor decreases the catalytic activity of an enzyme without influencing the binding relationship between substrate and

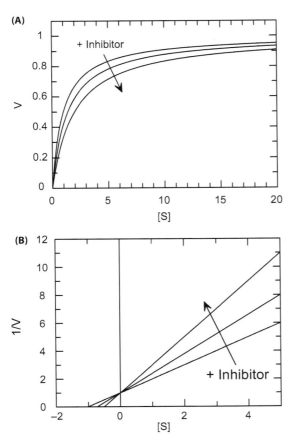

Figure 3 Plots showing competitive enzyme inhibition. (**A**) V versus [S]. Increasing concentrations of inhibitor (shown by the *arrow*) increase K_M but have no effect on V_{max}. This is readily apparent in the Lineweaver–Burk plot in (**B**).

enzyme. This means that inhibitor and substrate can bind simultaneously to an enzyme molecule to form ES, EI, or ESI complexes. Noncompetitive inhibition is dependent solely on the inhibitor concentration and is not overcome by high substrate concentration. This is shown in Figure 4. An example is the blocking of a catalytically essential cysteine residue by such heavy metals as copper or mercury.

Uncompetitive Inhibition. The inhibitor reacts only with the enzyme–substrate complex. An example is the reaction of azide with the oxidized form of cytochrome oxidase. Plots are shown in Figure 5. Note that V_{max} and K_M decrease concomitantly.

Substrate Inhibition. High concentrations of a substrate (or coenzyme) may decrease the catalytic activity of an enzyme. This can happen when the

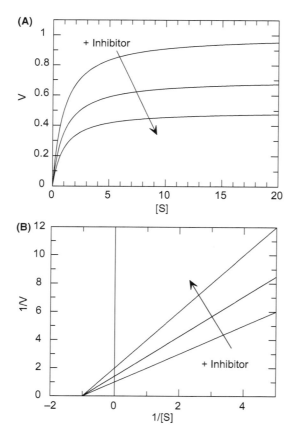

Figure 4 Plots showing noncompetitive enzyme inhibition. (**A**). V versus [S]. Increasing concentrations of inhibitor (shown by the *arrow*) decrease V_{max} but have no effect on K_M. This is readily apparent in the Lineweaver–Burk plot in (**B**).

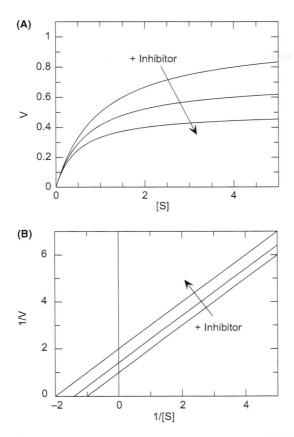

Figure 5 Plots showing uncompetitive enzyme inhibition. (**A**) V versus [S]. Increasing concentrations of inhibitor (shown by the *arrow*) cause a concomitant decrease in both K_M and V_{max}. This is readily apparent in the Lineweaver–Burk plot in (**B**).

substrate has an alternate, inhibitory, nonproductive mode of binding. Examples are the action of adenosine triphosphate (ATP) on phosphofructokinase and urea on urease. Plots showing substrate inhibition are shown in Figure 6.

End-Product Inhibition. In many multienzyme systems, such as an intracellular metabolic pathway, the end product of the reaction sequence may act as a specific inhibitor of an enzyme at or near the beginning of the sequence. Thus the flux through the pathway is regulated by its end product; the pathway produces more product when it is in short supply and less when it is plentiful. This type of inhibition, which acts as a feedback control loop, is also called feedback inhibition or retroinhibition. Many other factors control metabolic pathways as well, such as protein biosynthesis, and availability of ATP, nicotinamide adenine dinucleotide phosphate, reduced form (NADPH) and so on.

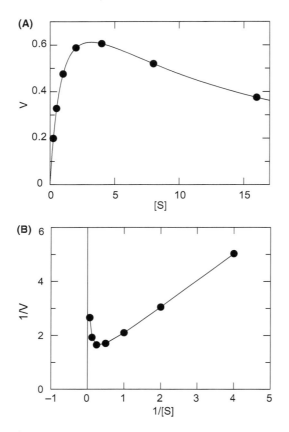

Figure 6 Plots showing substrate inhibition. (**A**) V versus [S]. Note that V decreases as [S] is raised to high levels. This results in the upward curvature at low 1/[S] in the Lineweaver–Burk plot in (**B**).

Kinetics of Reaction with Solid Substrates

Conventional enzyme kinetics concerns enzymes in solution acting on substrates in solution. This is sometimes not the case, particularly in personal care applications. An interesting variation on the kinetic equations presented above arises when an enzyme in solution acts on an insoluble substrate by adsorbing onto the surface of the substrate. In contrast to the previous cases, where the reaction rate increases in direct proportion to total enzyme concentration, a limiting rate is approached as enzyme concentration is increased. So to develop a kinetic model, we assume the enzyme adsorbs onto the substrate, rather than vice versa as in the previous section (7). One arrives at the converse of the previous model where activity levels out at high substrate concentration. In this case, enzyme activity is linear with respect to substrate concentration, and activity saturates with respect to enzyme concentration:

$$d[P]/dt = V_{max}[E]/(K + [E]) \tag{13}$$

Please refer to Figure 7. The mathematical difference between this result and the previous derivation is that now the enzyme concentration is much greater than the concentration of available adsorption sites, whereas in the previous, more conventional analysis, the substrate concentration is much greater than the enzyme concentration. These are limiting cases, and intermediate situations are encountered as well.

Well-known examples of enzymes functioning at the solid–liquid interface include cellulases acting on cellulose, amylases acting on starch granules, and protease enzymes, such as those in laundry detergents, acting on protein adsorbed to the surface of soiled fabric.

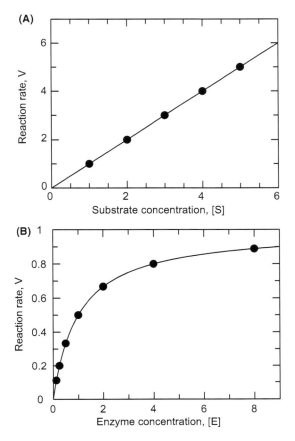

Figure 7 Plots of the kinetics of an idealized enzyme acting on an insoluble substrate. (**A**) V is linear with respect to substrate concentration. (**B**) V reaches a plateau at high enzyme concentration.

Enzyme Kinetics in Personal Care Applications

Enzyme kinetics in personal care applications will most likely be more complex than the idealized situations discussed above. A starting point for modeling the process will in many cases probably be based on the kinetics of reaction with a solid substrate. Steps in the reaction may involve (*i*) partitioning from the delivery formulation into the biological milleu, (*ii*) binding to the substrate, (*iii*) diffusion along the substrate surface to the chemical bond to be acted upon, (*iv*) the chemical reaction itself, and (*v*) release of product and enzyme. The rate-limiting step in this process will dominate the kinetics and efficiency of enzyme action.

ENZYME ACTIVITY—ITS MEASUREMENT AND INFLUENCE OF ENVIRONMENTAL FACTORS

Introduction

Measuring or assaying enzyme activity is generally central to the use and study of enzymes. For further information on this important topic there are a number of recent references available, including Ref. 8. To determine the catalytic activity of an enzyme, one usually measures the appearance of product, P, or the disappearance of substrate, S. It is generally desirable to adjust reaction conditions so the substrate is not significantly depleted during the course of the experiment. This is termed *initial rate conditions*. Thus, for a soluble enzyme-substrate system, substrate concentration is assumed to be constant, and Michaelis–Menten kinetics are valid with respect to the dependence of V on substrate concentration, and V is linearly dependent on enzyme concentration.

Units of Enzyme Activity

The units of activity of a particular enzyme are often defined by the investigators who first characterize its catalytic activity. In the literature, enzyme activity may be expressed in arbitrary units, for instance, changes in absorbance, increase of reducing groups, or amount of converted substrate expressed in milligrams or micromoles. These parameters are related to various time units, which can range from seconds to hours or perhaps days. This lack of standardized units of enzyme activity must be kept in mind when comparing results between various laboratories and the literature and source of enzyme.

Typical Enzyme Assays

Absorption spectrophotometry is a very common analytical technique for enzyme assays. Spectrophotometry is one of the preferred methods of enzyme assay because of its simplicity and the availability of reliable, reasonably priced instruments. In the simplest form of spectrophotometric assay, one monitors the appearance of a colored product or the disappearance of a colored substrate. The wavelength used can be in the visible or ultraviolet region of the electromagnetic spectrum.

Spectrofluorometry is also commonly used for enzyme assays. Because of its high sensitivity, it permits the assay of small amounts of enzymes. This technique often uses a fluorogenic substrate, that is, a substrate that becomes fluorescent when converted to product. The activity of enzyme systems that depend on nicotinamide adenine dinucleotide (NAD) and nicotinamide adenine dinucleotide phosphate (NADP) can be readily monitored by fluorometry. As a rule of thumb, the sensitivity of fluorometric assays is approximately 1000 times that of absorption spectrophotometry.

When radioactively labeled substrates are used, the activities of some enzymes can be determined with high sensitivity. This technique is widely employed in the field of molecular biology to monitor (*i*) the incorporation of radioactively labeled nucleotides into nucleic acids or polynucleotides (DNA and RNA polymerases), (*ii*) the decomposition of radioactively labeled DNA (exonuclease III), (*iii*) the transfer of a radioactively labeled phosphate group from γ-^{32}P-ATP to the 5'-hydroxyl end of a polynucleotide (polynucleotide kinase), or (*iv*) the exchange of radioactively labeled pyrophosphate on a carrier matrix (T4 DNA ligase). The most common isotopes for labeling are ^{32}P, ^{14}C, ^{3}H, and ^{35}S.

Other standard enzyme assay methods include: monitoring concentration changes of substrate or product in the reaction by gas or liquid chromatography, monitoring the uptake or release of protons (if this occurs on the reaction mechanism) with a "pH-stat," luminometry, conductometry, calorimetry, polarimetry, viscometry, and turbidimetry.

General Enzyme Assay Considerations

A reliable assay is of paramount importance for working with a particular enzyme. It allows one to measure enzyme production (during fermentation, for example), follow the enzyme recovery during purification, and monitor enzyme stability during storage. It allows one to measure the enzyme concentration in a sample to be used in an experimental application and, of course, is central to studying enzyme inhibition. Several aspects of achieving reliable enzyme assays include: using reproducible physical manipulations, preferably working within the range of enzyme concentrations where activity is linear with respect to both time and enzyme concentration, and determination of "blank" activities—determining apparent product formation by eliminating (in separate experiments) the presence of enzyme and substrate.

The reaction temperature must be controlled when measuring enzyme activity. As a general rule, the rate of enzyme-catalyzed reactions is approximately doubled by increasing the temperature by 10°C in the range of 0 to 40°C. Thus temperature must be kept constant to achieve reproducible results.

One important quality criterion of an enzyme preparation is its specific activity, for instance, the catalytic activity related to the protein content. Specific activity is usually expressed as units of enzyme activity per milligram of total protein. Specific activity of a given enzyme preparation is then compared with that of a highly purified enzyme sample of the same origin. For this purpose, catalytic activities and the determination of protein concentration must be measured under consistent conditions.

Effect of Environmental Variables on Enzyme Activity

(1) *Temperature*. The temperature dependence of enzyme-catalyzed reactions exhibits an optimum (Fig. 8). Activity increases with temperature at lower temperatures because of Arrhenius behavior of the reaction kinetics; as mentioned earlier, enzyme activity generally doubles for each 10°C increase in temperature. Activity decreases at higher temperatures because of thermal denaturation of the enzyme (loss of functional three-dimensional structure). The optimum is generally between 40 and 60°C. However, enzymes from thermophilic microbes, such as those that live in hot springs, may have temperature optima exceeding 100°C. A technologically important member of this class of enzymes is the DNA polymerase from *Thermus aquaticus*, which catalyzes DNA amplification via the polymerase chain reaction (9).

(2) *pH*. All enzymes have an optimum pH range for activity. The optimum depends on ionic strength and type of buffer, and may be influenced by temperature, substrate, and coenzyme concentrations. The pH dependence of enzyme catalysis often reflects the titration of amino acid side chains involved in

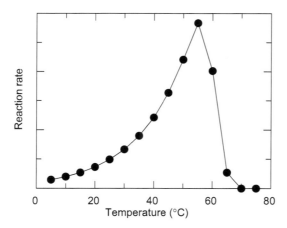

Figure 8   Effect of temperature on the reaction rate of an enzyme. The rate initially increases with temperature, and then falls off sharply as the enzyme denatures at high temperatures.

enzyme structure, in substrate binding, or in the chemical mechanism of the reaction itself. For many enzymes, the pH optimum lies in the neutral range. Extreme optimum values of 1.5 and 10.5 have been found for pepsin and for alkaline phosphatase, respectively. Figure 9 shows an example of ribonuclease, which has two histidine residues responsible for its mechanism (3). The action of ribonuclase requires that one of the histidine side chains is protonated and the other is not. The pKa of the protonated residue (histidine-12) is 5.8, whereas the other (histidine-119) has a pKa of 6.2. At low pH values, the enzyme is inactive because both histidines are protonated, and at high pH values the enzyme is inactive because both histidines are unprotonated. The optimum is at pH 6.0, where the ionization states of the histidines are balanced.

(3) *Ionic strength.* Because electrostatic interactions play a major role in substrate binding and catalysis, the ionic strength and types of ions present can have a significant influence on enzyme activity. Ionic strength can also affect protein aggregation, enhancing or preventing it, depending on the solutes and enzymes involved. It is essential to investigate the effect of salts and to mimic in the laboratory the actual conditions under which a particular enzyme will be applied.

(4) *Implications for the use of enzymes in personal care.* The strong dependence of enzyme activity on environmental conditions has benefits and drawbacks for personal care applications. On one hand, it may be possible to formulate an enzyme to optimize its activity, and on the other hand, the site of application of the enzyme and the nature of the biological milieu in which it functions may place severe constraints on the enzyme's environment. These factors must be carefully considered and studied when an enzyme is applied to a personal care opportunity.

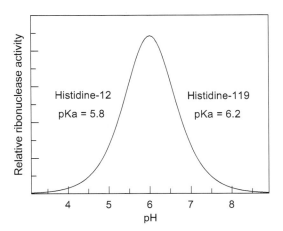

Figure 9   Effect of pH on enzyme activity. The case of ribonuclease is illustrated. See text for details.

ENZYME ENGINEERING

Enzyme engineering is a subdiscipline of protein engineering, which is the design, construction, and use of structurally modified proteins. The modifications in the structure of the protein of interest are achieved through genetic engineering, that is, modification of the DNA comprising the gene coding for the protein. Protein engineering was made possible in the early 1980s by breakthroughs in DNA manipulation technology.

Protein Structure and Biosynthesis

Changes in the amino acid sequence of a protein will affect its three-dimensional structure and function. Alteration of the amino acid sequence is accomplished by changing the DNA sequence of the gene. This allows the insertion of additional amino acids, the deletion of amino acids, or the substitution of one or more amino acids with others selected from the 20 amino acids available. These procedures are analogous to the mechanisms of mutation in nature, which also lead to altered proteins, some of which occasionally give rise to improved traits in the organism. This is, of course, central to the process of evolution.

Technologies Required for Protein Engineering

DNA cloning. This is the isolation and propagation of a particular DNA sequence; in the present case, the gene coding for the target protein. DNA cloning is now fairly easy and routinely performed (see chap. 1).

Mutagenesis techniques. This involves manipulating cloned DNA in order to insert or delete DNA or to change the DNA sequence in a highly specific or predictable and controlled fashion. There has been an explosion in mutagenesis techniques in the past few years; many of the methods take advantage of the ability to create many (not necessarily exact) copies of DNA through the polymerase chain reaction (PCR). Entire books have recently been published on mutagenesis techniques.

Protein expression. This consists of producing the protein of interest from its cloned DNA, generally in a microorganism, in quantities readily amenable to protein functional analysis. This generally requires placing the foreign DNA into the host DNA such that the context dictates that the host's transcription (conversion to messenger RNA) and translation (conversion of the messenger RNA to protein) mechanisms are co-opted to produce the foreign protein.

Protein functional analysis. This entails analyzing the properties of the target protein to determine which aspects require alteration, as well as analyzing the results of the protein engineering experiments to understand their underlying basis and provide hypotheses for further work. Protein functional analysis is an underappreciated aspect of protein engineering.

Enzyme/Protein structure determination. Rational protein engineering often requires knowledge of the three-dimensional molecular structure of the protein of interest. This is usually accomplished by X-ray crystallography. It is also often very useful to know the amino acid sequences of proteins that are structurally or functionally related to the target protein. This is achieved by experimentally determining DNA sequences and searching databases of known protein and DNA sequences. The methodologies for comparing and analyzing protein and DNA sequences are central to the rapidly growing field of bioinformatics.

Applications of Protein Engineering

Protein engineering can be used to solve a variety of different problems. Some of the major motivations for protein engineering are listed below. These are often interrelated and can be addressed simultaneously in well-designed enzyme engineering experiments.

Improving a property of an existing protein. This is the case where a protein, such as an enzyme, is found to be reasonably well suited for a particular application, but one or more of its functional properties require alteration. Typical examples include improving resistance of an enzyme to degradation at elevated temperatures or shifting its pH optimum.

Substantially altering the function of an existing protein. This is the case where a protein does not have a certain functional property required for a particular application. The goal is to introduce a new functional property into the protein by altering its structure. An example is changing an enzyme so that it acts on a different substrate than the one for which it evolved naturally.

Studying protein function. In this case, changes are made to the protein, and its functional response is analyzed. This approach can lead to deeper understanding of the underlying basis of the protein's function and builds on the knowledge base of the relation between protein structure and function.

Evolutionary Approaches to Protein Engineering

Protein engineering is not proper engineering in the strictest sense, because the physical and chemical principles that underlie the structure and function of proteins are not completely understood. We cannot readily predict the consequences of changes in the amino acid sequence of a protein, nor can we predict which changes will lead to a desired outcome. The size and complexity of proteins prevent us from using computational approaches in all but the simplest cases.

We are, however, able to take advantage of powerful techniques for efficient DNA manipulation in order to produce many altered proteins simultaneously. These proteins can then be screened for the property of interest by using the appropriate assay. Often, it is the development of a predictive assay that is the limiting factor in this approach; if large numbers of altered proteins are involved, then throughput becomes crucial as well (10).

Directed evolution of a protein in the laboratory involves (*i*) making amino-acid changes in a protein, often randomly throughout the sequence, (*ii*) subjecting the resulting large collection of protein variants to biological natural selection or a screening assay, and (*iii*) repeating the process with the fittest variant through a number of iterations.

CURRENT ENZYME APPLICATIONS IN PERSONAL CARE

Over the years, enzymes have been used for many applications, including dissolving blood clots in the body. The therapeutic use of enzymes has benefited significantly from biotechnology as evidenced by the increasing number of drugs that are currently designed based on enzymes. On the contrary, the use of enzymes within industrial settings is old. Many uses of enzymes for industrial applications, including personal care applications, are very well documented in various books (11–13). The use of enzymes for personal care applications is heavily patented. For example, if the U.S. Patents Database (patents issued from 1976 to 2004) is searched for the key words "enzyme" and "skin care," "hair care" or "oral care," it shows more than 600, 270 and 95 patents listed, respectively. These patents cover the direct use of enzymes, use of enzymes to make specific ingredients and modulation of enzyme activities in vivo to deliver a personal care benefit. In the personal care business, the use of enzymes as digestive aid and contact lens cleaning has grown, however, the use of enzymes in skin care, hair care, oral care, and for other personal care applications has been limited, despite the large number of patents existing in the area.

The section below describes the use of enzymes for specific benefits or claims in skin-care, hair-care, and oral-care applications. In addition, enzymes are also used as preservatives in cosmetic products. There are two enzyme systems used for this purpose: One is lysozyme (mostly from hen egg white), and the other system includes lactoperoxidase in conjunction with other enzymes and proteins (14–16).

Skin Care

The use of proteases in skin-care applications has been increasing over the last few years. It is claimed that proteases provide smoother skin through gentle exfoliation. The proposed mode of action of proteases is to cleave the proteins, which adhere dead cells and in turn make skin look younger and smoother by removing the keratinous dead cell layer (17). Therefore, proteases are used in one or more products of a typical skin-care regimen. To name a few product categories, proteases are included in cleansers, masks, exfoliating scrubs, peels, acne creams, and skin moisturizers. Proteases of plant origin, such as papain from papaya and bromelain from pineapple, have been the most widely used so far. Recently, proteases from bacterial and fungal origin are coming into greater favor. The reason behind the shift is that the bacterial and fungal protease products are available with a consistent quality and are more economical to produce as they are manufactured by fermentation rather than extracted from plants. In addition, there are a number of bacterial and fungal proteases with different attributes available to select from, for the personal care formulators. Bacteria and fungi produce a number of proteases that differ due to their preference for a specific protein substrate(s), pH profile, and ability to function in specific formulations and under other varied conditions (18,19).

Various bacterial ferments (which include enzymes) are also used in skin-care products. Bacteria and/or enzymes have been used in bathing products in Japan and around the world, and many times these are referred to as "enzyme bath." Such products contain proteases as well as other enzymatic activities.

In recent years, oxidative damage has been postulated as a major cause of skin aging, therefore enzymes (e.g., catalase and superoxide dismutase) implicated in relieving oxidative damage are used in skin-care products. Catalase hydrolyzes hydrogen peroxide to oxygen and water and is found in all cells and organs. Superoxide dismutase catalyzes the removal of oxygen-free radicals and protects cells against the harmful effects of superoxide-free radicals (20). Another enzyme implied for use in the skin care applications is T4 nuclease. It is shown to repair DNA damage caused by UV exposure (21).

Hair Care

One of the current applications of enyzmes in hair care is in lice egg removal. The key enzyme activity employed in this application is a protease (22,23). In addition, use of enzyme mixtures containing various families of enzymes, such as lyases, oxidoreductases, and hydrolases (includes proteases), is patented for nits removal from hair (24).

Hair dyeing is another application where enzymes may have utility. Use of enzymes in hair coloring is heavily patented, but there are no enzyme-based products currently on the market. The current processes of hair coloring are based on oxidative chemistry initiated by hydrogen peroxide (see chap. 12 of this book, Refs. 11,25). It is possible to substitute hydrogen peroxide with such oxidative enzymes as oxidases, peroxidases, and laccases in order to achieve a milder process. Use of these enzymes in the hair coloring process is described in detail elsewhere (11,26–28). Oxidases produce hydrogen peroxide in presence of oxygen by oxidizing their substrates; for example, glucose oxidase oxidizes glucose, whereas uricase (urate oxidase) acts on nitrogenous compounds (29–30). Peroxidases (31) generate more potent species from hydrogen peroxide. There are patents (32–34) claiming combined use of oxidases and peroxidases to color hair with the use of very small amount of hydrogen peroxide. However, in recent years, many patents are proposing the use of laccases in hair coloring. Laccases are copper-containing oxidases that act on diphenol and related substrates (35).

Other uses of enzymes for hair care applications are based on hair biochemistry. The primary component of hair is keratin proteins (see details in chap. 10 of this book). Keratins are rich in cysteines and have alpha helical structure, which coil around each other to form dimers. Cysteines from neighboring polypeptides form disulfide bonds. The amount of cysteines and the degree of cross-linking (disulfides) among them influences the physical properties of hair (36). Hair with higher disulfide bonds tends to curl, whereas hair with lower number of disulfide is straight. Therefore, an enzyme that can reshuffle cysteines can alter hair properties and can be used in hair waving or straightening products. Enzyme protein disulfide-isomerase (sometimes referred as thioredoxin or thioredoxin reductase), found in nature, has such enzymatic activities (37,38). In addition, transglutaminase that cross-links lysines is also proposed in hair waving application (39).

Oral Care

Dextranase and mutanase enzymes have been used in toothpastes in the past. These enzymes were used to hydrolyze or remove the dextran and mutan containing adhesive molecules produced by bacteria in the mouth cavity (40–42). In 1973, use of invertase along the same line was proposed for oral care application (43). However, the use of these enzymes in oral care products did not proliferate in those days, probably due to their limited availability and cost.

Currently other enzymes are used in toothpastes, as well as chewing gums, dental floss, and mouthwashes. These include a protease, glucoamylase, glucose oxidase, lactoperoxidase, and lysozyme (44–49). Starch hydrolyzing (glucoamylase) and protein-hydrolyzing (protease) enzymes are used to break down food residues to facilitate its removal and hydrolyze the bacterial film formed on teeth. As mentioned above, glucose oxidase oxidizes glucose (included with dentifrice in the presence of oxygen) and generates hydrogen peroxide, which is known to clean and whiten teeth. Many oral care products use glucose oxidase in conjunction with lactoperoxidase to generate active oxygen species from hydrogen peroxide (48).

INTRINSIC ENZYMES AS TARGETS IN PERSONAL CARE

Most biological processes involve one or more enzymatic reactions. This means that such enzymes present themselves as targets to develop personal care ingredients that could modulate them. Three examples of enzymes targeted in personal care applications are highlighted below. First, tyrosinase catalyzes the first critical step of melanin synthesis (see details in chap. 8 and Refs. 50,51) and, in turn, skin pigmentation. Therefore, there are many skin whitening/lightening products on the market containing ingredients that claim to inhibit tyrosinase (52,53).

The second group of targets includes proteases. By mid-2003, various teams around the world had annotated 553 genes that encode proteases or proteases homologue in the human genome (54)—which means close to 2% of the human genome codes for proteases. It seems that 93 of these proteases are catalytically inactive, meaning in the human body there are more than 400 active proteases. There are reports on the involvement of proteases that range from skin desquamation (54) to skin aging and firmness (see details in chap. 7, Refs. 55–59). However, very different proteases are involved in these processes. In skin desquamation, the stratum corneum chymotrypsin is involved, whereas a slew of metalloproteinases with collagenase and elastase activities that hydrolyze specific elastin or collagens play a role in skin aging and firmness. Our bodies also have many protease inhibitors that modulate the proteases that are implied in skin aging (see details in chap. 7 and Refs. 60–62). This wide range of proteases and their varied roles exhibit the potential for proteases to be targeted in skin-care applications. In addition, a protease is implicated in skin pigmentation (63). A protease-activated receptor (referred as PAR-2) of keratinocytes is involved in regulating skin pigmentation (see details in chap. 8, Refs. 64). In turn, soybean extract that inhibits proteases is used to inhibit the PAR-2 pathway for skin depigmentation (65).

Third example is related to hair growth. Androgenic alopecia, a common form of baldness in both sexes. As the name suggests, it is associated with androgens (chaps. 10 and 11, Ref. 66). Key hair growth inhibiting androgen, dihydrotestosterone is produced from testosterone by the enzymatic activity of 5-alpha-reductases. Therefore, reductase inhibitor like finasteride are used in hair-growth products (67).

THE FUTURE OF ENZYMES IN PERSONAL CARE

As biotechnology tools continue to improve and expand, development of enzymes as cosmetic ingredients or targets for cosmetic ingredients and products should increase. The impact of biotechnology will occur in multiple ways. First, biotechnology will make available the rare enzymes for testing and application development. Second, once the enzyme benefit is proven, biotechnology will help to produce it within the cost structure of a personal care ingredient industry. If an enzymatic activity delivers a benefit, but is unsuitable for the formulation or application, enzyme engineering (discussed earlier) will enable overcoming such difficulties. Use of enzyme engineering for stability, substrate specificity, application conditions like pH, temperature and so on has been demonstrated for other applications, such as starch processing and use in detergents (11,68,69). In addition, biotechnology enables targeting of enzymes to specific sites by adding specific sequences to them. Targeting of enzymes, thus, can be used to further enhance the benefits delivered. The efficacy of a laccase that bleaches a stain was improved tenfold by targeting it to the stain using a specific peptide (70).

Biotechnology would also aid in making available new enzyme targets. This has been evident in case of skin enzymes in the last few years. For example, besides proteases mentioned above, there are additional proteases and other class of enzymes that are critical in skin biology. The studies show involvement of five stratum corneum enzymes in establishing stratum corneum permeability barrier: chymotrypsin (stratum corneum chymotryptic enzyme or SCCE), its activator enzyme—trypsin (stratum corneum tryptic enzyme or SCTE), acid phosphatase, beta-glucocerebrosidase and phospholipase (71–73). There are reports of molecular cloning of the human stratum corneum chymotrypsin (SCCE) (74) and trypsin (SCTE) (75). Biotechnology tools (cloning and expression of enzymes and substrate proteins) allowed scientists to study both these proteases for their ability to act on the adhesive proteins of the extracellular part of the corneodesmosomes: desmoglein 1, desmocollin 1, and corneodesmosin (76). It is reported that chymotrypsin (SCCE) cleaved corneodesmosin and desmocollin 1; and upon mixing of trypsin (SCTE), all three proteins were degraded (76). In case of SCCE, it is expressed in *Aspergillus*, so a large amount of it is available for further studies (77). Once such human enzymes are available in enough quantity, screening and developing ingredients that specifically modulate them should become easier.

In earlier sections, targeting of skin tyrosinase for skin-lightening products is discussed. However, targeting of tyrosinase for hair-pigmentation products has not been a major research area. Hair pigmentation is an active research area and tyrosinase is a key enzyme in hair melanogenesis also (chap. 12, Ref. 78). Hair melanogenesis is also coupled with hair-growth cycle. As enzymatic processes involved in hair pigmentation and hair growth are elucidated, many of these enzymes will become targets for hair-care products. Similarly, not much is known about enzymes and enzymatic processes associated with nail. As the type and number of biotechnology and microscopy tools expand, enzymes will become target for hair-care and nail-care products. Enzyme steroid sulfatase and its substrate, cholesterol sulfate, were assayed in the nails of children being screened for X-linked ichthosis (79,80).

In future, oral care products will be based on the knowledge of oral cavity enzymes and enzymes produced by oral cavity microorganisms. Saliva enzymes, such as lysozyme and peroxidase, are implied in inhibition of microbial growth in mouth (81). However, intense area of research involves enzymes from oral bacteria. First, enzymes from oral cavity bacteria are implied in malodor (bad breath) generation (82,83). In future, these enzymes could become target for oral-care product developments. Second, interesting futuristic product concepts are based on the bacterial enzyme: glucosyltransferase (glucansucrase or dextransucrase). Glucosyltransferase enzymes play a key role in colonization of bacteria of *Streptococcus* species (many times referred as mutans streptococcia), plaque formation, and caries (chap. 13, Refs. 84,85). Bacteria adhere relatively poorly to tooth pellicle, however, they adhere strongly and in larger numbers to glucan that is formed from sucrose in the pellicle by glucosyltransferase from mutans streptococci. Glucosyltransferases have been an intense area of oral-care research, which has been using biotechnology tools for a while. There are at least three glucosyltransferases present in mutans streptococci (86–88) that play a key role in plaque formation. Mutational inactivation techniques have shown that each of these gene products (enzymes) is important to the cariogenicity of the respective strain. These enzymes are being explored to develop oral care product concepts in various ways. The initial studies used potential inhibitors of these enzymes: tea extracts and propolis secreted by bees (89–91). These materials report reduced incidence of caries in animal models. Furthermore, based on the biotechnology tools and knowledge of these enzymes, an intriguing way to battle dental plaque and caries is also being explored and tested in animals: immunization, either active or passive (see reviews 92–95). Induction of salivary IgA antibody in human by oral or topical administration of glucosyltransferase enzyme, that in turn is reported to reduce the colonization of mutans streptococci (92–96). Passive administration of antibody to glucosyltransferase in the diet also reported to protect rats from experimental dental caries (92–94,97). There is also work done with peptides from glucosyltransferase (from active site region or substrate binding region). Immunization of rats with such peptides provided protection against caries (98). In addition, scientists are exploring use of mutans streptococci with mutated or deleted enzyme genes to colonize mouth, so bad bacteria do not bind to teeth (92). Studies have shown that in comparison with their parent strains, mutants that are unable to synthesize water-insoluble glucans have a decreased ability to adhere to the teeth and induce a lower rate of caries in animals (99,100).

This gives a flavor of what is possible and coming up with enzymes in conjunction with biotechnology tools in personal care.

REFERENCES

1. Kuhn P, Knapp M, Soltis SM, Ganshaw G, Theoene M, Bott R. The 0.78 A strutcture of a serine protease: *Bacillus lentus* sutilisin. Biochem 1998; 39:13446–13452
2. Lehninger AL. Biochemistry. 2d ed. New York: Worth Publishers, Inc., 1975.
3. Fersht AR. Enzyme Structure and Mechanism. 2d ed. New York, NY: W.H. Freeman and Co., 1985.
4. Michaelis L, Menten ML. Kinetik der Invertinwirkung. Biochem Z 1913; 49:333.
5. Segel IH. Enzyme Kinetics. New York: John Wiley and Sons, 1993.
6. Lineweaver H, Burk D. The determination of enzyme dissociation constants. J Am Chem Soc 1934; 56:658.
7. Bailey JE, Ollis DF. Biochemical Engineering Fundamentals. 2d ed. New York: McGraw-Hill, Inc. 1986; 148–152.
8. Eisenthal R, Danson MJ, eds. Enzyme Assays. 2d ed. Oxford, UK: Oxford University Press, 2002.
9. White BA, ed. PCR Cloning Protocols. New Jersey: Humana Press, Inc., 1997.
10. Arnold FH, Georgiou G, eds. Directed Enzyme Evolution. New Jersey: Humana Press, Inc., 2003.
11. Wolfgang A, ed. Enzymes in Industry: Production and Applications. KgaA, Berlin, Germany: Wiley-Vch Verlag GmbH & Co., 2003.
12. Godfrey T, West S, eds. Industrial Enzymology. 2d ed. Basingstoke Hampshire, England: Macmillan Press Ltd., 1996.

13. Wiseman A, ed. Handbook of Enzyme Biotechnology. West Sussex, England: Ellis Horwood Limited, 1986.
14. Meyer A. Antimicrobial enzymes. In: Zeuthen P, Bogh-Sorensen L, eds. Food Preservation Techniques. USA: Woodhead Publishing Ltd., 2003.
15. Galley E, Godfrey DC, Guthrie WG, Hodgkinson DM, Linnington HL. Antimicrobial compositions 1997; US Patent 5,607,681.
16. Guthrie WG. A novel adaptation of a naturally occurring antimicrobial system for cosmetic protection. SOFW-J 1992; 118:556–562
17. Masunaga T. Enzymes in cleansers. In: Leyden JJ, Rawlings AV, eds. Skin Moisturization. New York, NY: Marcel Dekker, Inc., 2002:385–403.
18. Barrett AJ, Rawlings ND, Woessner JF. Handbook of Proteolytic Enzymes. London: Academic Press, 1998.
19. Visse R, Nagase H. Matrix metalloproteinases and tissue inhibitors of metalloproteinases: structure, function, and biochemistry. Circ Res 2003; 92(8):827–839.
20. White JS, White DC. Source Book of Enzymes. Boca Raton: CRC Press, 1997: 176–179.
21. Yarosh DB, O'Connor A, Alas L, Potten C, Wolf, P. Photoprotection by topical DNA repair enzymes: molecular correlates of clinical studies. Photochem Photobiol 1999; 69(2):136–140.
22. Tvedten SL. The Best Control II Book on CD-ROM Intelligent Pest Management. Marne, MI: Safe Solutions, Inc., 2004:767–770.
23. Jones SC, Bozick JV. Head Lice. Bulletin 893-01 2001, Ohio State University Extension.
24. Upton HF. Method for removing nits from hair 1996; U.S. Patent 5,547,665.
25. Corbett JF. Hair Colorants: Chemistry and Toxicology (Cosmetic Science Monograph No. 2), Port Washington, NY: Micelle Press, 1998.
26. Soloway S. Method for coloring human hair with polyhydric aromatic compound, aromatic amine and an oxidation enzyme 1996; U.S. Patent 3,251,742.
27. Lang G, Cotteret J. Mixture for the oxidation tinting of keratin fibers containing a laccase and tinting methods using said mixture 2003; U.S. Patent 6,626,962.
28. Sorensen NH, McDevitt JP. Method for treating hair 2000; U.S. Patent 6,572,843.
29. White JS, White DC. Source Book of Enzymes. Boca Raton: CRC Press, 1997: 129–132.
30. Tsujino Y, Kitayama K, Yokoo Y, Sakato K. The application of oxidases to hair dyeing and permanent waving. J Soc Cos Chem 1991; 24:220–223.
31. Zeffren E, Sullivan JF. Enzyme-activated oxidative process for coloring hair 1976; U.S. Patent 3,957,424.
32. Kunz M, Le Cruer. Oxidation hair dye composition and method of dyeing hair using same, 1997; EP 795313 A2.
33. Saettler A, Kleen A, Weiss A, Rose D. Colouring Agents With Enzymes, 2000; WO 0021497.
34. Dornbusch K, Lorenz A, Olt A, Tennigkeit J. Process and composition for oxidative dyeing of human hair using catalase-free peroxidase, 1993; EP-A 548620.
35. White JS, White DC. Source Book of Enzymes. Boca Raton: CRC Press, 1997: 139.
36. Fuchs E. Keratins and the skin. Annu Rev Cell Dev Biol 1995; 11:123–153.
37. Schreiber W. Mittel Zur Formveraenerung Von Skelroproteinen, 1973; Patent DE 2141764, 19730301.

38. Pigiet VP. Use of thioredoxin, thioredoxin-derived, or thioredoxin-like dithiol peptides in hair care preparations 1991; U.S. Patent 5,028,419.

39. Gardner JM, Swanson PE, Torres-Lopez B. An investigation into the action of transglutaminase on human hair. Virg J Soc Cosmet Chem 1995; 46:11–28.

40. Barker SA, Wiggins LF. Pharmazeutisch annehmbare Zubereitungen zur Anwendung an den Zaehnen, 1971; Patent DE 1965043.

41. Harth H, Rau K, Scheer K. Zahnreinigungsmittel, 1971; Patent DE 1948468.

42. Schilling K.M, Bowen WH. Glucans synthesized in situ in experimental salivary pellicle function as specific binding sites for *Streptococcus mutans*. Infect Immun 1992; 90:284–295.

43. Becker JG, Mitchell RL, Pierson WG. Oral composition containing an enzyme 1973; U.S. Patent 3,733,399.

44. Glace WR, Ibsen RL. Toothpaste having low abrasion 1991; U.S. Patent 4,986,981.

45. Sauer J, Sigurskjold BW, Christensen U, Frandsen TP, Mirgorodskaya E, Harrison M, Roepstorff P, Svensson B. Glucoamylase: structure/function relationships, and protein engineering. Biochim Biophys Acta-Protein Structure and Molecular Enzymology 2000; 1543:275–293.

46. Pellico MA, Montgomery RE. Stabilized enzymatic dentrifice containing beta-D-glucose and glucose oxidase 1985; U.S. Patent 4,537,764.

47. Fridh G, Koch G. Effect of mouthrinse containing amyloglucosidase and glucose oxidase on recurrent aphthous ulcers in children and adolescents. Swed Dent J 1999; 23:49–57.

48. Pellico MA, Montgomery RE. Di-enzymatic dentrifrice 1986; U.S. Patent 4,578,265.

49. Lenander-Lumikari M, Tenovuo J, Mikola H. Effects of a lactoperoxidase system-containing toothpaste on levels of hypothiocyanite and bacteria in saliva. Caries Res 1993; 27:285–291.

50. Prota G. Melanins and Melanogenesis. San Diego: Academic Press, 1992.

51. Sturm RA, Fox NF, Ramsay M. Human pigmentation genetics: the difference is only skin deep. BioEssays 1998; 20:712–721.

52. Petit L, Pierard GE. Skin-tightening products revisited. Int J Cosmet Sci 2003; 25:169–181.

53. Bauman L. Depigmenting agents. In: Bauman L, ed. Cosmetic Dermatology: Principles and Practice. Hong Kong: The McGraw-Hill Companies, 2002.

54. Puente XS, Sanchez LM, Overall CM, Lopez-Otin C. Human and mouse proteases: a comparative genomic approach. Nature Rev(Genetics) 2003; 4: 544–558.

55. Sato J. Desquamation and the role of stratum corneum enzymes. In: Leyden JJ, Rawlings AV, eds. Skin Moisturization. Marcel Dekker, Inc., 2002:81–94.

56. Kahari V, Saarialho-Kere U. Matrix metallproteinases in skin. Exp Dermatol 1997; 6(5):199–213.

57. Rittie L, Fisher GJ. UV-induced signal cascades and skin aging. Ageing Res Rev 2002; 1(4):705–720.

58. Hornebeck W. Down-regulation of tissue inhibitor of matrix metalloprotease-1 (TIMP-1) in aged human skin contributes to matrix degradation and impaired cell growth and survival. Pathol Biol (Paris) 2003; 117(5):569–573.

59. Chung JH, Seo JY, Choi HR, Lee MK, Youn CS, Rhie G, Cho KH, Park KC, Eun HC. Modulation of skin collagen metabolism in aged and photoaged human skin in vivo. J Invest Dermatol 2001; 117(5):1218–1224.

60. Gomez DE, Alanso DF, Yashiji H, Thorgeirson UP. Tissue inhibitors of metalloproteinases: structure, regulation and biological functions. Eur J Cell Biol 1997; 74(2):111–122.
61. Voegeli R, Meier J, Doppler S, Sturzebeeher J, Girad P. Elastase and tryptase determination on human skin surface. Cosmet & Toilet 1996; 111(7):51–55.
62. Trojanowska M, LeRoy EC, Eckes B, Krieg TC. Pathogenesis of fibrosis: type 1 collagen and the skin. J Mol Med 1998; 76(3–4):266–274.
63. Babiarz-Magee L, Chen N, Seiberg M, Lin CB. The expression and activation of protease-activated receptor-2 correlate with skin color. Pigment Cell Res 2004; 17:241–251.
64. Seiberg M, Paine C, Sharlow E, Andrade-Gordon P, Costano M, Eisinger M, Shapiro SS. The protease-activated receptor-2 regulates pigmentation via keratinocyte–melanocyte interactions. Exp Cell Res 2000; 254:25–32.
65. Paine C, Sharlow E, Liebel F, Eisinger, Shapiro S, Seiberg M. An alternative approach to depigmentation by soybean extracts via inhibition of the PAR-2 pathway. J Invest Dermatol 2001; 116:587–595.
66. Randall VA. Androgens and human hair growth. Clin Endocrinol 1994; 40: 439–457.
67. Dallob AL, Sadic NS, Unger W, Lipert S, Geissler LA, Gregoire SL, Nguyen HH, Moore EC, Tanaka WK. The effect of finasteride, a 5 alpha-reductase inhibitor, on scalp skin testosterone and dihydrotestosterone concentrations in patients with male pattern baldness. J Clin Endocrinol Metab 1994; 3:703–706.
68. Graycar TP, Bott RR, Caldwell RM, Dauberman JL, Lad PJ, Power SD, Sagar IH, Silva RA, Weiss GL, Woodhouse LR, Estell DE. Altering the proteolytic activity of subtilisin through protein engineering. Enzyme Engineering XI. Annals N.Y. Acad Sci 1992; 672:71–79.
69. van Ee JH, Misset O, Baas EJ, eds. Enzymes in Detergency. Surfactant Science Series, Vol. 69. Boca Raton, FL: CRC Press, 1997.
70. Janssen GG, Baldwin TM, Winetzky DS, Tierney LM, Wang H, Murray CJ. Selective targeting of a laccase from Stachybotrys chartarum covalently linked to a carotenoid binding peptide. J Peptide Res 2004; 64(1):10–24.
71. Redoules D, Tarroux R, Perie JJ. Epidermal enzymes: their role in homeostasis and their relationships with dermatoses. Skin Pharmacol Appl Skin Physiol 1998; 11: 183–192.
72. Redoules D, Tarroux R, Assalit MF, Perie JJ. Characterization and assay of five enzymatic activities in the stratum corneum using tape-strippings. Skin Pharmacol Appl Skin Physiol 1999; 12:182–192
73. Elias PM. The epidermal permeability barrier: from early days at Harvard to emerging concepts. J Invest Dermatol 2004; 122(2):XXXVI–XXXIX.
74. Hansson L, Stromqvist M, Backman A, Wallbrandt P, Carlstein A. Egelrud T. Cloning, expression, and characterization of stratum corneum chymotryptic enzym: a skin-specific human serine proteinase. J Biol Chem 1994; 269:19420–19426.
75. Brattsand M, Egelrud T. Purification, molecular cloning and expression of a human stratum corneum trypsin-like serine protease with possible function in desquamation. J Biol Chem 1999; 274(42):30033–30040.
76. Caubet C, Jonca N, Brattsand M, Guerrin M, Bernard D, Schmidt R, Egelrud T, Simon M, Serre G. Degradation of coneodesmosome proteins by two serine proteases of the Kallikrein family, SCTE/KLK5/hK5 and SCCE/KLK7/hK7. J Invest Dermatol 2004; 122(5):1235–1244.

77. Baldwin T, Barnett C, Granshaw G, Bower B. Abstract from the conference: recombinant protein production with prokaryotic and eukaryotic host cells. Hosted by European Federation of Biology, in Italy, Nov 14–16, 2002.

78. Jimbow K, Park JS, Kato F, Hirosaki K, Toyofuku K, Hua C. Yamashita T. Assembly, target-signaling and intracellular transport of tyrosinase gene family proteins in the initial stage of melanosome biogenesis. Pigment Cell Res 2000; 13(4):10698–10703.

79. Matsumuto T, Sakura N, Ueda K. Steroid sulphatase activity in nails: screening for X-linked ichthyosis. Pediatr Dermatol 1990; 7:266–269.

80. Serizawa S, Nagai T, Ito M, Sato Y. Cholesterol sulphate levels in the hair and nails of patients with recessive X-linked ichthyosis. Clin Exp Dermatol 1990; 15:13–15.

81. Marcotte H, Lavoie MC. Oral microbial ecology and the role of salivary immunoglobulin A. Microbiol Mol Biol Rev 1998; 62:71–109.

82. Monita M, Wang H. Association between oral malodor and adult periodontis: a review. J Clin Periodontol 2001; 28(9):813–819.

83. Ratcliff PA, Johnson PW. The relationship between oral malodor, gingivitis, and periodontitis. A review. J Periodontol 1999; 7:485–489.

84. Yamashita Y, Bowen WH, Burne RA, Kuramitsu HK. Role of the *Strptococcia mutans gtf* in caries induction in the specific-pathogen-free rat model. Infect Immun 1993; 61:3811–3817.

85. Schilling KM, Bowen WH. Glucans synthesized in situ in experimental salivary pellicle function as specific binding sites for *Streptococcus mutans*. Infect Immun 1992; 60:284–295.

86. Aoki H, Shiroza T, Hayakawa M, Sato S, Kuramitsu HK. Cloning of a *Streptococcus mutans* glucosyltransferase gene coding for insoluble glucan synthesis. Infect Immun 1986; 53(3):587–594.

87. Hanada N, Kuramitsu HK. Isolation and characterization of the *Streptococcus mutans gtfC* gene coding for synthesis of both soluble and insoluble glucans. Infect Immun 1988; 56:1999–2005.

88. Hanada N, Kuramitsu HK. Isolation and characterization of the *Streptococcus mutans gtfD* gene coding for primer-dependent soluble glucan synthesis. Infect Immun 1989; 57:2079–2085.

89. Hamilton-Miller JM. Anti-cariogenic properties of tea (Camellia sinensis). J Med Micribiol 2001; 50(4):299–302.

90. Koo H, Rosalen PL, Cury JA, Park YK, Ikegaki M, Sattler A. Effect of *Apis mellifera* propolis from two Brazalian regions on caries development in desalivated rats. Caries Res 1999; 33:393–400.

91. Koo H, Pearson SK, Scott-Anne K, Abranches J, Cury JA, Rosalen PL, Park YK, Marquis RE, Bowen WH. Effects of apigenein and *tt*-farnrsol on glucosyltransferase activity, biofilm viability and caries development in rats. Oral Microbiol Immunol 2002; 17(6):337–343.

92. Kuramitsu HK. Molecular genetic analysis of the virulence of oral bacterial pathogens: an historical perspective. Crit Rev Oral Biol Med 2003; 14(5):331–344.

93. Smith DJ. Dental caries vaccines: Prospects and concerns. Crit Rev Oral Biol Med 2002; 13(4):335–349.

94. Russell MW, Childers NK, Michalek SM, Smith DJ, Taubman MA. A caries vaccine? Caries Res 2004; 38:230–235.

95. Smith DJ, Taubman MA. Oral immunization of humans with *Streptococcus sorbinus* glucosyltransferase. Infet Immun 1987; 55:2562–2569.
96. Childers NK, Zhang SS, Michalek SM. Oral immunization of humans with dehydrated liposomes containing *Streptococcus mutans* glucosyl transferase induces salivary immunoglobulin A2 antibody responses. Oral Microbiol Immunol 1994; 9:146–153.
97. Hamada S, Horikoshi T, Minami T, Kawabata S, Hiraoka J, Fujiwara T, Ooshima T. Oral passive immunization against dental caries in rats by use of hen egg yolk antibodies specific for cell-associated glucosyltransferase of *Streptococcus mutans*. Infect Immun 1991; 59:4161–4167.
98. Taubman MA, Holmberg CJ, Smith DJ. Immunization of rats with synthetic peptide constructs from the glucan-binding or catalytic region of mutans streptococcal glucosyltransferase protects against dental caries. Infect Immun 1995; 63:3088–3093.
99. de Stoppelaar JD, Konig K, Piasschaert A, van der Hoeven. Decreased cariogenicity of a mutant of *Streptococcus mutans*. Arch Oral Biol 1971; 16:971–975.
100. Tanzer JM, Freedman ML, Fitzgerald RJ, Larsan RH. Diminished virulence of glucan synthesis-defective mutants of *Streptococcus mutans*. Infect Immun 1974; 10:197–203.
101. International Union of Biochemistry and Molecular Biology Nomenclature Committee, Enzyme Nomenclature 1992. California: Academic Press, Inc.

5

Biotechnology in Skin Care (I): Overview

Susanne Iobst, Uma Santhanam, and Ronni L. Weinkauf

Unilever Research U.S., Edgewater, New Jersey, U.S.A.

SKIN STRUCTURE, PROPERTIES, AND PHYSIOLOGY

Structure of Skin

Skin is the largest organ in the body, constituting about 12% of body weight and covering an area of up to 2 sq.m. in an average adult. The thickness of skin ranges from 2 mm in such areas as palms and soles to 0.5 mm on the eyelids. Skin comprises two major layers—the outer epidermis and the underlying dermis—which are distinct in architecture, physiology, and function. Embedded in the dermis are several types of appendages such as the hair follicle, sweat glands, and sebaceous glands that are unique to skin. Skin also contains systems that are common to other organs, such as elements of the vasculature and nerve fibers (1).

Epidermis forms the external surface of skin. Its thickness varies from 75 to 150 μm, except on soles and palms where it is about 0.4 to 0.6 mm. The epidermis is a stratified epithelium that is composed of four layers: *stratum basale, stratum spinosum, stratum granulosum*, and the outermost *stratum corneum*. These layers are formed by the differentiation of the major cell in the epidermis called the keratinocyte.

A single layer of cuboidal keratinocytes attached to a basement membrane forms the *stratum basale*. Above the basal layer is the spinous layer, so called for the prickly appearance of cells caused by the abundance of desmosomes. The next layer up is the *stratum granulosum*, consisting of keratinocytes containing basophilic keratohyalin granules. This layer is also marked by the presence of lamellar granules that are extruded into the intercellular compartment.

The outermost layer is the S*tratum corneum* or the corneal layer, which is made up of anucleated, fully keratinized, flat, and fused cells called corneocytes and is several cells thick. The protein involucrin forms a tough, cross-linked layer on the inner surface of the plasma membrane and confers mechanical resistance to this outermost layer of skin. The intercellular space is occupied by ordered lipid lamellae, consisting of cholesterol, its esters, and ceramides. The stratum corneum resembles a brick-and-mortar arrangement with corneocytes forming the bricks and the intercellular lipids and proteins forming the mortar (Fig. 1).

The main cell type that forms the epidermis is the keratinocyte, named for its key function of synthesizing the intermediate filament keratin. Keratinocytes in the basal layer proliferate and undergo differentiation as they migrate upward toward the surface, ending up as terminally differentiated cornified cells that are then sloughed off. The migration process usually takes about 28 days and is perturbed in disease states such as psoriasis. The process of differentiation is accompanied by increased expression of different types of keratin as well as other proteins, such as involucrin and filaggrin and the enzyme transglutaminase I,

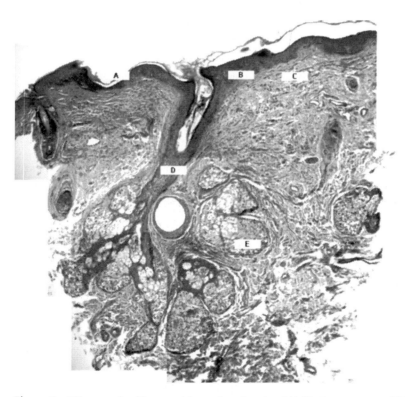

Figure 1   Micrograph of human skin section showing (**A**) Stratum corneum (**B**) Epidermis (**C**) Dermis (**D**) Hair follicle, and (**E**) Sebaceous gland.

compared to the cells in the basal layer. A gradient of calcium exists in the epidermis, with concentration increasing toward the outer layer, and this is believed to be the physiological driver of the differentiation process.

Melanocytes are also present in the basal layer, these cells synthesize the pigment melanin, which imparts color to the skin. Skin color is generally determined by the amount and type of melanin produced by the melanocytes and not by the number of melanocytes, which is believed to be fairly constant in all races. Melanocytes originate in the neural crest and migrate to the epidermis during development. The ratio of melanocytes to keratinocytes in the basal layer is about 1:36. Melanocytes contact the surrounding keratinocytes through dendritic processes and transfer melanosomes, which are pigment-containing granules. Melanosomes form a cap over the nuclei of keratinocytes, protecting them from ultraviolet radiation. Melanin synthesis is controlled by Melanocyte Stimulating Hormone (MSH) secreted by the pituitary gland and is increased in response to UV exposure.

Besides keratinocytes and melanocytes, specialized cells derived from the bone marrow called Langerhans cells are interspersed throughout the epidermis; these are dendritic antigen-presenting cells involved in the immunological responses in the skin. Merkel cells are specialized cells that occur in combination with a nerve terminal in the basal layer; these are believed to function as slow-acting mechanoreceptors for touch.

Dermis lies below the epidermis, separated by a basement membrane. The dermis is a dense fibroelastic connective tissue that provides a strong and flexible foundation for the epidermis. The thickness of the dermis is variable from 1 to 5 mm. The dermis consists of cells, ground substance, and a fibrous network. Collagen forms the majority of the fibrous component, comprising about 77% of the dry weight of the skin. Type I collagen is the major collagen, followed by collagen III (15%) and lesser amounts of V and VI. Elastic fibers are interwoven among the bundles of collagen; these are made up of elastin surrounding an inner fibrillin fiber. This fibrous network confers mechanical properties to the skin, collagen provides tensile strength and elastic fibers restore shape after deformation by mechanical forces.

Fibroblasts are the major cell type in the dermis, and their primary function is to elaborate the fibrous network. Also present are perivascular mast cells and tissue macrophages. Surrounding the cells and the fibers is a visco-elastic gel that consists mainly of mucopolysaccharides, (also called glycosaminoglycans) salts, and water. The major types of glycosaminoglycans are hyaluronic acid, chondroitin 4-sulfate, dermatan sulfate, and heparan sulfate; examples include decorin, biglycan, and versican. These compounds are metabolized and degraded by the cells in the dermis and serve as a repository and conduit for nutrients and growth factors.

The dermis is divided into two regions, the papillary dermis and the reticular dermis. The papillary dermis conforms to the overlying epidermis, forming rete ridges and papillae. The reticular dermis lies below the papillary dermis and forms the bulk of the dermal layer. The papillary dermis contains a smaller and less dense network of fibers compared to the reticular dermis and also has a higher proportion of cells and ground substance. The papillary dermis also encloses the vast array of microcirculatory blood and lymphatic vessels just beneath the papillary projections. The reticular dermis is relatively acellular and avascular and has much thicker collagen bundles that range from 10 to 40 μm in diameter.

The junction between the epidermis and dermis is occupied by a basement membrane, divided into a clear zone called *lamina lucida* and the darker *lamina densa*. The basal lamina consists of a network of filamentous glyco-proteins; type IV and type VII collagen have been identified as well as a micro-fibrillar component that is continuous with the elastic fiber network in the dermis. Many of the basement membrane components are synthesized by basal keratinocytes.

The hypodermis or the subcutis layer lies below the dermis. It is composed of adipose tissue and serves to attach the dermis to underlying tissues and provide protection and insulation.

Different types of appendageal structures are also present in the skin; they are of epidermal origin but extend into the dermis. These include the pilosebac-eous unit consisting of a hair follicle, sebaceous glands, and arrector pili muscle. Hair follicles make a keratinized structure, hair. Hair follicles are present every-where on the body except for palms and soles. Different types of follicles are present on different body parts, small follicles that give rise to fine vellus hairs are present on female faces and large follicles that grow thick hair are present on such areas as the scalp. Hair follicles go through cycles of growth through anagen (active growth), catagen (regression), and telogen (rest). The length of this cycle determines the length of the hair and is characteristic of an individual and the body site. Hair is believed to play a role in beauty, with no obvious phys-iological function.

The sebaceous glands are attached to the hair follicles, and they secrete an oily substance called sebum, which is extruded to the skin surface through the follicles. The face and the back have a high concentration of sebaceous glands and, consequently, can get oily. Sebum contains unique lipids, such as squalene, besides triglycerides. Sebum is believed to lubricate and protect the skin. More recently, it has been proposed that sebaceous gland secre-tions may be a source of antioxidants that can protect the top layers of the skin (2).

Two distinct types of sweat glands also exist in skin; the eccrine sweat gland and the apocrine sweat gland. The eccrine sweat gland is mainly respon-sible for secretion of sweat in response to physiological stimuli. There are several million of these distributed over the entire body and are particularly prevalent on underarms, palms, soles, and forehead. The apocrine gland is responsible for producing body odor, and is present in the underarms, around the nipples, navel, and genital areas.

Physiology and Function of the Skin

The skin acts as the primary interface between the body and the environment and plays a fundamental protective role. It protects the body from injuries, pathogens, the sun, and extremes of temperature. It helps to stabilize the internal environment of the body and keeps organs in place and acts as a sensor of the surroundings.

The epidermis, though thin as a paper, is elegantly designed to withstand everyday mechanical stress. The outermost layer of the epidermis is made up of sheets of dead cells that are imperceptibly shed and replaced with newer layers. This layer is also tightly packed with flattened cells and cemented with lipids and proteins, which serve as the major waterpoof barrier to the environment. The continuous process of proliferation of basal keratinocytes followed by maturation and differentiation and eventual shedding of dead cells provides a means of renewal of the epidermis every four weeks. In the long term, this minimizes the accumulation of damaged cells in the skin and serves to keep it healthy and mostly disease free. In addition to the keratinocytes, melanocytes play a key role in protecting cells from DNA damage and oxidative stress due to exposure to ultraviolet light, by transferring melanin to basal keratinocytes.

Langerhans cells, residing in the epidermis function in immune surveillance and make skin an immunological defense organ. Upon exposure to contact allergens, tumor antigens, and microorganisms, Langerhans cells provide a sensitizing signal to initiate a T-cell mediated immune response.

Underlying the epidermal layer, the dermis serves as a cushion and a physical as well as a physiological support for the epidermis. It imparts firmness, tensile strength, extensibility, and elastic properties to the skin. It provides structural support for embedded appendages as well as the vascular and nerve networks. The epidermis, being avascular, is supplied with nutrients solely via the dermis. The dermis also acts as a repository for growth factors, enzymes, nutrients, and so on.

Another important function of the skin is thermoregulation, which is achieved by the combined action of the eccrine sweat gland and the microcirculatory system. When exposed to hot environments or strenous physical activity, the eccrine glands secrete sweat, a dilute salt solution, which cools the skin when it evaporates from the surface.

In addition, the microcirculatory system also helps to regulate heat. The skin is supplied by cutaneous arteries that give rise to a small vessel plexus running parallel to skin surface deep in the dermis, which branch into ascending arteries and arterioles that reach the papillary dermis. These further give rise to capillary loops directed toward the epidermis. In a hot environment, the blood vessels dilate, causing the skin to flush and give off heat. In colder environments, they constrict to conserve heat, causing pallor. The blood vessels are responsible for nourishing the dermis as well as the epidermis and also play a very important role in the healing of wounds.

The microcirculatory system as well as the eccrine glands also act in response to emotional stress.

The skin is the sensory organ for touch, pressure, pain, itch, and temperature. Myelinated cutaneous nerves lie parallel to the skin surface in the subcutaneous layer and branch extensively in two main plexuses in the dermis. Ascending branches end in free nerve endings, whose ultrastuctural morphology suggests that they are C fibers that function as polymodal nociceptors. They are generally associated with pain and itch. Free nerve endings have been shown to come up almost into the granular layer of skin (3). Besides the free nerve endings, another kind of sensory terminal, the Merkel cell–neurite complex, lies at the base of epidermal ridges. The Merkel cell has attachment to keratinocytes and is associated with a flattened axon terminal plate. They are believed to function as slowly adapting mechanoreceptors for touch. Meissner's touch corpuscles, found predominantly in the dermal papillae on palms and soles, also sense touch. Pacinian corpuscles, lying in the deep part of the dermis, transduce vibratory stimuli. In addition to the sensory nerves, sympathetic motor nerves innervate the sweat glands, pilomotor apparatus and muscle (responsible for causing "goosebumps"), and the microvasculature. These fibers may be of cholinergic, adrenergic, or purinergic types.

The skin is also home to myriads of microorganisms that are normal residents on the surface and in the follicles of skin. A majority of these microbes are gram-positive, and they are in dynamic equilibrium with the host tissue. Local skin anatomy, availability of nutrients, hydration level, and presence of inhibitors of various types dictate the types and dominance of particular groups of microbes. The microflora may be considered as an integral component of skin and cause few problems in healthy hosts. It is important to ensure that long-term use of cosmetics or other skin-care products does not disturb the natural balance of the skin microflora (4).

In summary, the skin is a very dynamic organ, complex in its architecture and organization, carrying out a multitude of critical functions and at the same time, imparting a definition to one's external appearance.

RECOMBINANT DNA TECHNOLOGY: THE IMPACT ON SKIN STRUCTURE AND FUNCTION

The last 10 years have seen the advent of several new methods to study global gene and protein expression. Several enabling technologies have made these methods possible. First, vast new amounts of sequence information have been generated from the Human Genome Project as well as the complete sequence identification of several other organisms. With this information, the function of these genes and the proteins they encode can be identified. Second, advances in computer capacity and new algorithm development has allowed for the rapid handling and interpretation of extremely large data sets. Third, the further development of high throughput platforms has enabled the construction of highly organized, multicomponent systems.

New gene expression methods provide an exciting opportunity for investigators to study the effects on multiple genes at the same time. As a result, scientists are able to generate testable hypotheses for target identification, target validation, as well as for mapping signaling pathways. These findings are contributing to the drug discovery process and enabling new approaches to scientific investigation, such as systems biology. The more commonly used methods to study gene expression are described below.

Methods of Gene Expression

(1) *Serial Analysis of Gene Expression* (SAGE). This technique was developed by scientists at Johns Hopkins University (5) to conduct quantitative and simultaneous global gene expression. In this method, RNA is reverse transcribed and tagged using a biotinylated primer. It is digested with a specific restriction enzyme, and the 3' end is isolated by binding to streptavidin and a second restriction fragment (tagging enzyme). The resulting tags are ligated and amplified. The resulting ditags are isolated, concatenated, cloned, and sequenced. The sequenced tags are then matched against a nucleic acid database to identify the corresponding gene. The advantage of this method is that global gene expression is measured without preselecting the genes.

Several groups have applied this method to identify the "transcriptome" of various conditions of skin. These studies include a comparison of gene expression in premalignant epidermis (6), a partial transcriptome of epidermis (7), a comparison of gene expression in differentiated versus undifferentiated cultures (8), and a comparison of photodamaged versus photoprotected skin (9). Several of these studies focus on identifying the primary drivers of skin cancer formation; however, they have applications in both the pharmaceutical and cosmetic arenas. The SAGE studies to date have been used to identify the global gene expression patterns within specific cell types. This data can then be used to identify genes that are only expressed in a given cell or tissue type and differentially expressed in developmental, disease, or normal states.

(2) *Differential display*. In this method, RNA isolated from the different conditions that are to be compared is reverse transcribed and amplified by the polymerase chain reaction (PCR) under low stringency conditions. The amplified DNA is then run on gels and quantitative comparisons made. The advantage of this technique is that these DNA fragments can then be isolated from the gel and cloned for functional studies. Like SAGE, the advantage of this method is that genes are not preselected. The main disadvantage of this method is getting good quantitative data; because PCR is only a semiquantitative method, small differences are harder to detect.

Differential display has been used in several skin studies related to psoriasis (10), skin cancer (11), and pheomelanogenesis (12). These studies have identified lists of genes that are modulated in these processes and have identified novel genes and novel signal transduction pathways that are involved in the control of the particular disease or cosmetic phenotype.

(3) *DNA/oligonucleotide arrays.* This method has become the most popular for gene expression studies. Typically cDNA or oligonucleotides are printed or attached to a solid matrix (membranes, glass, chips). From a single sample of RNA, the gene expression profile of thousands of genes can be assessed simultaneously. The advantages are clear as the technique is relatively quick and can yield a tremendous amount of information from a single RNA experiment. However, analysis of the information, including normalization and handling of replicates, has posed challenges to the interpretation of the data. The other disadvantage is that only those genes that are on the array are tested. Manufacturers of the arrays are attempting to overcome this bias by developing arrays of higher density that cover the entire genome of the organism of interest. A second issue is the amount of RNA that is needed to run an array. Although amplification techniques have been established to deal with the issue of low sample availability, there still are situations where the sample is limited. Microarrays have been used in many studies relating to skin, particularly in the following: toxicological studies (13), comparisons of in vitro models versus in vivo conditions (14), and the effects of environmental stresses (15). The data has been used for chemical toxicology, new tissue gene expression, identification of new signal transduction pathways, target identification, and validation for new pharmaceutical applications. This method has also shown potential to be used in addition to histology to differentiate different cancer types (16).

(4) *Quantitative real-time PCR.* The polymerase chain reaction (PRC) has been used very successfully in molecular biology in a semiquantitative manner. The advent of real-time PCR has provided an avenue for a more quantitative analysis of PCR data. PCR is based on doubling of the amount of RNA at each step, eventually due to reagent depletion during the reaction, the curve reaches a plateau after an exponential response. This response curve is captured in real time, using a fluorescent signal. Using this method, fewer numbers of genes are studied at one time, however the formats are amenable to running hundreds or thousands of samples. Another clear advantage of real-time PCR over microarrays is that it can be performed using a very low amount of sample without the need of additional amplification techniques prior to running the method. Normalization is one remaining issue with the PCR quantitation that is similar to that of arrays. Different approaches have been adopted to address this issue, including normalizing to the original starting quantity, making a DNA probe of a gene of interest and running as a standard, or using a "housekeeping" gene or gene sets. Real-time PCR has been used primarily to confirm the results obtained from microarray experiments.

(5) *Single Nucleotide Polymorphisms* (SNPs). SNPs are changes in an individual's gene that occur as a single nucleotide difference in the genome sequence. These polymorphisms can either be "silent" or result in a change in

the protein coded for by that gene. Each individual has a set of polymorphisms, that then become their individual DNA blueprint. SNPs are being studied intensely as a possible route to understanding the basis of human disease. In addition, SNPs may be indicators not only of specific disease types but also potentially as a predisposition to both clinical and cosmetic conditions. Recently, one of the susceptibility factors for psoriasis has been traced to SNPs in or near the gene SLC9A3R1 on chromosome 17q25; this leads to loss of a transcription factor (RUNX1) binding site and thereby affecting the regulation of this gene (17). It is envisioned that sometime in the future, we may walk around with our own SNP chip, so that treatment of disease may be more tailored to our specific genetic profile. In addition to selecting the appropriate course of treatment, this can also potentially give physicians the opportunity to prescribe different medications to reduce side effects.

In conclusion, regardless of the method selected, one of the major outputs of gene expression studies is to provide new sets of testable hypotheses that can be used for mechanistic understanding as well as translation into drug technologies. One of the prime examples of application of this process is in the treatment of breast cancer. Gene expression studies revealed that her-2 (epidermal growth factor) receptor expression is indicative of a subtype of breast cancers. This identification led to the development of a monoclonal antibody approach (Herceptin) that specifically targets the cancer and is being recommended for patients whose breast cancer is her-2 positive. This is one example of how these techniques can be used in the pharmaceutical and biotech industry, and it may be applicable to consumer product development as well.

Methods of Protein Expression

(1) *Proteomics*. In addition to expression profiling at either the DNA or RNA level, it is important to determine how many of these differences manifest in changes in protein expression. Analyzing the proteome of many tissues, including skin, will help us toward understanding biological functions (18). The largest amount of information on the skin proteome, particularly in keratinocytes, has been assembled by the Celis Group, who have published numerous studies on protein expression in skin under various conditions (19).

The method that has been traditionally used to study protein expression is two-dimensional (2D) gel electrophoresis. These gels separate the proteins first by molecular weight and then in the second dimension by charge. The spots on the gel can be cut out and be analyzed by Mass Spectrometry (MS) methods for further identification. Clearly, the advantages of this method are that you can get both quantitative information and a positive identification of the protein. The disadvantage is the limit of sensitivity. In addition, absolute identification requires expertise in MS analytical capability. More recently, such techniques as Matrix-Assisted Laser Desorption Ionization–Time of Flight (MALDI TOF) have increased the throughput and sensitivity of MS methods.

(2) *Antibody arrays.* Another tool that is being developed for large-scale proteomics is the use of antibody arrays. The idea is to immobilize antibodies on a solid matrix in a similar manner to oligonucleotides or cDNA for DNA arrays. The disadvantage is that there are a limited number of antibodies available, which limits the number of proteins that can be detected. Another limitation is that the antibodies have to remain available for binding to the protein epitope after they have been bound to the solid support.

Although many of the studies that have been reported have been "list" oriented, these studies are beginning to reveal potential mechanisms related to processes in skin, such as inflammation, pigmentation, and photodamage. Furthermore, using the genome and the proteome information, protein–protein interaction maps, or "interactomes," are being charted (20). This emerging field of interactomics is laying the foundation for systems biology, which holds the promise of being able to explain the workings of the cell and eventually the organism.

HOW WILL BIOTECHNOLOGY IMPACT SKIN CARE IN FUTURE?

Advances in biotechnology can be expected to impact the business of skin care at least in two major ways—one is through providing a better understanding of the structure, function, and physiology of the substrate, that is, skin, and the other is in the area of identifying efficacious technologies for care and treatment of skin. It is anticipated that using many of the techniques and tools that have been developed in the field of biotechnology, such as genomics and proteomics, as outlined in the previous section, will result in deep insights into the function of skin and its components, at the cellular and tissue levels.

This will lead to a superior appreciation of the workings of skin both in normal as well as abnormal conditions. Skin physiology and function can be better characterized, using the tools of biotechnology, as the skin evolves through various stages and ages starting from in utero development through middle and old age. Such tools can also be extremely helpful in characterizing differences in physiology and function of skin of various ethnic origins, for example, in identifying drivers of pigmentation differences. These methods can be applied to studying variations of skin function across body sites; this knowledge can be built into development of products more appropriately suited to various parts of the body ranging from face to feet. Recently developed techniques in molecular biology and proteomics will further add to the knowledge of the processes that are dysregulated in abnormal skin either in diseases, such as psoriasis, or in such conditions as acne or eczema and can lead to the development of effective treatments.

Another area that advances in biotechnology will impact is the development of in vitro models of skin that are more representative of in vivo behavior. Considerable progress has been made in the area of three-dimensional models of skin or living skin equivalents. Some models only have the epidermal component, typically generated by seeding keratinocytes on a suitable matrix and allowing them to grow and stratify when exposed to an air–liquid interface. A dermal equivalent can be generated by seeding fibroblasts in a collagen gel. Some models have the epidermal as well as the dermal components.

The most attractive use of skin equivalents is in the area of toxicology and prediction of irritation potential of chemicals and products. Recently, several models were compared for their usefulness in predicting skin irritation (21). These models can also serve in answering fundamental questions regarding the function of skin and its components and the communication process between different cell types and components, for instance, by examining the effects of perturbing specific proteins (22). The artificial skin models have also proven to be extremely useful in treating burn patients.

Overall, the current in vitro models have been found to be somewhat, though not entirely, predictive of in vivo situations. The area of in vitro models will be most useful in the development of skin-care products as it may overcome the necessity of animal testing, and personal product companies can benefit greatly from this advance. It is expected that use of biotechnology methods, such as gene expression profiling, will significantly aid in refining these in vitro models.

Another area that can benefit from applying some of the methods developed for biotechnology is that of optimizing skin penetration. Although skin is an organ that has low permeability in general to topically applied chemicals, there is a growing interest in developing transdermal routes to drug delivery. The efforts invested in understanding the rules and constraints of delivering into skin can be advantageous to the development of better-performing products, with the ability to deliver actives when and where necessary and in the desired amounts (23). The structures of active ingredients—such as small molecules, lipids, peptides, sugars, as well as co-solvents—can be designed and optimized for delivery using advanced modeling in combination with high throughput experimentation. It is expected that advances in this area can lead to products with greater efficacy and minimum side effects.

As consumers seek to fulfill the need for products that go beyond the hype and truly deliver the benefits promised, whether it be cleaning pores or improvement in fine lines or providing relief from dry skin, companies that are in the business of selling skin-care products are equally anxious to help fulfill that need. This has led to increased effort in identifying skin-care technologies that border on the "cosmeceutical" rather than simply cosmetic. Recombinant DNA and other synthetic techniques may be applied to identifying and developing superior ingredients to be included in skin-care products, for instance, active ingredients targeted against such various conditions as acne or pigmentation, as well as preservatives, antioxidants, and sun protection ingredients. Advances in biotechnology in the area of fermentation and bioreactors may be applied in producing ingredients of better quality and/or quantity, in a cost-effective manner. Recombinant proteins and peptides could one day be used as active ingredients for cosmetic applications. In the case of natural plant-based products, suppliers currently have to contend with crop variations due to numerous factors, such as climate, soil nutrition, and so on, that can affect the properties or activities of such products. Novel ways to grow plants in the laboratory under controlled conditions may yield more consistency in the quality and activity of natural products used in skin care.

Even pharmaceutical giants are shifting more resource to biotechnology as a route to identify therapeutics. Furthermore, it will not be surprising if pharmaceutical companies with significant consumer health care businesses start applying approaches that are employed in drug discovery to identifying technologies that impact conditions, which are currently in the realm of cosmetic claims. This would be in keeping with the trend of pharmaceutical companies expanding their focus beyond treating disease to improving lifestyles. Suppliers to the cosmetic industry are also becoming savvy in their adaptation of advances geared toward drug discovery, such as high throughput screening, and applying it to identify technologies that are biologically active, at least in vitro.

As a result of these developments, it is expected that the list of active ingredients that have superior benefits for improving the appearance of skin will be expanded beyond the handful that are available today and can enable customized skin care as described in the following section.

PERSONALIZED SKIN CARE: IS IT A DREAM OR REALITY?

It is well known that both drugs and personal care products are not equally efficacious across a population. With this awareness and the techniques we have described earlier, the movement within the medical field is toward personalized medicine. The benefits are clearly evident as each individual would get the therapeutic effects without or with minimal negative side effects. The question remains as to what the advantages of personalized skin care are and is it a realistic goal.

Current Status/Activities in the Marketplace

There are already several types of offerings available today that consumers can use to get product recommendations tailored to their particular needs. Web sites offer consumers the opportunity to fill out questionnaires about their skin-care habits and about their skin types and then recommend a product offering. More recently, there is a company that asks consumers to submit cheek swabs, and after testing several markers by SNP analysis, a customized product is returned to the consumer. The critique from dermatologists primarily is that these personalized products are not very different from what can be purchased in the mass market or in departmental stores. The question remains as to what needs to change to make critics into believers and what other potential hurdles need to be overcome.

What Can Make It a Reality?

In our Internet world, personal care product companies have very real ways to get in close contact with the consumer. Consumers of all ages are becoming technically savvy, thanks to the greater growth in using the Internet. Skin-care companies now have a personalized way to reach individual consumers. They also have the ability to store information about their consumers and provide them feedback in return.

In addition to communicating with and receiving information from consumers, new marketing channels such as mall kiosks and direct Internet sales make the opportunity to provide personalized skin-care products much more in the realm of reality than the traditional marketing channels that mass products in particular are limited to.

Finally, new scientific techniques that were outlined in the earlier portion of this chapter can make personalized skin care a reality. Many envision a future in which everyone carries their SNP and/or DNA profile with them. In that environment, feeding that chip in and getting a less irritating or more customized product may be a possibility.

Potential Hurdles

In addition to the enabling technologies, there are several potential hurdles. The first are the economic ones. Skin-care companies will have to learn to market to mass in a personalized way that does not adversely affect the overall price and profitability. Consumers have already shown a willingness to pay a high premium for skin care. Cosmetic procedures that usually come with a much higher price tag are continuing to grow in popularity. The cost of personalized skin care may be acceptable to consumers as long as the benefits that they desire are delivered.

If the development of designer cosmetics involves using personalized information gained from an individual's genetic material, then ethical issues enter the picture. If personal skin markers are identified, does a company limit its information to those markers? What happens if one of those markers, thought only to contribute toward a skin condition today, also becomes indicative of a much more serious disorder in the future? What is the obligation of the company that holds this information? Would a consumer value a cosmetics company having this information for a relatively trivial purpose as opposed to a serious medical condition? Will they be subject to discriminatory practices?

A much larger challenge is in the development of sufficient number of active ingredients that will actually deliver the customized service. In color cosmetics, where there is a plethora of colors, a personalized skin-care line is quite realistic as the technology already exists. In terms of skin care, however, there are fewer active ingredients that actually have an effect. Until the range of active ingredients is expanded, there is little confidence that the solutions for skin-care products are broad enough to credibly provide the personalization that consumers seek. What can be offered are a range of formulations that may be more esthetically pleasing to individual consumers. This, in and of itself, may be a large enough benefit to make it worthwhile for the consumer to share personal information. The question is—can this be combined with enough efficacy to present a clearly superior product? In addition, in order to make personalized skin care a reality, the current manufacturing capabilities geared toward producing large amounts of the same product will need to be reconfigured to produce smaller amounts of lots of different products. Even if personalized skin care becomes a reality, it remains to be seen whether this will just be a fad, or a sustainable proposition.

Overall, the prospect of personalized skin care is very exciting and could be market displacing and rewarding to the company that best determines the correct formula for success.

REFERENCES

1. Odland GF. Structure of the skin. In: Goldsmith LA, ed. Physiology, Biochemistry, and Molecular Biology of the Skin. New York: Oxford University Press, 1991:3–62.
2. Thiele JJ, Weber SU, Packer L. Sebaceous gland secretion is a major physiologic route of vitamin E delivery to skin. J Invest Dermatol 1999; 113:1006–1010.
3. Reilly DM, Ferdinando D, Johnston D, Shaw C, Buchanan KD, Green MR. The epidermal nerve fiber network: characterization of nerve fibers in human skin by confocal microscopy and assessment of racial variations. Br J Dermatol 1997; 137:163–170.
4. Holland KT, Bojar RA. Cosmetics: what is their influence on the skin microflora? Am J Clin Dermatol 2002; 3:445–449.
5. Velculescu VE, Zhang L, Vogelstein B, Kinzler KW. Serial analysis of gene expression. Science 1995; 270:484–487.
6. van Ruissen F, Jansen BJ, de Jongh GJ, van Vlijmen-Willems IM, Schalkwijk J. Differential gene expression in premalignant human epidermis revealed by cluster analysis of serial analysis of gene expression (SAGE) libraries. FASEB J 2002; 16:246–248.
7. van Ruissen F, Bastiaan JH, Jansen BJ, de Jongh GJ, Patrick LJ, Zeeuwen M, Schalkwijk J. A partial transcriptome of human epidermis. Genomics 2002; 79:671–678.
8. Bastiaan JH, Jansen BJ, van Ruissen F, de Jongh GJ, Zeeuwen PLJM, Schalkwijk J. Serial analysis of gene expression in differentiated cultures of human epidermal keratinocytes. J Invest Dermatol 2001; 116:1–12.
9. Urschitz J, Iobst S, Urban Z, Granda S, Souza KA, Lupp C, Schilling K, Scott I, Csiszar K, Boyd CD. A serial analysis of gene expression in sun-damaged human skin. J Invest Dermatol 2002; 119:3–13.
10. Mirmohammadsadegh A, Tartler U, Gunter M, Baer A, Walz M, Wolf R, Ruzicka T, Hengge U. HAX-1, Identified by differential display reverse transcription polymerase chain reaction, is overexpressed in lesional psoriasis. J Invest Dermatol 2003; 120:1045–1051.

11. Welss T, Papoutsaki M, Michel G, Reifenberger J, Chimenti S, Ruzicka T, Abts HF. Molecular basis of basal cell carcinoma: analysis of differential gene expression by differential display PCR and expression array. Int J Cancer 2003; 104:66–72.

12. Furumura M, Sakai C, Potterf SB, Vieira WD, Barsh GS, Hearing V. Characterization of genes modulated during pheomelanogenesis using differential display. Proc Natl Acad Sci USA 1998; 95:7374–7378.

13. Huang O, Jin X, Gaillard ET, Knight BL, Pack FD, Stoltz JH, Jayadev S, Blanchard KT. Gene expression profiling reveals multiple toxicity endpoints induced by hepatotoxicants. Mutat Res 2004; 549:147–167.

14. Bernard FX, Pedretti N, Rosdy M, Deguercy A. Comparison of gene expression profiles in human keratinocyte monolayer cultures, reconstituted epidermis and normal human skin; transcriptional effects of retinoid treatments in reconstituted human epidermis. Exp Dermatol 2002; 11:59–74.

15. Sesto A, Navarro M, Burslem F, Jorcano JL. Analysis of the ultraviolet B response in primary human keratinocytes using oligonucleotide microarrays. Proc Natl Acad Sci USA 2002; 99:2965–2970.

16. Khan J, Wei JS, Ringner M, Saal LH, Ladanyi M, Westerman F, Berthold F, Schwab M, Antonescu CR, Peterson C, Meltzer PS. Classification and diagnostic prediction of cancers using gene expression profiling and artificial neural networks. Nat Med 2001; 6: 673–679.

17. Helms C, Cao L, Krueger JG, Wijsman EM, Chamian F, Gordon D, Heffernan M, Daw JA, Robarge J, Ott J, Kwok PY, Menter A, Bowcock AM. A putative RUNX1 binding site variant between SLC9A3R1 and NAT9 is associated with susceptibility to psoriasis. Nat Genet 2003; 35:349–356.

18. Goldstein AM. Changing paradigms in dermatology: proteomics: a new approach to skin disease. Clin Dermatol 2003; 21:370–374.

19. Gromov PS, Ostergaard M, Gromova I, Celis JE. Human proteomic databases: a powerful resource for functional genomics in health and disease. Prog Biophys Mol Biol 2002; 80:3–22.

20. Tucker CL, Gera JF, Uetz P. Toward an understanding of complex protein networks. Trends Cell Biol 2001; 11:102–106.

21. Faller C, Bracher M. Reconstructed skin kits: reproducibity of cutaneous human irritancy testing. Skin Pharmacol Appl Skin Physiol 2002; 15(suppl):74–91.

22. Maas-Szabowski N, Szabowski A, Stark HJ, Andrecht S, Kolbus A, Schorpp-Kistner M, Angel P, Fusenig NE. Organotypic cocultures with genetically modified mouse fibroblasts as a tool to dissect molecular mechanisms regulating keratinocyte growth and differentiation. J Invest Dermatol 2001; 116:816–820.

23. Prausnitz MR, Mitragotri S, Langer R. Current status and future potential of transdermal drug delivery. Nature Rev Drug Discov 2004; 3:115–124.

6

Biotechnology in Skin Care (II): Moisturization

Shintaro Inoue

Basic Research Laboratory, Kanebo Cosmetics Inc., Odawara, Kanagawa, Japan

INTRODUCTION

Biotechnology is a vital field for the cosmetics industry. Its many roles in the industry extend from the discovery, manufacture, and evaluation of the raw materials for cosmetics to the development of skin science, the basis of cosmetics itself. The use of biotechnology has thus led to the development of many ingredients to improve the skin and protect it against undue conditions such as dryness. Recent biotechnologies, such as transgenic mice generation, artificial skin engineering, and comprehensive mRNA expression analysis, have engendered new proposals for skin functions and mechanisms for dry skin. After reviewing the skin structure and functions involved in moisturization, this chapter describes how biotechnology has been used to develop new skin-care concepts and ingredients to regulate skin hydration.

SKIN STRUCTURE AND FUNCTIONS INVOLVED IN MOISTURIZATION

Structure

The skin, the largest organ of the body, is primarily composed of three layers: the epidermis, the dermis, and the subcutaneous tissue. The epidermis, the most superficial layer of the skin, plays a very important role in both providing and maintaining moisture. Though no more than 0.1 to 1.0 mm thick itself, the epidermis is covered with an even thinner but mechanically and functionally sophisticated layer called the stratum corneum (SC), or horny layer (Fig. 1).

In spite of its extreme thinness (less than 20 μm), the SC prevents transepidermal water loss (TEWL) and protects the body from various physical, chemical, and biological stimuli outside the skin (1). Structurally, the SC is composed of 10 to 20 layers of cornified cells (corneocytes), most of them mature and keratinized, derived through terminal differentiation from the keratinocytes born at the base of the epidermis. The protective and retentive functions of the SC are achieved by the strict arrangement of these layered cells in what is known as a "bricks-and-mortar" structure (2) (Fig. 1). The "bricks" are composed of corneocytes endowed with rigid cornified envelopes but lacking organelles, and the "mortar" is composed of specialized proteins and intercellular lipids, such as ceramides (40–60%), fatty acids (20–30%) and cholesterols (20–30%), excreted from the lamellar granules in the stratum granulosum. The lipids and water join to form a characteristic lamellar structure (Fig. 1).

Water Folding Capacity

The SC imparts the important moisturizing effect by retaining the water on the skin surface and preventing water loss.

The water content of the SC is an important determinant of the appearance and physical properties of the skin, including its suppleness and flexibility. Corneocytes can hold water within cells through the action of the natural moisturizing factor (NMF), which is composed of amino acids, ions, lactic acid, urea, and other ingredients that confer humectant qualities to the SC (3–5).

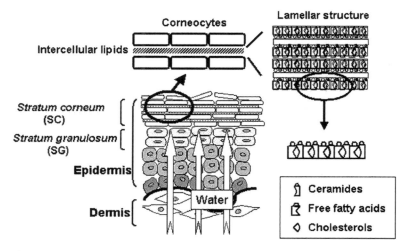

Figure 1   Skin structure involved in moisturization.

The constituents of the NMF are by-products formed from the breakdown of filaggrin processed from profilaggrin during the terminal differentiation of keratinocytes. Profilaggrin is synthesized and pooled in keratohyalin granules in the granular layer. Processed filaggrin binds keratin filament to form a structural matrix in the SC, whereupon it completely degrades at the top layer of the SC. The amino acid composition of NMF is consistent with that deduced from the DNA sequence of profilaggrin (4,6).

Skin surface lipids (sebum)—including triglycerides, fatty acids, squalene, wax esters, diglycerides, cholesterol esters, and cholesterol in order of abundance—are derived from the sebaceous glands and also play a significant role in the hydration of the skin (7). Decreased skin surface lipids may contribute to dry skin in the elderly people (8).

Epidermal Permeability Barrier Function

The bricks-and-mortar structure plays a crucial role in protecting against TEWL. In fact, transgenic and knockout mice are lethal when SC formation is perturbed by knocking out genes essential for keratinocyte differentiation (9,10). Moreover, the intercellular lipids making up the mortar of the SC are known to play an essential role in maintaining the epidermal permeability barrier function, as their removal with organic solvent has been found to dramatically increase TEWL (11,12). Ultraviolet (UV) irradiation to the skin has also been found to induce alterations in the epidermal permeability barrier function with an increased TEWL for a few days (13,14).

The most important of the intercellular lipids are thought to be ceramides (ceramides 1–7, of which 1 and 4 are acylceramides) (15). In the granular layer, the ceramides are synthesized and pooled in the lamellar bodies as either of the two forms, that is, as glucosylceramides (or acylglucosylceramides) or sphingomyelins (Fig. 2). The (acyl)glucosylceramides and sphingomyelins are both secreted from the lamellar bodies into the intercellular spaces at the interface of the stratum granulosum and the SC, where they are hydrolyzed to each ceramide by the enzymes β-glucocerebrosidase or sphingomyelinase. Both ceramides 1 and 4 are specifically derived from acylglucosylceramides (16). As a result, the ceramides form the lamellar structure in combination with free fatty acids and cholesterols (Fig. 1). Atopic dermatitis, a disorder characterized by dry skin with an increase in TEWL, has been reported to occur in skin with decreased levels of ceramide, especially ceramide 1 of the SC (17).

EVOLUTION OF BIOTECHNOLOGY FOR SKIN MOISTURIZATION

As biotechnology advances, pharmaceutical and skin-care manufacturers have continued to apply it more intensively to personal care for skin functions mentioned earlier. Inquiries into the physiological events of the skin from biotechnological perspectives have advanced the evolution of skin science as well

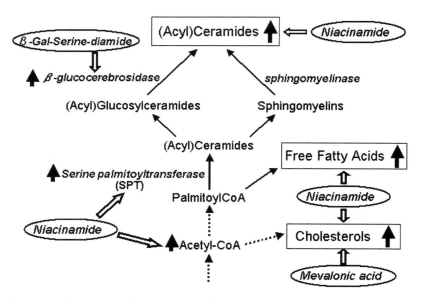

Figure 2   Schematic pathway of intercellular lipid biosynthesis and stimulating agents.

as the field of biotechnology itself. In the process of this evolution, skin-care strategies have come to place more emphasis on "regulating" the skin function with biologically active agents rather than on "supplementing" the skin with moisturizing ingredients.

Evolution of Biotechnology (Four Types of Method)

Skin-care specialists have come to tap the functions of living organisms using four technological approaches. The first approach involves (*i*) "technologies utilizing natural products." This includes techniques for extracting, separating, and purifying useful moisturizers from living organisms. The second approach involves (*ii*) "technologies for producing natural products and useful substances." This includes production techniques using fermentation, gene manipulation, and cell fusion, as well as animal and plant cell-culture techniques. The third approach, the evolutionary type, involves (*iii*) "technologies for improving and modifying natural products and useful substances." This approach includes immobilization and gene modification techniques, such as the technique now applied to produce collagen with reduced antigenicity by protease treatment.

The fourth methodological approach involves (*iv*) "technologies that add new value to (non)natural products and (non)useful substances." These can be regarded as advanced value-creating technologies that represent an integration of the technologies described earlier. Technologies (*i*), (*ii*), and (*iii*) may be sufficient to supply moisture to the skin surface, but technology (*iv*) is required for "regulating" the skin function. Technology (*iv*) can help us understand "water metabolism in the skin" scientifically and evaluate the effects of developed ingredients or skin-care treatment on changes in skin conditions. As described in further detail in this section, this approach to skin care will ultimately lead to new proposals of scientifically supported products for protecting and improving the various types of dry skin.

The Mechanisms Responsible for Dry Skin

Dry skin, a condition called xerosis when severe, is characterized by decreased water content of the SC followed by abnormal desquamation of the corneocytes (18). As the corneocytes lose their cohesiveness, they begin to curl up at the edges, leaving the skin rough to the touch and less supple than normal. Recent studies have revealed that dry skin may result from both internal mechanisms associated with aging, genetics, and physiology, and such external factors as UV exposure, environmental temperature, humidity, and harmful chemicals.

Dry Skin with Decreased SC Water Content and Increased TEWL

Dry skin with decreased SC water content and increased TEWL is typically seen when the skin is frequently washed with soap and water. The loss of SC intercellular lipids and NMF reduces the transepidermal permeability barrier (increased TEWL) and water-holding activity (decreased water content). In this case, the dryness is simply due to a loss of SC components (19).

Prolonged low humidity and low temperature in the winter season also leads to dry skin (20). These environmental conditions impair the formation of complete corneocytes by inducing a continuous loss of the SC water content and enhanced proliferation of keratinocytes in the epidermis (21,22). The ceramide level of the SC has also been reported to fall during the winter (23).

UV irradiation also decreases the hydration of the SC by depleting the SC lipids in the lamellar bodies, a process that destroys the epidermal barrier function and leads to a hyperproliferation of basal keratinocytes that prevents newly generated SC from completely forming (13,14).

In the disease atopic dermatitis, a decrease in the SC ceramide 1 level apparently impairs the epidermal barrier function, even though the nonlesional regions consist of atopic dry skin (17,24). The alterations in immunoresponsiveness and inflammatory reaction seen in dermatitis are probably associated with skin phenotypes. Common symptoms of dry skin are seen in contact dermatitis, ichtchyosis, and psoriasis, suggesting the involvement of inflammatory-induced keratinocyte hyperproliferation in the SC phenotypes with immature corneocytes.

Dry Skin with Decreased SC Water Content but Normal TEWL

Dry scaled skin seen in the elderly is also characterized by decreased hydration of the SC, but the TEWL is only sometimes decreased in this type of skin or it remains unchanged (25). The decreased turnover of the epidermis results in an accumulation of cornified layers (20 layers or less), a process that may lower the TEWL and reduce the supply of water to the top layer of the SC. Judging from the TEWL, the epidermal permeability barrier function in this type of skin seems to be normal or even improved. Yet damaged barrier function recovers more slowly in aged skin (26). This reduction in barrier resistance has been ascribed to impairment in cholesterol synthesis. In fact, a precursor of cholesterol, mevalonic acid (Fig. 2), has been demonstrated to recover the barrier resistance against acetone treatment of the SC, although cholesterol itself exhibited no such effect (26).

In experimentally induced diabetes, the SC water content drops to extremely low levels, yet the levels of SC amino acids, intercellular ceramides, free fatty acids, and cholesterols remain unchanged, or even increased (27), leaving the TEWL itself completely unaltered. A recent study by our group confirmed that the SC water content in diabetic patients decreased when their blood glucose levels rose (28). These findings suggest that factors other than NMF and intercellular lipids might be involved in the regulation of SC hydration. This aspect will be described later in the present and next sections in connection with the application of progressing biotechnology.

Regulating the Skin Function from Within the Skin

Thus far, most cosmetic researchers working on the problem of dry skin have sought to develop ingredients that "supplement the skin with water" when topically applied. The classical approach to prevent water loss has been to apply oily materials, such as Vaseline or olive oil, and the more recent approach is to apply (pseudo)ceramides in combination with free fatty acids and cholesterols (29). Some cosmetics contain formulations that retain the water of the SC through the use of hydrophilic materials, such as glycerol, amino acids, collagen, and hyaluronan. Biotechnology now plays a greater role in the development of these ingredients through the application of such methods as enzyme engineering and fermentation technology with recombinant DNA techniques. Recent progress in skin science and biotechnology allows us to develop active ingredients that can regulate SC hydration from within the skin, although these ingredients still lack a water-holding capacity and the ability to protect against TEWL by themselves.

Niacinamide (nicotinamide), one of the B vitamins, is a typical example of these active ingredients. Though deficiency in niacinamide (NA) is known to result in the disease pellagra, the role of NA in the epidermis and the mechanism by which NA induces dermatitis have not been determined. In studies on the roles of NA in human keratinocytes using an in vitro culture system, our group has found that NA ($1.0-10$ μM) dose-dependently increases the biosynthesis of ceramides (fourfold to sixfold), glucosylceramides (sevenfold), and sphingomyelins (threefold) in cultured human keratinocytes (30) (Fig. 2). In addition, a series of gene expression analyses revealed that NA increases the level of human long chain base 1 (*LCB1*) and *LCB2* mRNA, both of which encode subunits LCB1 and LCB2 respectively of serine palmitoyltransferase (SPT), the rate-limiting enzyme in sphingolipid synthesis. This increase of SPT activity was also confirmed in NA-treated cells. Moreover, NA was suggested to play an important role in synthesizing precursor lipids for the intercellular lamellar structure, as its application augmented the synthesis of free fatty acids and cholesterol as well as that of the ceramides. In fact, the topical application of NA increased the intercellular lipids in the SC and decreased TEWL in human dry skin without any side effects (30). NA was thus confirmed to improve the epidermal permeability barrier by stimulating de novo synthesis of the ceramides and other intercellular lipids. As such, it can be grouped as one of the new cosmetic ingredients, unique for its ability to regulate the SC hydration from within the skin.

NA is just one of many new ingredients being rapidly developed by biotechnology. Henceforth, our group is developing a new amino acid derivative, β-galactosyl-L-serine-diamide (31), as an analogue of β-galactosylceramide (32) that increases the β-glucocerebrosidase activity essential for the conversion of β-glucosylceramides to the ceramides, including acylceramides (ceramides 1 and 4) (Fig. 2).

NEW ASPECTS TO REGULATE THE WATER BALANCE IN THE SKIN AND DEVELOP NEW PRODUCTS USING BIOTECHNOLOGY

Recent techniques in biotechnology, such as transgenic mice studies, artificial skin engineering, and highly sensitive quantitative mRNA expression analyses, have led to many new proposals for skin function and effective ingredients to maintain the water balance of the skin. This section reviews recent topics and summarizes several new concepts for developing ingredients targeting the regulation of SC hydration.

Determination of the Function of a Skin Water Channel, Aquaporin (AQP) Using a Nonradioactive RNase Protection Assay and AQP-Deficient Knockout Mice

Moving beyond our earlier studies seeking to retain water in the SC and protect against TEWL, our group has also sought to develop ingredients that directly regulate the water metabolism of the skin. Having observed from earlier studies that the epidermal barrier function fails to recover normally when damaged skin is covered with an occlusive membrane (33), we speculated that the "movement of water" may be important to maintain skin homeostasis. Thus we took a great interest in the aquaporins (AQPs), a family of water channel proteins expressed in diverse tissues.

To date, 11 AQPs (AQP0–AQP10) have been cloned in mammals. Seven of them are permeable only by water, whereas the other four (AQP3, AQP7, AQP9, and AQP10) can be permeated by glycerol and urea as well as water

(34). We embarked on our investigation of AQP with good background knowledge from earlier research, although we had almost no information on which AQPs were expressed in the skin or the functions they served there.

Nonradioactive RNase Protection Assay

Our group began its AQP research by establishing the nonradioactive RNase protection assay (RPA), a new and quantitatively stronger method to simultaneously compare the expression levels of the different AQP genes in the skin (35). The nonradioactive RPA contains a peculiar process of hybridization of target gene mRNAs with unlabeled probes followed by an RNase treatment (Fig. 3). The resultant RNase-resistant mRNAs are subjected to an electrophoresis and a second hybridization with biotin- or digoxigenin (DIG)-labeled probes. This technique gives sharp bands with a high sensitivity comparable to that obtained by ^{32}P-labeled probes.

Characterization of AQPs in the Skin

Using our nonradioactive RPA, we found that *AQP3* and *AQP9* were expressed in cultured normal human keratinocytes (Fig. 4), and, further, that the *AQP3* expression was upregulated by an osmotic pressure induced by physiological stimulation (35). The same results were obtained in an artificial skin-equivalent model composed of human fibroblasts and keratinocytes. Moreover, the immunostaining of the artificial skin with a specific antihuman AQP3 antibody revealed the location clearly at cell membranes of epidermal keratinocytes (Fig. 4).

Transgenic or knockout mouse systems might be capable of elucidating the AQP functions in the skin. Our group collaborated with Dr. A. S. Verkman of

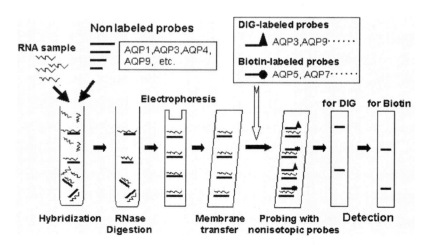

Figure 3   Nonradioactive RNase protection assay (RPA). *Abbreviations*: AQP, Aquaporin; DIG, digoxigenin.

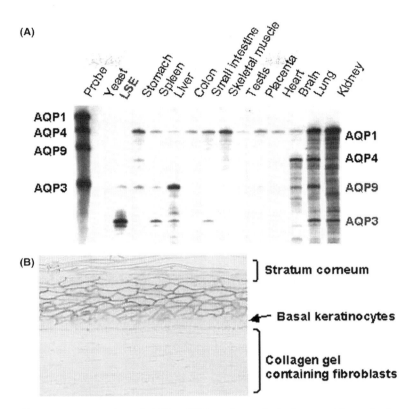

Figure 4 Expression of AQP mRNA and protein in human skin-equivalent cultures: (**A**) Simultaneous nonradioactive RNase Protection Assay of *AQP1*, *AQP3*, *AQP4*, and *AQP9*. LSE; epidermis from human skin-equivalent cultures. (**B**) Immunostaining of AQP3 protein of the cultured artificial skin using a specific antihuman AQP3 antibody.

UCSF in a detailed study of the skin phenotypes of hairless *AQP3* knockout mice. Skin lacking AQP3 showed an apparent decrease in SC hydration associated with decreased permeability of both water and glycerol (36). It was also interesting to find that the *AQP3*-deficient mice exhibited a loss of skin elasticity and delays in both wound healing and the recovery of barrier function after barrier disruption. Thus, it appeared that the decreased water and/or glycerol permeability not only triggered dry skin and low elasticity, but also altered physiological skin functions such as the recovery of disrupted epidermal barrier and wound healing (37,38).

These findings, in combination with studies by others, clearly prove that "the movement of water" is an important process in maintaining the skin homeostasis. Provided that adequate ingredients can be found, this new concept might be useful for skin care.

Screening for Selecting Active Ingredients to Upregulate AQP3

Original evaluation systems designed to prove working hypotheses in skin science will also be generally useful as original screening systems. In the search for biologically active substances, the necessary stages of cell cultivation will prevent most screening systems from becoming high throughput. Our group is screening active ingredients for cosmetic application by visually examining 96-well dot blots obtained by a reaction of keratinocyte lysates with a specific anti-AQP3 antibody. The dot blots are visualized by the reaction of a chemiluminescent substrate with horseradish peroxidase conjugated with a second anti-IgG antibody. Once the candidates are selected, their effects on cultured keratinocytes and artificial skin cultures are examined in a second evaluation using technologies such as Western blotting, Northern blotting, and in situ hybridization.

Estimation of Active Ingredients Using an Artificial Skin-Equivalent Model with Microarray Techniques

This is an example of the application of biotechnology to investigate the mechanism of a cosmetic ingredient. Some years ago, our group developed an active ingredient, γ-amino-β-hydroxybutyric acid (Bisamin), as a quasi-drug. Bisamin improved clinically both xerosis and asteatosis. Though the clinical efficacy of this agent was confirmed, we were unable to identify any mechanisms other than the improvement of skin blood circulation. More recently, this prompted our group to study the effects of Bisamin on cultured human keratinocytes.

Initial studies on the effects of Bisamin on keratinocyte proliferation and differentiation revealed no effect. Next, we obtained mRNAs from a Bisamin-treated monolayer culture of human keratinocytes and examined about 8×10^3 genes by a microarray analysis. As none of the genes exhibited any change in expression significant enough to implicate them causally, it appeared that Bisamin might be inert for keratinocytes at the monolayer condition. Next, we added Bisamin to the artificial skin-equivalent model and performed a microarray analysis of mRNAs obtained from the dissected epidermal layer. This time, we found changes in the expressions of 12 genes and were able to use Northern blot analysis to confirm the results for two of the genes, namely, α-catenin (upregulated) and corneodesmosin (downregulated) (Fig. 5). Interestingly, the expression levels of the two genes were confirmed to remain unchanged when Bisamin was added to the monolayer keratinocyte cultures (Fig. 5). This is not altogether surprising, however, as both gene products contribute to the cell–cell adhesion required for the construction of the three-dimensional network (39,40). Although further investigation will be required, these findings lead us to two hypotheses: first, that Bisamin may strengthen the intercellular adhesion of keratinocytes by α-catenin upregulation, and, second, that it may weaken the interaction of cornified cells by downregulating corneodesmosin, thereby promoting normal desquamation and improving the condition of dry skin.

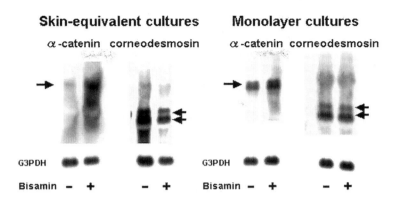

Figure 5 Northern blot analyses of α-catenin and corneodesmosin mRNAs. Both mRNAs obtained from the dissected epidermis of the artificial skin-equivalent culture (*left*) and from the monolayered keratinocyte culture (*right*) in the presence or absence of Bisamin were subjected to Northern blot analyses. *Abbreviation*: G3PDH, glyceraldehyde-3-phosphate dehydrogenase.

Regulation of HA Synthesis in the Epidermis and Dermis by the Different HA Synthase Gene Locus

Hyaluronan (HA) is a high-molecular-weight glycosaminoglycan composed of *N*-acetylglucosamine and glucuronic acid. In addition to its main functions of holding water, maintaining the extracellular space, and facilitating the transport of ion solutes and nutrients, HA alters the structure of the extracellular matrix and modulates cell adhesiveness by influencing the processes of cell growth, cell migration, cell differentiation, angiogenesis, and immune regulation (41). HA is widely distributed over a range of diverse tissues, though by far the largest amount, about 50% of all HA in the body, resides in the skin (0.5–1.0 mg/g wet tissue weight). The HA in the skin is produced mainly by fibroblasts and keratinocytes, and the relatively fast turnover of 2 to 4.5 days in mammalians indicates that HA synthesis and degradation are controlled both strictly and dynamically in the skin (41). The HA content is reported to decline during aging (42), and its loss may be one of the factors contributing to dryness, wrinkle formation, and the decreased elasticity of aging skin. For this reason, the regulation of the HA metabolism in the skin is very important for moisturization (41).

Genes Responsible for Synthesis of Skin HA

HA is synthesized by the HA synthase (HAS) proteins, a family of membrane-bound enzymes encoded by three genetically distinct genes: *HAS1*, *HAS2*, and *HAS3* (41) (Fig. 6). Much has yet to be learned of these enzymes, and in mammals they have yet to be purified and characterized. The in situ functions

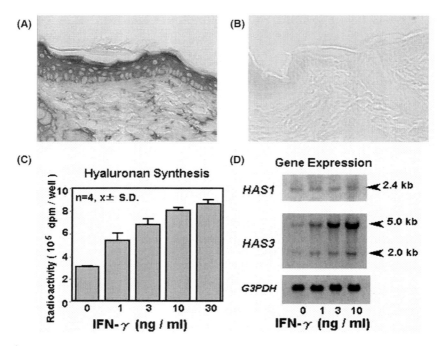

Figure 6 *HAS3* mRNA expression and regulation in epidermal keratinocytes. (**A**) and
(**B**) in situ hybridization of *HAS3* mRNA in mouse skin. (**A**) DIG-labeled antisense
RNA probe; (**B**) DIG-labeled sense RNA probe (control). (**C**) Dose-dependent HA production enhanced by IFN-γ in cultured human keratinocytes. (**D**) Dose-dependent *HAS3*
mRNA expression enhanced by IFN-γ in cultured human keratinocytes. *Abbreviations*:
DIG, digoxigen; G3PDH, glyceraldehyde-3-phosphate dehydrogenase; HAS, hyaluronan
synthase.

of HA and the regulation of *HAS* gene expressions in the skin remain unclear,
though HAS is known to be important for synthesizing HA (41).

In a recent examination of the expressions of *HAS1*, *HAS2*, and *HAS3*
mRNAs in the skin by our group, an in situ mRNA hybridization technique
showed that mouse skin expressed all HAS mRNAs in the dermis and epidermis
(43,44). More recently, however, we found that each *HAS* gene was independently and characteristically regulated by intrinsic bioactive factors. In Northern
blot analyses, cultured human skin fibroblasts expressed *HAS1* and *HAS2*
mRNAs (43), and stimulation with TGF-β induced the upregulation of both.
Human keratinocytes, on the other hand, expressed mainly *HAS3* mRNA,
while stimulation by IFN-γ and TGF-β conferred opposing effects on *HAS3*
(i.e., upregulation by IFN-γ and downregulation by TGF-β), without exerting
any effect on *HAS1* and *HAS2* whatsoever (44). The changes in the degree of
HAS3 expression in response to IFN-γ and TGF-β were consistent with the

amounts of HA secreted into the culture media, suggesting that HA is regulated by *HAS3* gene expression in human epidermal keratinocytes (Fig. 6). These findings suggest that every HAS gene is regulated independently, and that synthesized HA may have different functions in the epidermis and dermis.

In addition to cytokines, histamine was found to stimulate HA synthesis in human skin fibroblast cells via both *HAS1* and *HAS2* mRNA expression but not via *HAS3* mRNA (45). These responses were blocked by a histamine H1 receptor antagonist but not by the histamine H2 receptor antagonist, suggesting that the H1 receptors may mediate the regulation of *HAS1* and *HAS2* expression in response to inflammation. In keratinocytes, we have also obtained evidence that retinoic acid and retinol upregulate *HAS3* mRNA expression to produce HA in the culture media (46). This suggests a possible development of cosmetic ingredients targeted for *HAS3* gene expression because retinoic acid, as used in medicine, has already been reported to improve wrinkles and thicken the epidermis while concomitantly increasing the levels of epidermal HA.

The Discovery of HA in the SC

In recent investigations using a new histochemical technique with a biotinylated HA-binding protein specific and sensitive to HA, HA localization has been confirmed in the epidermis as well as the dermis (47,48). The technique revealed the presence of HA in the epidermal intercellular spaces, especially the middle spinous layer, but not in the SC or stratum granulosum. Based on these results, HA is generally considered to be absent in the normal SC.

In the in situ mRNA hybridization of the epidermis described earlier, we observed several strong signals of HAS mRNAs within the stratum granulosum (Fig. 6). To determine whether HA may be important within this layer or the SC, we decided to check for the presence of HA in the SC. If HA did exist in the SC, we speculated, its extremely high water-holding capacity might have made it crucial as an NMF. Using high-performance liquid chromatography to quantify HA content, we demonstrated the presence of HA in the normal SC of mice (49). The observed dry weights of HA in the SC, epidermis, and dermis were 22.3 ± 3, 15.1 ± 2, and 739 ± 32 µg/g, respectively, and a tracer experiment using $[^3H]$-glucosamine in a skin organ culture revealed the transfer of $[^3H]$-labeled HA from the epidermal layer to the SC. Based on these results, we confirmed for the first time that HA is supplied from keratinocytes beneath the SC layer and exists in the normal SC. We speculate that HA may play roles in moisturizing the SC and/or regulating its mechanical properties.

Screening of Active Ingredients to Upregulate *HAS3*

Our previous study found that N-methyl-L-serine (NMS), an amino acid derivative, enhanced HA production in dermal fibroblasts (50). Having performed well in trials on topical application to human skin, NMS is now widely used in skin-care products. Screenings by fibroblast cell cultures have confirmed that NMS increases the enzyme activity of the membrane fraction, but it has never been found to upregulate *HAS* genes.

Retinoic acid (RA) is a potent inducer of HA production in the epidermis (46,51), and clinical trials have proved that topically applied RA reduces wrinkles (52). Although RA has become one of the first antiwrinkle agents to be introduced as an ethical drug, its topical application induces irritation, scaling, and itching of the skin, side effects that make it unsuitable as a cosmetic ingredient. In the hope of finding alternatives, our group searched for natural substances that enhance HA production without inducing the same adverse effects. Ultimately, we discovered that *N*-acetylglucosamine (NAG), a monosaccharide derived from crab chitin by enzymatic degradation, exhibited a stimulatory effect in human keratinocytes (46). NAG, a major component of complex carbohydrates, is a product of lysosome-induced degradation of oligosaccharides from glycoprotein and glycolipids. In our experiments, the addition of exogenous NAG increased HA production in cultured keratinocytes with a concomitant increase of an intracellular UDP (uridine 5′-diphospho)–NAG pool as a HAS substrate, whereas *HAS3* gene expression and HAS activity both remained unaffected.

In Northern blot analyses, we were interested to find that β-carotene demonstrated an effect similar to RA in inducing the *HAS3* gene expression (46). Although this result supports the hypothesis that β-carotene converts into RA within the keratinocytes, this has yet to be confirmed. We observed that the copresence of NAG and RA conferred a synergistic effect on HA production (46). Similar synergy was obtained by adding NAG with retinal or NAG with β-carotene (46). Both β-carotene and NAG are now used in cosmetic products.

Epidermis-Specific Conditional Knockout Mice to Study New Factors Involved in the Regulation of the Skin Water Balance

Recent advances in biotechnology have made it possible to establish various mouse models with modulated target genes, including technologies for establishing conditional knockout mice specific for targeted organs, sites, and cells (9), as well as gene-targeted transposon-generated knockout or knock-in mice (53), and oligonucleotide-based RNA-knock-down mice (54). These technologies are powerful tools in functional genomics and have been applied in studies to elucidate and target physiological events. In the field of skin care, epidermis-specific conditional knockout mice will allow researchers to examine new factors involved in the regulation of skin water balance, especially when systemic knockout of the target gene results in embryonic lethal phenotypes in mice.

A Principle of Epidermis-Specific Knockout of the Targeting Gene

This technology is based on the unique property of an enzyme called Cre recombinase (Cre). Cre is a gene splicing enzyme in bacteriophage P1 that binds to a specific site "loxP" with a 34-nucleotide DNA sequence. The enzyme can splice out the DNA sequences located between two loxP sites by intramolecular site-specific recombination (9). This Cre/loxP system is available for tissue-specific deletion of targeted DNA sequences between the loxP sites if an active promoter functioning tissue-specifically can be designed as a regulator of the Cre expression. In the case of epidermal-specific recombination with Cre/loxP system, a K5 promoter from the keratin-5 gene can be used to induce the Cre expression specifically in the epidermis (9,55,56). The findings described later in this chapter were obtained in collaborative work performed with Dr. J. Takeda of Osaka University.

Epidermal-Specific Knockout of the ARNT Gene

Aryl hydrocarbon receptor nuclear translocator (ARNT), a transcription factor of the Per/AHR/ARNT/Sim gene family, regulates gene expression in response to environmental stimuli such as xenobiotics and hypoxia. Epidermal-specific ARNT gene-disrupted newborn mice appeared almost normal but died neonatally due to severe dehydration caused by water loss (56). The detailed characterization of the *ARNT-null* epidermis revealed significant alterations in the compositions of ceramides with a severe decrease in the amounts of ceramides with 4-hydroxysphinganine, suggesting deficiency of the dihydroceramide desaturases that catalyze the formation of both 4-sphingenyl and 4-hydroxysphingayl moieties. These results confirm that the epidermal barrier function cannot be maintained without proper ceramide compositions through the 4-desaturation regulated by ARNT (56).

Epidermal-Specific Depletion of GPI-Anchored Proteins

Proteins anchored by Glycosylphosphatidylinositol (GPI) are widely distributed on external plasma membranes of eukaryotes. *Pig-a*, an X-linked gene, is involved in the first step of GPI–anchor biosynthesis. Disruption of this gene causes cessation of GPI biosynthesis on the endoplasmic reticulum, leading to embryonic lethality with the absence of GPI-anchored proteins on the cell surface (57). A study on epidermal-specific GPI-anchor-deficient mice (*Pig-a null* mice) generated by *Pig-a* gene disruption has suggested that the GPI anchor or GPI-anchored proteins play an important role in skin development (9). The mice were born with wrinkled, dry, and hyperkeratotic skin with abnormal differentiation and died within a few days after birth. In another study, *Pig-a null* mice displayed abnormal permeability barrier function, evidenced by a significant elevation in TEWL with abnormal lamellar membrane structures in the SC (58). Western blot analyses showed a defect of filaggrin monomer with normal expression of profilaggrin in the epidermis of *Pig-a null* mice, indicating impaired conversion of profilaggrin to the monomeric form (59). These findings are consistent with the dry skin phenotypes. *Pig-a null* mice may be a useful animal model for understanding the process of acquiring barrier function and water-holding capacity in the epidermis.

BIOINFORMATICS FOR UNDERSTANDING AND PREDICTING SKIN PHENOTYPES AFTER EXTERNAL STIMULATION OR DURING AGING

The complete sequencing of the human genome now makes it possible to gather information on the DNA sequence, as well as the deduced amino acid sequences of candidate proteins. The functions of candidate proteins are still elusive, however. Though it will remain important to collect raw data through experiments, further progress of personal skin care will hinge on our ability to gather more functional information on the skin, to select the most useful data from the vast stores of information now recorded, and finally to construct new scientific knowledge for understanding skin physiology. Bioinformatics is expected to prove useful, though the development of valuable tools using informatics may require better communication between biologists and bioinformaticians.

Microarray Analyses of Gene Expression in Human Skin Tissues or Skin Cells

New technologies for comprehensive gene expression analyses have been developing, for instance, dot hybridization-based DNA microarray (60,61), sequencing-based serial analysis of gene expression (SAGE) (62), and polymerase chain reaction (PCR)-based adaptor-tagged competitive PCR (ATAC-PCR) (63,64), introduced amplified fragment length polymorphism (iAFLP) (65), and high coverage expression profiling (HiCEP) (66). Among them, abundant array data on human skin tissues and skin cells have been reported in dermatological journals as the quality of microarray technology continues to improve (Table 1) (67–90). Notwithstanding, difference in materials (whole skin, parts of skin, age, sex, race, artificial skin, or cultured cells), conditions (dose and time in UV-irradiation, skin lesion, or confluency of cells), and accuracy might hinder quantitative evaluations and comparisons of these data arrays. The difficulties are also mathematic. One set of array data, for example, contains information of 10^4 or more gene expressions. Bioinformatics will clearly be an essential tool.

Another impediment to the application of microarray technology for personal care is the limited amount of skin that can be obtained from healthy volunteers for analyses. This requires quantitative copy amplification of mRNA in the samples (91–94) or an improvement of microarray sensitivity with a higher S/N ratio (95–98). The recent technologies used to approach these problems are shown in Tables 2 and 3.

Bioinformatics for Understanding Comprehensive Gene Expression Data

Database Organization for UV-Regulated Genes

The intensity of UV irradiation on the surface of the earth is now increasing, posing a serious environmental risk for skin cancer and photoaging. To

Table 1 Microarray Analyses of Gene Expression Profile in Normal Human Skin Cells and Tissues

Type of array	Cell/Tissue	Genes[a]	Target	No. of genes with different expression levels	Refs.
Oligo-nucleotide	NHEK; REp; skin	12,000	Transcriptom	>70 (keratinocyte-specific)	(67)
	Skin	12,000	Scleroderma	2776	(68)
	Skin	12,000	Atopic dermatitis; psoriasis	Not determined	(69)
	Skin	12,000	Atopic dermatitis; psoriasis	80	(70)
	Skin	12,000	Wound healing	35	(71)
	NHEK; SCC	12,000	UV-B response	1039 (NHEK); 244 (SCC)	(72)
	NHEK	6,800	UV-B response	539	(73)
	NHEK	6,800	UV-B response	187	(74)
	NHEK	6,800	UV-B response	198	(75)
cDNA	Epi	588	Stress response	37 (tape stripping)	(76)
	REp	1,176	Barrier function	154	(77)
	NHEK; NHOK	3,063	Replicative senescence	83 (NHEK); 92 (NHOK)	(78)
	Skin	8,400	Wound healing	402 (keloid)	(79)
	NHEK; REp; Epi	475	Retinoid effect	44	(80)
	NHEK; MC; FB	4,405	Cell-type specificity	158	(81)

(Continued)

Table 1 Microarray Analyses of Gene Expression Profile in Normal Human Skin Cells and Tissues (*Continued*)

Type of array	Cell/Tissue	Genes[a]	Target	No. of genes with different expression levels	Refs.
	NHEK	588	UV-B response	64	(82)
	NHEK	IMAGE[b]	UV-B response	19	(83)
	HaCaT	588	UV-B response	Not determined	(84)
	HaCaT	1,200	UV-A; apoptosis	77	(85)
	MC	9,000	UV response	198	(86)
	MC	588	UV-A response	11	(87)
	Skin	4,000	Wound healing	>310	(88)
	REp	3,600	Skin irritation	Not determined	(89)
	Skin	4,400	Wound healing	192 (normal scar)	(90)
				178 (hypertrophic scar)	

[a]The number of genes on the array.
[b]IMAGE cDNA arrays were used (Ref. 83).
Abbreviations: NHEK, normal human epidermal keratinocytes; REp, reconstituted epidermis; Epi, epidermis; SCC, squamous carcinoma cells; NHOK, normal human oral keratinocytes; MC, normal human melanocytes; FB, normal human dermal fibroblasts.

Table 2 mRNA Amplification Methods Prior to Microarrays

Method	T7-promoter site	Characteristics	Refs.
SMART[a]	5' end	Products: sense RNA same size as the starting mRNA template. Sample: >100 ng of total RNA	(91) (92)
T7-based amplification	3' end	Products: antisense RNA shorter size than the starting mRNA template. Sample: >20 ng of total RNA	(93) (94)

[a]Switch Mechanism At the 5' end of RNA Transcription.

understand the physiological effects of UV on the skin, the expression patterns of the genes related to UV response must be analyzed on a genome-wide scale. To use the comprehensive results more efficiently, our analyses of the expression data should refer to information on gene functions and previous experimental results. Though no database of all of the known information on UV-regulated genes is yet completed, our group is working to construct one in collaboration with Intec Web and Genome Informatics Corporation and Dr. T. Takagi of the University of Tokyo. This database will provide reference data useful for (cosmetic) dermatologists.

As we place great importance on its quality, the database contains hybridization- and PCR-based expression data from published papers (99,100). Consulting researchers can refer to this information as they evaluate microarray data. We have also developed a simple Web-based browsing system and search functions with Perl and CGI (Common Gateway Interface). Gene ontology (specifications of a relational vocabulary for gene products to understand their functions) annotation and links to major databases, such as OMIM (Online Mendelian Inheritance in Man, the NCBI database of human genes and genetic disorders developed by staff at Johns Hopkins) and LocusLink (the NCBI database to provide a single query interface to curated sequence and descriptive information about genetic loci), are assigned when available. Users can examine the visible time course of gene expression after UV irradiation and search for genes with patterns resembling those of examined gene (hits sorted by the degree of similarity). Summarized information on experimental results and conditions can also be obtained directly from the database before users access the cited papers. The database contains our original keratinocyte data obtained by microarray analyses.

Extraction of Information on UV-Regulated Gene Interactions with Other Genes

To investigate the function of UV-regulated genes, our group has also been attempting to extract information on their interactions with other genes from

Table 3 Performance Comparison of Microarrays According to Published Reports

Method	Probes	Sample[a] (μg)	Detection	Image analysis	Sensitivity[b]	Refs.
Glass microarrays	cDNA clones (PCR products)	50	FL[c]	Confocal scanning	1/100,000	(95)
	Oligo-nucleotides (80mer)	20	FL	Confocal scanning	>1/300,000	(96)
	Oligo-nucleotides (30mer)	2	FL	Non-confocal scanning	1/300,000	(97)
Oligonucleotide chips (Photolithography)	Oligo-nucleotides (25mer)	15	FL	Confocal scanning	1/300,000	(96) (98)
Nylon microarrays	cDNA clones (PCR products)	0.1	^{33}P	Phosphorimager	1/10,000	(98)

[a]Total RNA.

[b]The abundance of mRNA in the sample.

[c]Fluorescence.

Abbreviation: PCR, polymerase chain reaction.

the MEDLINE (the NLM bibliographic database covering the fields of medicine, nursing, dentistry, veterinary medicine, the health care system, and the preclinical sciences) by natural language processing (101–103). This work also is being performed in collaboration with Dr. T. Takagi of the University of Tokyo. As the naming of genes has thus far been arbitrary, gene names and abbreviations often include redundancies that lead to false hits (noise) in searches for specific genes (abstracts containing no mention of the gene in question). In order to extract accurate sentences describing the gene interactions, our database employs an efficient system to eliminate irrelevant hits from PubMed (the NLM search service that provides access to over 11 million citations in MEDLINE and other related databases, with links to participating online journals) search returns. The system exploits the fact that an abstract usually includes both a query (gene name) and a keyword derived from synonyms. The system also employs an effective algorithm to identify abbreviations and their expansions automatically (104). In the future, this will provide a powerful tool for automatically extracting sentences that describe gene interactions.

Continuing efforts to complete the comprehensive database described earlier will allow us to apply new knowledge obtained by biotechnology and bioinformatics for further progress in personal care.

Tailor-Designing Skin Care by Predicting Lifestyle-Related Risk Factors

Biotechnology and the bioinformatics tools described earlier will help cosmetic dermatologists ascertain the expression profiles and functions of UV-regulated genes. It will be possible to compare the individual profiles of targeted genes or UV-regulated genes with the profiles of others, for example, UV-hypersensitive patients or photoaged donors. Individual single nucleotide polymorphism (SNP) information on target genes will also become available when ethical problems are resolved.

Our group has also taken a great interest in the DNA repair system for DNA damaged by internal and external agents, such as UV irradiation and reactive oxygen species. A reduction in the post-UV DNA repair capacity is associated with age and probably with skin carcinogenesis and photoaging as well (105,106). In another collaborative study, our group confirmed a significant age-related decrease in the ability to restore damaged DNA. The experiments were performed using a cell reactivation assay to evaluate the functional recovery of transfected reporter genes damaged by UV light, in collaboration with Drs. S. Moriwaki and M. Takigawa of Hamamatsu University School of Medicine and Dr. T. Mori of Nara Medical University. Our results indicated the reduced post-UV DNA repair capacity in aging results from an impairment in the latter step of nucleotide excision repair due to a decrease in the expression of factors in DNA repair synthesis (107). Additional results were obtained by a DNA damage evaluation by an enzyme-linked immunosorbent assay (ELISA) using lesion-specific monoclonal antibodies, and by a series of quantitative

Gene function

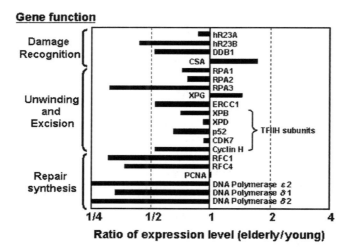

Ratio of expression level (elderly/young)

Figure 7   Aadaptor-tagged competitive PCR (ATAC-PCR) analyses of the constitutive expression of 20 NER (a nucleotide excision repair) genes in cultured fibroblasts. The expression level of NER genes in confluent fibroblasts from the elderly (95 years old) was compared to those from the young (3 years old). β-Actin and glyceraldehyde-3-phosphate dehydrogenase genes were employed as standards to normalize gene expression.

mRNA expression analyses of 20 genes involved in nucleotide excision repair using the ATAC-PCR technique (63,64) (Fig. 7) (107). The enzymes involved in this repair step might be candidates for target genes for personal care against UV and aging risks.

As bioinformatics tools grow more powerful, it will become possible to build a comprehensive database that combines all of these findings with data on cosmetic characteristics. When such a database becomes available, it may enable cosmetic researchers to predict risk and tailor skin-care regimens for individuals based on their lifestyles.

Biotechnology will surely play an indispensable role in the development of personal care and the enhancement of quality of life.

REFERENCES

1. Kligman AM. The biology of the stratum corneum. In: Montagna W, Lobitz Jr WC, eds. The Epidermis. New York: Academic Press, 1964:387–433.
2. Elias PM, Friend DS. The permeability barrier in mammalian epidermis. J Cell Biol 1975; 65:180–191.
3. Middleton JD. The mechanism of water binding in stratum corneum. Br J Dermatol 1968; 80:437–450.
4. Rawlings AV, Scott IR, Harding CR, Bowser PA. Stratum corneum moisturization at the molecular level. J Invest Dermatol 1994; 103:7331–741.

5. Horii I, Nakayama Y, Obata M, Tagami H. Stratum corneum hydration and amino acid content in xerotic skin. Br J Dermatol 1989; 121:587–592.

6. Presland RB, Haydock PV, Fleckman P, Nirunsuksiri W, Dale BA. Characterization of the human epidermal profilaggrin gene. Genomic organization and identification of an S-100-like calcium binding domain at the amino terminus. J Biol Chem 1992; 267:23772–23781.

7. Downing DT, Strauss JS, Pochi PE. Variability in the chemical composition of human skin surface lipids. J Invest Dermatol 1969; 53:322–327.

8. Nazzaro-Porro M, Passi S, Boniforti L, Belsito F. Effects of aging on fatty acids in skin surface lipids. J Invest Dermatol 1979; 73:112–117.

9. Tarutani M, Itami S, Okabe M, Ikawa M, Tezuka T, Yoshikawa K, Kinoshita T, Takeda J. Tissue-specific knockout of the mouse *Pig-a* gene reveals important roles for GPI-anchored proteins in skin development. Proc Natl Acad Sci USA 1997; 94:7400–7405.

10. Zeeuwen PL, van Vlijmen-Willems IM, Hendriks W, Merkx GF, Schalkwijk J. A null mutation in the cystatin M/E gene of ichq mice causes juvenile lethality and defects in epidermal cornification. Hum Mol Genet 2002; 11:2867–2875.

11. Elias PM, Menon GK. Structural and lipid biochemical correlates of the epidermal permeability barrier. Adv Lipid Res 1991; 24:1–26.

12. Matoltsy AG, Downes AM, Sweeney TM. Studies of the epidermal water barrier. II. Investigation of the chemical nature of the water barrier. J Invest Dermatol 1968; 50:19–26.

13. Haratake A, Uchida Y, Schmuth M, Tanno O, Yasuda R, Epstein JH, Elias PM, Holleran WM. UVB-induced alterations in permeability barrier function: roles for epidermal hyperproliferation and thymocyte-mediated response. J Invest Dermatol 1997; 108:769–775.

14. Holleran WM, Uchida T, Halkier-Sorensen L, Haratake A, Hara M, Epstein JH, Elias PM. Structural and biochemical basis for the UVB-induced alterations in epidermal barrier function. Photodermatol Photoimmunol Photomed 1997; 13:117–128.

15. Schreiner V, Gooris GS, Pfeiffer S, Lanzendorfer G, Wenck H, Diembeck W, Proksch E, Bouwstra J. Barrier characteristics of different human skin types investigated with X-ray diffraction, lipid analysis, and electron microscopy imaging. J Invest Dermatol 2000; 114:654–660.

16. Uchida Y, Hara M, Nishio H, Sidransky E, Inoue S, Otsuka F, Suzuki A, Elias PM, Holleran WM, Hamanaka S. Epidermal sphingomyelins are precursors for selected stratum corneum ceramides. J Lipid Res 2000; 41:2071–2082.

17. Imokawa G, Abe A, Jin K, Higaki Y, Kawashima M, Hidano A. Decreased level of ceramides in stratum corneum of atopic dermatitis: an etiologic factor in atopic dry skin? J Invest Dermatol 1991; 96:523–526.

18. Wildnauer RH, Bothwell JW, Douglass AB. Stratum corneum biomechanical properties. I. Influence of relative humidity on normal and extracted human stratum corneum. J Invest Dermatol 1971; 56:72–78.

19. Hashimoto-Kumasaka K, Horii I, Tagami H. In vitro comparison of water-holding capacity of the superficial and deeper layers of the stratum corneum. Arch Dermatol Res 1991; 283:342–346.

20. Cooper MD, Jardine H, Ferguson J. Seasonal influence on the occurrence of dry flaking facial skin. In: Marks R, Plewig G, eds. The Environmental Threat to the Skin. London: Martin Dunitz, 1992:159–164.

21. Egawa M, Oguri M, Kuwahara T, Takahashi M. Effect of exposure of human skin to a dry environment. Skin Res Technol 2002; 8:212–218.
22. Denda M, Sato J, Tsuchiya T, Elias PM, Feingold KR. Low humidity stimulates epidermal DNA synthesis and amplifies the hyperproliferative response to barrier disruption: implication for seasonal exacerbations of inflammatory dermatoses. J Invest Dermatol 1998; 111:873–878.
23. Rogers J, Harding C, Mayo A, Banks J, Rawlings A. Stratum corneum lipids: the effect of ageing and the seasons. Arch Dermatol Res 1996; 288:765–770.
24. Yamamoto A, Serizawa S, Ito M, Sato Y. Stratum corneum lipid abnormalities in atopic dermatitis. Arch Dermatol Res 1991; 283:219–223.
25. Hara M, Kikuchi K, Watanabe M, Denda M, Koyama J, Nomura J, Horii I, Tagami H. Senile xerosis: functional, morphological, and biochemical studies. J Geriatr Dermatol 1993; 1:111–120.
26. Haratake A, Ikenaga K, Katoh N, Uchiwa H, Hirano S, Yasuno H. Topical mevalonic acid stimulates de novo cholesterol synthesis and epidermal permeability barrier homeostasis in aged mice. J Invest Dermatol 2000; 114:247–252.
27. Sakai S, Endo Y, Ozawa N, Sugawara T, Kusaka A, Sayo T, Tagami H, Inoue S. Characteristics of the epidermis and stratum corneum of hairless mice with experimentally induced diabetes mellitus. J Invest Dermatol 2003; 120:79–85.
28. Sakai S, Kikuchi K, Satoh J, Tagami H, Inoue S. Functional properties of the stratum corneum in patients with diabetes mellitus: similarities to senile xerosis. Br J Dermatol 2005; 153:319–323.
29. Berardesca E, Barbareschi M, Veraldi S, Pimpinelli N. Evaluation of efficacy of a skin lipid mixture in patients with irritant contact dermatitis, allergic contact dermatitis or atopic dermatitis: a multicenter study. Contact Dermat 2001; 45:280–285.
30. Tanno O, Ota Y, Kitamura N, Katsube T, Inoue S. Nicotinamide increases biosynthesis of ceramides as well as other stratum corneum lipids to improve the epidermal permeability barrier. Br J Dermatol 2000; 143:524–531.
31. Fukunaga K, Yoshida M, Nakajima F, Uematsu R, Hara M, Inoue S, Kondo H, Nishimura S. Design, synthesis, and evaluation of beta-galactosylceramide mimics promoting beta-glucocerebrosidase activity in keratinocytes. Bioorg Med Chem Lett 2003; 10; 13:813–815.
32. Hara M, Uchida Y, Haratake A, Mimura K, Hamanaka S. Galactocerebroside and not glucocerebroside or ceramide stimulate epidermal beta-glucocerebrosidase activity. J Dermatol Sci 1998; 16:111–119.
33. Grubauer G, Elias PM, Feingold KR. Transepidermal water loss: the signal for recovery of barrier structure and function. J Lipid Res 1989; 30:323–333.
34. Ishibashi K, Morinaga T, Kuwahara M, Sasaki S, Imai M. Cloning and identification of a new member of water channel (AQP10) as an aquaglyceroporin. Biochim Biophys Acta 2002; 1576:335–340.
35. Sugiyama Y, Ota Y, Hara M, Inoue S. Osmotic stress up-regulates aquaporin-3 gene expression in cultured human keratinocytes. Biochim Biophys Acta 2001; 1522:82–88.
36. Ma T, Hara M, Sougrat R, Verbavatz JM, Verkman AS. Impaired stratum corneum hydration in mice lacking epidermal water channel aquaporin-3. J Biol Chem 2002; 277:17147–17153.
37. Hara M, Ma T, Verkman AS. Selectively reduced glycerol in skin of aquaporin-3-deficient mice may account for impaired skin hydration, elasticity, and barrier recovery. J Biol Chem 2002; 277:46616–46621.

38. Hara M, Verkman AS. Glycerol replacement corrects defective skin hydration, elasticity, and barrier function in aquaporin-3-deficient mice. Proc Natl Acad Sci USA 2003; 100:7360–7365.

39. Vasioukhin V, Bauer C, Degenstein L, Wise B, Fuchs E. Hyperproliferation and defects in epithelial polarity upon conditional ablation of alpha-catenin in skin. Cell 2001; 104:605–617.

40. Guerrin M, Simon M, Montezin M, Haftek M, Vincent C, Serre G. Expression cloning of human corneodesmosin proves its identity with the product of the S gene and allows improved characterization of its processing during keratinocyte differentiation. J Biol Chem 1998; 273:22640–22647.

41. Inoue S. Skin hyaluronan: its metabolism and roles in skin physiology. Connect Tissue Res 2001; 33:235–243.

42. Ghersetich I, Lotti T, Campanile G, Grappone C, Dini G. Hyaluronic acid in cutaneous intrinsic aging. Int J Dermatol 1994; 33:119–122.

43. Sugiyama Y, Shimada A, Sayo T, Sakai S, Inoue S. Putative hyaluronan synthase mRNA are expressed in mouse skin and TGF-beta upregulates their expression in cultured human skin cells. J Invest Dermatol 1998; 110:116–121.

44. Sayo T, Sugiyama Y, Takahashi Y, Ozawa N, Sakai S, Ishikawa O, Tamura M, Inoue S. Hyaluronan synthase 3 regulates hyaluronan synthesis in cultured human keratinocytes. J Invest Dermatol 2002; 118:43–48.

45. Yoshida H, Sakai S, Sayo T, Sugiyama Y, Inoue S. Histamine upregulates putative hyaluronan synthase mRNAs via H1 receptors to accumulate low-molecular-mass hyaluronan in human skin fibroblasts. In preparation, 2006.

46. Sayo T, Sakai S, Inoue S. Synergistic Effect of N-acetylglucosamine and retinoids on hyaluronan production in human keratinocytes. Skin Pharmacol Physiol 2004; 17:77–83.

47. Tammi R, Ripellino JA, Margolis RU, Tammi M. Localization of epidermal hyaluronic acid using the hyaluronate binding region of cartilage proteoglycan as a specific probe. J Invest Dermatol 1988; 90:412–414.

48. Meyer LJ, Stern R. Age-dependent changes of hyaluronan in human skin. J Invest Dermatol 1994; 102:385–389.

49. Sakai S, Yasuda R, Sayo T, Ishikawa O, Inoue S. Hyaluronan exists in the normal stratum corneum. J Invest Dermatol 2000; 114:1184–1187.

50. Sakai S, Sayo T, Kodama S, Inoue S. N-Methyl-L-serine stimulates hyaluronan production in human skin fibroblasts. Skin Pharmacol Appl Skin Physiol 1999; 12:276–283.

51. Tammi R, Ripellino JA, Margolis RU, Maibach HI, Tammi N. Hyaluronate accumulation in human epidermis treated with retinoic acid in skin organ culture. J Invest Dermatol 1989; 92: 326–332.

52. Weiss JS, Ellis CN, Headington JT, Voorhees JJ. Topical tretinoin in the treatment of aging skin. J Am Acad Dermatol 1988; 19:169–175.

53. Westphal CH, Leder P. Transposon-generated knock-out and knock-in gene-targeting constructs for use in mice. Curr Biol 1997; 7:530–533.

54. Tiscornia G, Singer O, Ikawa M, Verma IM. A general method for gene knockdown in mice by using lentiviral vectors expressing small interfering RNA. Proc Natl Acad Sci USA 2003; 100:1844–1848.

55. Sano S, Itami S, Takeda K, Tarutani M, Yamaguchi Y, Miura H, Yoshikawa K, Akira S, Takeda J. Keratinocyte-specific ablation of Stat3 exhibits impaired

skin remodeling, but does not affect skin morphogenesis. EMBO J 1999; 18: 4657–4668.

56. Takagi S, Tojo H, Tomita S, Sano S, Itami S, Hara M, Inoue S, Horie K, Kondoh G, Hosokawa K, Gonzalez FJ, Takeda J. Alteration of the 4-sphingenine scaffolds of ceramides in keratinocyte-specific Arnt-deficient mice affects skin barrier function. J Clin Invest 2003; 112:1372–1382.

57. Nozaki M, Ohishi K, Yamada N, Kinoshita T, Nagy A, Takeda J. Developmental abnormalities of glycosylphosphatidylinositol-anchor-deficient embryos revealed by Cre/loxP system. Lab Invest 1999; 79:293–299.

58. Inoue S, Hara M, Takeda J, Tarutani M, Uchida Y, Elias PM, Holleran WM. A GPI anchor is required for the epidermal permeability barrier (abstr). J Invest Dermatol 2001; 117:415.

59. Hara-Chikuma M, Takeda J, Tarutani M, Uchida Y, Holleran WM, Endo Y, Elias PM, Inoue S. Epidermal-specific defect of GPI anchor in *Pig-a null* mice results in Harlequin ichthyosis-like features. J Invest Dermatol 2004; 123:464–469.

60. Schena M, Shalon D, Davis RW, Brown PO. Quantitative monitoring of gene expression patterns with a complementary DNA microarray. Science 1995; 270: 467–470.

61. Chee M, Yang R, Hubbell E, Berno A, Huang XC, Stern D, Winkler J, Lockhart DJ, Morris MS, Fodor SP. Accessing genetic information with high-density DNA arrays. Science 1996; 274:610–614.

62. Velculescu VE, Zhang L, Vogelstein B, Kinzler KW. Serial analysis of gene expression. Science 1995; 270:484–487.

63. Saito S, Matoba R, Kato K. Adapter-tagged competitive PCR (ATAC-PCR)—a high-throughput quantitative PCR method for microarray validation. Methods 2003; 31:326–331.

64. Kato K. Adaptor-tagged competitive PCR: a novel method for measuring relative gene expression. Nucleic Acids Res 1997; 25:4694–4696.

65. Kawamoto S, Ohnishi T, Kita H, Chisaka O, Okubo K. Expression profiling by iAFLP: a PCR-based method for genome-wide gene expression profiling. Genome Res 1999; 9:1305–1312.

66. Fukumura R, Takahashi H, Saito T, Tsutsumi Y, Fujimori A, Sato S, Tatsumi K, Araki R, Abe M. A sensitive transcriptome analysis method that can detect unknown transcripts. Nucleic Acids Res 2003; 31:e94.

67. Gazel A, Ramphal P, Rosdy M, De Wever B, Tornier C, Hosein N, Lee B, Tomic-Canic M, M Blumenberg. Transcriptional profiling of epidermal keratinocytes: comparison of genes expressed in skin, cultured keratinocytes, and reconstituted epidermis, using large DNA microarrays. J Invest Dermatol 2003; 121:1459–1468.

68. Whitfield ML, Finlay DR, Murray JT, Troyanskaya OG, Chi JT, Pergamenschikov A, McCalmont TH, Brown PO, Botstein D, Connolly MK. Systemic and cell type-specific gene expression patterns in scleroderma skin. Proc Natl Acad Sci USA 2003; 100:12319–12324.

69. Nomura I, Goleva E, Howell MD, Hamid QA, Ong PY, Hall CF, Darst MA, Gao B, Boguniewicz M, Travers JB, Leung DY. Cytokine milieu of atopic dermatitis, as compared to psoriasis, skin prevents induction of innate immune response genes. J Immunol 2003; 171:3262–3269.

70. Nomura I, Gao B, Boguniewicz M, Darst MA, Travers JB, Leung DY. Distinct patterns of gene expression in the skin lesions of atopic dermatitis and psoriasis: a gene microarray analysis. J Allergy Clin Immunol 2003; 112:1195–1202.
71. Paddock HN, Schultz GS, Baker HV, Varela JC, Beierle EA, Moldawer LL, Mozingo DW. Analysis of gene expression patterns in human postburn hypertrophic scars. J Burn Care Rehabil 2003; 24:371–377.
72. Dazard JE, Gal H, Amariglio N, Rechavi G, Domany E, Givol D. Genome-wide comparison of human keratinocyte and squamous cell carcinoma responses to UVB irradiation: implications for skin and epithelial cancer. Oncogene 2003; 22:2993–3006.
73. Sesto A, Navarro M, Burslem F, Jorcano JL. Analysis of the ultraviolet B response in primary human keratinocytes using oligonucleotide microarrays. Proc Natl Acad Sci USA 2000; 99:2965–2970.
74. Takao J, Ariizumi K, Dougherty II, Cruz Jr. PD Genomic scale analysis of the human keratinocyte response to broad-band ultraviolet-B irradiation. Photodermatol Photoimmunol Photomed 2002; 18:5–13.
75. Li D, Turi TG, Schuck A, Freedberg IM, Khitrov G, Blumenberg M. Rays and arrays: the transcriptional program in the response of human epidermal keratinocytes to UVB illumination. FASEB J 2001; 15:2533–2535.
76. Marionnet C, Bernerd F, Dumas A, Verrecchia F, Mollier K, Compan D, Bernard B, Lahfa M, Leclaire J, Medaisko C, Mehul B, Seite S, Mauviel A, Dubertret L. Modulation of gene expression induced in human epidermis by environmental stress in vivo. J Invest Dermatol 2003; 121:1447–1458.
77. Koria P, Brazeau D, Kirkwood K, Hayden P, Klausner M, Andreadis ST. Gene expression profile of tissue engineered skin subjected to acute barrier disruption. J Invest Dermatol 2003; 121:368–382.
78. Baek JH, Lee G, Kim SN, Kim JM, Kim M, Chung SC, Min BM. Common genes responsible for differentiation and senescence of human mucosal and epidermal keratinocytes. Int J Mol Med 2003; 12:319–325.
79. Chen W, Fu X, Sun X, Sun T, Zhao Z, Sheng Z. Analysis of differentially expressed genes in keloids and normal skin with cDNA microarray. J Surg Res 2003; 113:208–216.
80. Bernard FX, Pedretti N, Rosdy M, Deguercy A. Comparison of gene expression profiles in human keratinocyte mono-layer cultures, reconstituted epidermis and normal human skin; transcriptional effects of retinoid treatments in reconstituted human epidermis. Exp Dermatol 2002; 11:59–74.
81. Curto EV, Lambert GW, Davis RL, Wilborn TW, Dooley TP. Biomarkers of human skin cells identified using DermArray DNA arrays and new bioinformatics methods. Biochem Biophys Res Commun 2002; 291:1052–1064.
82. Murakami T, Fujimoto M, Ohtsuki M, Nakagawa H. Expression profiling of cancer-related genes in human keratinocytes following non-lethal ultraviolet B irradiation. J Dermatol Sci 2001; 27:121–129.
83. Becker B, Vogt T, Landthaler M, Stolz W. Detection of differentially regulated genes in keratinocytes by cDNA array hybridization: Hsp27 and other novel players in response to artificial ultraviolet radiation. J Invest Dermatol 2001; 116:983–988.
84. He YY, Huang JL, Sik RH, Liu J, Waalkes MP, Chignell CF. Expression profiling of human keratinocyte response to ultraviolet A: implications in apoptosis. J Invest Dermatol 2004; 122:533–43.

85. Catani MV, Rossi A, Costanzo A, Sabatini S, Levrero M, Melino G, Avigliano L. Induction of gene expression via activator protein-1 in the ascorbate protection against UV-induced damage. Biochem J 2001; 356:77–85.
86. Valery C, Grob JJ, Verrando P. Identification by cDNA microarray technology of genes modulated by artificial ultraviolet radiation in normal human melanocytes: relation to melanocarcinogenesis. J Invest Dermatol 2001; 117:1471–1482.
87. Jean S, Bideau C, Bellon L, Halimi G, Meo MD, Orsiere T, Dumenil G, Berge-Lefranc JL, Botta A. The expression of genes induced in melanocytes by exposure to 365-nm UVA: study by cDNA arrays and real-time quantitative RT-PCR. Biochim Biophys Acta 2001; 1522:89–96.
88. Cole J, Tsou R, Wallace K, Gibran N, Isik F. Early gene expression profile of human skin to injury using high-density cDNA microarrays. Wound Repair Regen 2001; 9:360–370.
89. Fletcher ST, Baker VA, Fentem JH, Basketter DA, Kelsell DP. Gene expression analysis of EpiDerm following exposure to SLS using cDNA microarrays. Toxicol In Vitro 2001; 15:393–398.
90. Tsou R, Cole JK, Nathens AB, Isik FF, Heimbach DM, Engrav LH, Gibran NS. Analysis of hypertrophic and normal scar gene expression with cDNA microarrays. J Burn Care Rehabil 2000; 21:541–550.
91. Gonzalez P, Zigler Jr JS, Epstein DL, Borras T. Identification and isolation of differentially expressed genes from very small tissue samples. Biotechniques 1999; 26:884–892.
92. Wang J, Hu L, Hamilton SR, Coombes KR, Zhang W. RNA anmplification strategies for cDNA microarray. Biotechniques 2003; 34:394–400.
93. Van Gelder RN, Von Zastrow ME, Yool A, Dement WC, Barchas JD, Eberwine JH. Amplified RNA synthesized from limited quantities of heterogeneous cDNA. Proc Natl Acad Sci USA 1990; 87:1663–1667.
94. Gomes LI, Silva RL, Stolf BS, Cristo EB, Hirata R, Soares FA, Reis LF, Neves EJ, Carvalho AF. Comparative analysis of amplified and nonamplified RNA for hybridization in cDNA microarray. Anal Biochem 2003; 321:244–251.
95. Duggan DJ, Bittner M, Chen Y, Meltzer P, Trent JM. Expression profiling using cDNA microarrays. Nat Genet 1999; 21:10–14.
96. Rogojina AT, Orr WE, Song BK, Geisert Jr. EE Comparing the use of Affymetrix to spotted oligonucleotide microarrays using two retinal pigment epithelium cell lines. Mol Vis 2003; 9:482–496.
97. Sendera TJ, Dorris D, Ramakrishnan R, Nguyen A, Trakas D, Mazumder A. Expression profiling with oligonucleotide arrays: technologies and applications for neurobiology. Neurochem Res 2002; 27:1005–1026.
98. Bertucci F, Bernard K, Loriod B, Chang YC, Granjeaud S, Birnbaum D, Nguyen C, Peck K, Jordan BR. Sensitivity issues in DNA array-based expression measurements and performance of nylon microarrays for small samples. Hum Mol Genet 1999; 8:1715–1722.
99. Yamazaki M, Ao H, Terai G, Kitamura N, Takagi T. Database for human UV-regulated genes (abstr). Genome Informatics 2001; 12:468–487.
100. Terai G, Yamazaki M, Sugiyama Y, Ao H, Inoue S, Takagi T. Database for human UV-regulated genes (abstr). Genome Informatics 2002; 12:506–507.

101. Ao H, Takagi T. An algorithm to select abstracts from MEDLINE concerning UV-regulated genes (abstr). 11th International Conference on Intelligent Systems for Molecular Biology 2003; p63.

102. Ao H, Yamamoto Y, Takagi T. PETER: A novel system to select PubMed results concerning human genes. In preparation, 2006.

103. Ao H, Takagi T. A simple method to extract information about interactions of UV-regulated genes from MEDLINE (abstr). Pacific Symposium on Biocomputing 2004; 52.

104. Ao H, Takagi T. ALICE: an algorithm to extract abbreviations from MEDLINE. J Am Med Inform Assoc 2005; 12:576–586.

105. Moriwaki S, Ray S, Tarone RE, Kraemer KH, Grossman L. The effect of donor age on the processing of UV-damaged DNA by cultured human cells: reduced DNA repair capacity and increased DNA mutability. Mutat Res 1996; 364:117–123.

106. Goukassian D, Gad F, Yaar M, Eller MS, Nehal US, Gilchrest BA. Mechanisms and implications of the age-associated decrease in DNA repair capacity. FASEB J 2000; 14:1325–1334.

107. Takahashi Y, Moriwaki S, Sugiyama Y, Endo Y, Yamsaki K, Mori T, Takigawa M, Inoue S. Decreased gene expression responsible for post-ultraviolet DNA repair synthesis in aging: a possible mechanism of age-related reduction in DNA repair capacity. J Invest Dermatol 2005; 124:435–442.

7

Biotechnology in Skin Care (III): Skin Aging

Anthony V. Rawlings

AVR Consulting Ltd., Kingsmead, Northwich, Cheshire, U.K.

INTRODUCTION

This chapter gives a short overview of the effects of aging on skin structure, function, and quality, together with the positive skin benefits and effects of a variety of anti-aging ingredients that have been derived using biotechnological approaches. It covers the effects of:

1. Ligands of specific cellular nuclear receptors that improve epidermal differentiation, that increase the levels of dermal matrix components, and that reduce melanogenesis.
2. The effects of peptides on dermal matrix remodeling.
3. The effects of enzymes on oxidation of skin components.
4. The effects of ceramides on stratum corneum function.

This is not meant to be an exhaustive review of all actives but my own personal choice of a selection of novel ingredients that have been derived by biotechnological means, or whose mechanisms of action have been determined using molecular biology approaches and have been tested on human skin in vivo.

PROCESSES OF SKIN AGING

General Aspects of Skin Aging

Skin aging is a complex process associated with changes in skin ultrastructure and biochemistry. These changes are a consequence of chronological aging, which is further exacerbated by UV irradiation (UVR) leading to photoaging. Superimposed on these are lifestyle factors (habits, diets, smoking), diseased states (e.g., diabetes), and the effect of gravity. Reductions in endogenous hormone levels can also contribute to the aging process during the menopause (e.g., reduced concentrations of estrogens). The clinical changes to skin associated with photoaging are age spots (freckles or ephelides, solar lentigines, and solar keratoses) and wrinkles (Fig. 1) (1). Sensitive subjects (e.g., skin phototypes I/II) can expect to have solar lentigines and freckles, especially in photoexposed areas earlier than more pigmented subjects. Acute clinical effects of UVR in the skin are erythema and inflammation (sunburn), which eventually lead to skin tanning, epidermal hyperplasia, and a thickening of stratum corneum, together with faulty desquamation. The skin can repair some of UVR-induced damage provided that UVR exposure is avoided or reduced (2). The histological changes in the skin due to chronic UVR exposure have been investigated extensively, and they precede the clinical signs of photoaging. The effects of gravity and further dermal remodeling events eventually take their toll, leading to the

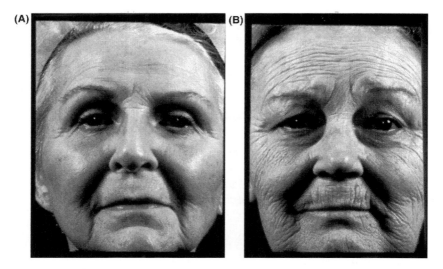

Figure 1   Photographs of two ladies, one from Chicago (**A**) and one (a farm worker) from Michigan (**B**). Both are 71 years old. Notice the extensive photodamage on the face of the farm worker (**B**). *Source*: Courtesy of Professor C. E. M. Griffiths, University of Manchester, Hope Hospital, Manchester, UK.

expression of sags and wrinkles, particularly on facial skin. In general terms, facial sagging and the presence of age spots are more apparent on Asian skin, whereas in Caucasian subjects age spots are largely found on the dorsal aspect of the hands and facial wrinkles are more apparent (3). In darker-skinned individuals, their skin is largely protected from these classical signs of aging due to the inherent UV photoprotection provided by melanin, but hyperpigmentary problems can occur in these individuals following skin irritation.

Aging of the Epidermis

The epidermis undergoes subtle but significant structural alterations during aging. There is an overall thinning of non-sun-exposed epidermis (4). Epidermal atrophy seems to affect mostly the spinous cell layers, whereas neither stratum corneum nor stratum granulosum seem to be greatly affected. A clear flattening of the dermo-epidermal junction (DEJ) occurs, and the intradermal villous cytoplasmic projections of basal layer keratinocytes are lost in aged skin (5). These changes explain the increased fragility of aged skin to shear stress and readiness to form blisters. It is the loss of these rete ridges that induces the loss of primarily spinous cells. The epidermis has a constant point where these cells differentiate into granular cells to then ultimately form the stratum corneum. In photoaging, despite the reduction in the rete ridges, the epidermis can also become appreciably thicker. Moreover, basal cells display an increased heterogeneity in size and volume. Increased keratinocyte proliferation is apparent, but in general there are also increased signs of apoptotic markers (6). Generally, the stratum corneum becomes slightly thicker due to reduced desquamation. Reduced levels of stratum corneum natural moisturizing factors derived from filaggrin and reduced levels of barrier lipids (ceramides, cholesterol, and fatty acids) are also known (7). Although baseline transepidermal water loss (TEWL) is not reduced, reduced barrier function occurs in older subjects, especially when the skin is challenged (8).

Aging occurs in other cell types found in the epidermis. The number of melanocytes decreases, and considerable heterogeneity in their morphology occurs (9). Foci of activated melanocytes forming lentigines ("liver" spots) are seen aside groups of small, inactive melanocytes (apparent white spots). This suggests that repeated sun exposure can lead to a dysregulation of melanocyte homeostasis and increased focal melanocyte density probably due to changes in basement membrane components. Lentigines have increased numbers of melanocytes that produce dense epidermal deposits of melanin, whereas ephelides (freckles) have a normal number of melanocytes but an increased number of melanosomes. Facial solar lentigines have a twofold increase in both the epidermal area and number of melanocytes compared with facial skin with a similar degree of photodamage, but they frequently lacked the rete ridge hyperplasia classically associated with lentigines from other anatomical sites (10).

Epidermal dendritic Langerhans cells are the single most important antigen presenting cell population in the skin. The number of Langerhans cells decreases significantly in elderly subjects. Langerhans cells undergo morphological alterations comprising less dendrite formation and reduced antigen trapping capacity. More importantly, aged Langerhans cells seem to be functionally impaired, which may explain diminished cutaneous immune function in the elderly.

Aging of the Dermis

Aging, Proteases, and Transcription Factors

UV irradiation can directly damage cellular membranes, leading to reactive oxygen species, which initiates the aging process. However, UV irradiation also leads to long-lived reactive oxygen species (ROS) by increasing the levels and activity of nicotinamide adenine dinucleotide (NADH) oxidase. Subsequently, activation of transcription factors, such as NFKb and AP-1, leads to increased levels of inflammatory cytokines (IL-1, TNF, etc.) accentuating the inflammatory state and also leads to an increase in such proteases as matrix metalloproteases (MMPs), resulting in a degradation of the dermal matrix (11). The MMPs also degrade dermoepidermal matrix proteins and the capillary network.

The AP-1 transcription factor is composed of homo- or heterodimer proteins of the leucine zipper family. The proteins in this family are Fos (Fra-1, Fra-2, FosB, FosB2, and c-Fos) and Jun (c-Jun, JunB, and JunD) (12). Different combinations of these proteins are important for the transcription of differentiation specific proteins. Following solar irradiation, c-Jun is inappropriately expressed in both the keratinocytes and fibroblasts, which lead to an upregulation of MMPs by both cells and to reduced collagen biosynthesis by fibroblasts. Retinoic acid (RA) appears to transrepress AP-1 activity.

C-Jun is activated by phosphorylation mechanisms by a specific enzyme called c-Jun terminal kinase (JNK), which is a member of the mitogen-activated protein kinase family (MAPK) (13). Solar irradiation leads to the activation of mitogen-activated protein kinases kinase kinase (MAPKKKs) that are capable of activating either MAP kinases kinase 4 or 7 (MAP2K4/MAP2K7). MAPK2K4 can activate either the JNKs or the p38-MAPKs. MAP2K7 selectively activates the JNKs. Phosphorylation of threonine residues triggers the specific interaction of activated JNKs with a number of substrates, including the c-Jun component of the AP-1 transcription factor. The resulting phosphorylation, of c-Jun then leads to enhanced transcriptional activity of complexes containing AP-1. In the absence of phosphorylation, c-Jun is degraded by a ubiquitin (Ub) dependent proteolytic pathway. MAPK phosphatases can dephosphorylate c-Jun, thereby leading to its degradation. In fact, RA leads to upregulation of phosphatases and c-Jun degradation.

The nuclear factor kappa beta (NF-κB) transcription factor belongs to the Rel family of proteins that primarily are composed of homo- or heterodimeric proteins (14). The most commonly found combinations are p50/p65 heterodimers and p50 homodimers. In the cytoplasm, this transcription factor is usually inactive where it is bound to its inhibitory protein inhibitory kappa B (IκB). Extracellular stimuli, such as solar stress, activates IκB kinases (IKK), which becomes phosphorylate IκB. Phosphorylated IKb then undergoes degradation by the 26S proteasome, releasing NK-κB, which translocates to the nucleus and initiates transcription. This action then increases the levels of inflammatory cytokines, such as IL-1 and TNF, which accentuate the aging process.

MMPs are synthesized as latent zymogens and can be activated proteolytically via cleavage of a cysteine containing proenzyme or can be activated oxidatively. The catalytic domain has a Histidine-Glutamic-X-Glycine-Histidine (HEXGH) motif responsible for zinc binding. They are inhibited by the tissue inhibitors of metalloproteinases (TIMP 1-4). As well as being involved in photoaging, they are also involved in wound healing.

There are five main families of MMPs:

1. Collagenases (MMP-1, -13 degrading collagen I, II, III, V, Elastin).
2. Gelatinases (MMP-2, -9 degrading Collagen IV, V, X, Elastin, Gelatin).
3. Stromelysins (MMP-3, -10, 11, -9 degrading Collagen IV, V, X, Elastin, Gelatin).
4. Matrilysins (MMP-7 degrading collagen IV, laminin, fibronectin).
5. Membrane-type (MMP-19 degrading gelatine, collagen IV, X elastin) (15).

Interstial collagenases (MMP-1 and to some extent MMP-2) are specific for collagen fibers, whereas gelatinases (MMP-2 and MMP-9) degrade basement membrane collagen, denatured collagens, and collagen fragments. MMP-1 is believed to be the major collagenase and is present as an active form. Only MMP-1 together with MMP-3 and MMP-9 are increased by UV. Elastin can be degraded by serine proteases from inflammatory cells (e.g., macrophage elastase: HME) and fibroblast elastase.

Although MMP-1, 2, and 9 are induced by UV irradiation, only the former two enzymes are significantly increased in aged skin; the largest increase in activity occurs for MMP-1, however. A significant increase in MMP-9 only occurs in skin greater than 80 years of age (16). Other studies indicate that only MMP-1, and not MMP-2 or 3, is increased in actinic keratosis.

Aging and Collagen

Collagen is the main proteinaceous component of the dermis, constituting 75% of its dry weight. More than 70% is type I collagen and approximately 15% type III collagen. The size and arrangement of the collagen fibers distinguishes two dermal main regions in adults. The papillary dermis, which interdigitates with the epidermis, is a well-vascularized area composed mainly of type III collagen. The collagen fibers are narrow in diameter, short, loosely interwoven, randomly oriented, and embedded within the ground substance, such as glycosaminoglycans (GAGs). The reticular dermis is composed mainly of type I collagen. The collagen fibers are large in diameter and tightly packed together in large, broad, and wavy bundles. These bundles are loosely interwoven, arranged parallel with the skin surface, and also embedded in a GAG matrix.

The most prominent microscopic alteration in the structure of photo-damaged dermis is replacement of the normal fibrillary protein fibers by large quantities of abnormal, thickened, fibers, which finally degenerate into a non-fibrous, heterogeneous, and amorphous mass. Biochemically, the elastotic material resembles elastin, although it is disorganized and abnormal. It is thought to be generated through transformation of both pre-existing normal collagen and elastic network as well as abnormal synthetic activities of the fibroblasts stimulated via cytokine release from epidermal keratinocytes acting on the NFκB and AP-1 pathways. Concomitantly, there is a decrease in collagen fibers and bundles. Findings of deformed collagen fibers of various diameters in the papillary dermis suggest that degradation and remodeling of collagen takes place in photo-damaged skin. The changes related to chronic UVR exposure (loss of collagen) is thought to be compensated for either by the increased levels of elastotic material or the GAGs. Changes in collagen composition might also play a role where the proportion of collagen type III is increased in photodamaged skin. In sun protected skin, collagens type I and III have been reported to decline only after the 8th decade of life, whereas it was reduced to approximately 50% of its original levels in the 1st decade to the 9th decade in photoaged skin. The collagen architecture was also disorganized after the 4th decade of life. Typical reductions in the levels of collagen can be seen in Figure 2 (16).

In photoaging, apart from the dermal distruction by MMPs, the fibroblasts now also synthesize less collagen, leading to a net reduction in total dermal collagen levels and associated skin changes due to the AP-1, suppression of collagen synthesis. The diminution in collagen biosynthesis occurs by AP-1, blocking the effects of TGFb and decreasing type II TGFb receptors (17,18). Supporting these findings, Chung et al. (19) recently demonstrated that the levels of mRNA message for collagen synthesis was much greater in photoaged skin than intrinsically aged skin, but collagen protein levels were lower. However, there is also a sustained reduction in collagen synthesis in severely photodamaged skin independent of recent UV exposure. This is due to a reduction in the number of cells producing collagen and also inhibition of synthesis by collagen fragments. Varani et al. (20) recently reported that inhibition of procollagen I synthesis occurs by the presence of high molecular weight collagen fragments in skin. So it appears that the initial collagen degradation by MMP-1 leads to fragments of collagen that, if not degraded further by other metalloproteases, especially MMP-9, lead to a downregulation of collagen synthesis. Nevertheless, a presumed collagen breakdown product is Gly-His-Lys, which is reported to stimulate collagen biosynthesis (see section on antiaging peptides).

The nonenzymatic glycosylation process of proteins, also known as the Maillard reaction, also occurs in skin. The products of the Maillard reaction are called the advanced glycosylation endproducts (AGEs). AGEs induce

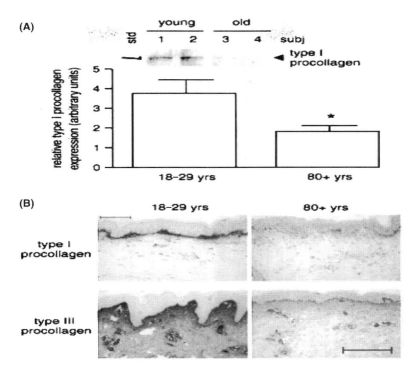

Figure 2 Type I and type III procollagen levels are decreased in aged skin. (**A**) Type I procollagen (α1 chain) levels in skin samples from 18- to 29-year-old persons and 80+ year-old persons (n = 16 per age group) were determined by western blot analysis. Values are mean ± SEM. *p < 0.001 versus 18- to 29-year-old individuals. (**B**) Representative immunohistology of type I procollagen (α1 chain) and type III procollagen (α1 chain) in skin from young and aged persons. Scale bar: 200 μm. *Source*: From Ref. 20.

molecular damage by forming cross-links in long-lived proteins, such as collagen. So far, only one AGE product, pentosidine (Pen) in collagen has been isolated and characterized; Pen is a cross-link formed between arginine and lysine residues in collagen and might be formed through a Maillard reaction with pentose. Pen has been shown to increase with age and in diabetes mellitus. Although Pen is only found in low concentration in the skin, it is regarded as a biomarker in the assessment of cumulative damage to proteins by nonenzymatic glycosylation.

Aging and Elastin

Elastin accounts for 2–4% of dermal proteins and forms an interconnecting network of elastin fibers that provide elasticity and resilience to normal skin. Elastic fibers have a central core of cross-linked hydrophobic elastin surrounded by fibrillin-rich microfibrils. Usually tropoelastin is deposited on a microfibrillar template during development of the elastic fibers. In skin, the elastic fiber network forms a continuum from the DEJ to the deep dermis. Although there are thick elastic fibers in the reticular dermis, a network of finer fibers with reduced elastin content is found in the upper papillary dermis and cascades of discrete microfibrillar bundles that do not contain elastin terminate at the DEJ. The staining intensity of elastin also decreased by 50% in 1st decade to the 9th decade in sun-protected skin, whereas in sun-exposed skin the intensity increased by 50% by the 9th decade (21). The accumulated morphologically abnormal elastin appears to occupy the areas of lost collagen. Thus, atrophy of elastic fibers occurs in chronological aging, but in photoaging, abundant dystrophic elastotic material (tropoelastin and fibrillin wrapped around distorted collagen fibers) is found in the reticular dermis. UV irradiation upregulates the synthesis of this material (22). In addition to this, elastosis in photoaged forearm skin, fibrillin-1 but not fibrillin-2 mRNA is reduced, and at the histological level microfibrils at the DEJ are also significantly reduced. These changes may contribute to known loss of elasticity that occurs with aging (23,24).

Tsukahara et al. (25) have demonstrated that selective inhibition of skin fibroblast elastase prevents UV-induced wrinkle formation (in rats). In normal nonerythemal skin there are usually no dermal infiltrates, so most of the elastolysis occurs as a result of fibroblast elastase activity. Using N-phenotylphosphonyl-leucyl-tryptophane, a reduction in formation of wrinkles was evident. When skin erythema occurs, then a dermal inflammatory infiltrate develops and neutrophil elastase activity can potentially degrade the elastin fibers. For instance, increased MMP-7 (matrilysin) and MMP-12 (human macrophage metalloelastase, HME) also accumulate in actinic damage (26,27). Although MMP-12 degrades elastin, it also degrades type IV collagen, laminin, fibronectin, vitronectin, and entactin together with heparan and chondroitin sulphates. Dermal fibroblasts but not keratinocytes also have the capacity to produce HME. Studies have shown that infiltrating macrophages in UV-irradiated skin did not show immunostaining for HME. HME was only increased in intrinsically aged photoprotected skin after 80 years of age, which may be due to c-JUN induction of AP-1 in old skin (19).

Increased MMP-7 levels have also been observed in the deeper dermal regions. MMP-7 is probably also derived from dermal macrophages and can be activated by stromelysin-1. MMP-7 has very broad substrate specificity in vitro, being able to degrade elastin, fibronectin, gelatins, type IV collagens, laminin, entactin, fibrulins, vitronectin, and aggrecan. Neutrophil elastase and cathepsin G activity are also found to be increased in sun-exposed skin but not in sun-protected skin and to be increased following UV-A irradiation (28).

Elastin peptides also induce elastin synthesis by fibroblasts, and, in addition to the UV stimulation of elastin synthesis, these probably contribute to the large amounts of the elastotic tissue in the dermis. Elastin peptides bind to receptors on fibroblasts, act as a chemotactic agent, and intensify the adhesion to elastin fibers.

This has implications for the oriented biosynthesis of elastin fibers. Laminin and lactose interfere with this receptor-mediated interaction. Equally fucose and fucose-rich polysaccharides also downregulate elastase activities (MMP-2 and -9). These act at the elastin–laminin receptor (or fucose–mannose receptor, 29). Elastin peptides also stimulate the known increase in GAG synthesis that occurs in photoaging and equally lead to the expression and activation of MMP-1, exacerbating the local connective tissue damage. Interestingly, hyaluronic acid also increases the activation of MMP-2 (30).

Aging and the Dermoepidermal Junction

The DEJ is a basement membrane that separates the epidermis and its appendages from the dermis, provides anchorage for adjacent cells, transmits information to neighbouring cells, and acts as a reservoir for growth factors. The lamina densa is composed of type IV collagen. The lamina fibroreticularis underlies the lamina densa and contains fine collagen fibrils and anchoring fibrils composed of type VII collagen. Keratinocytes are bound by the hemidesmosomes, which are composed of the collagenous BP180 antigen, and integrins, which interacts with the laminin 5 one component of the anchoring filaments of the lamina lucida. The beta integrins also connect with the underlying extracellular matrix proteins (collagen type IV) in the lamina densa, and this whole complex is attached to the underlying stroma by anchoring fibrils composed of type VII collagen. There is a general flattening of the DEJ during aging. However, it has been established (31) that the levels of integrins, collagen type IV and VII together with fibrillin-1 and other associated elastic fibril proteins are reduced cellular adhesion and leaves the skin less resistant to shearing forces.

The importance of the balance between extracellular matrix synthesis and degradation in basement membrane formation has also been studied in vitro. MMP-2 (gelatinase A) and MMP-9 (gelatinase B) digest type IV and VII collagens and MMP-3 & -10 (stromelysins) degrade laminins of the BM (32). In LSE's the epidermal basement membrane components laminin 5 and type IV & VII collagens were not detected at the DEJ. This was considered to be a result of increased proteolysis. However, broad spectrum MMP inhibitors augmented their deposition, resulting in formation of a continuous epidermal basement membrane.

Aging and the Microcirculation

Another important aspect of aging is the reduction in the capillary network. Chung et al. (33). demonstrated, using image analysis of biopsies stained for platelet endothelial adhesion molecule (CD31 or PECAM-1), that age dependent reductions in cutaneous vessel size were found in Koreans and that photoaged skin, in particular, exhibited significantly reduced numbers of dermal vessels in areas that display extensive matrix damage. Linear regression analysis showed an inverse relationship of vessel numbers with age in skin that was sun-damaged but not photoprotected. Therefore, photodamaged skin has fewer vessels, and both types of aged skin had reduced vessel size.

Using in vivo confocal measurements Huzaira et al. (34) demonstrated that the enface numerical density of perfused blood vessels at a depth of 58 to 65 μm appear to be greater on sun exposed areas, but these are of smaller diameter (3–5 μm vs. 4–10 μm) and grouped in small clusters. On sun-protected sites, the capillaries are larger, fewer in number, and arranged in isolated loops.

Aging and Immune Cells

Although photoaging shows histological features of chronic skin inflammation, it has been reported that this occurs without clinical abnormalities (35). Increased mast cells, macrophages, T helper cells (CD4+), and memory or activated T (CD45RO) cells as well as a higher number of CD1+ dendritic cells (Langerhan cells) are present. CD8 T cells decreased slightly (T suppressor cells). Despite this, inflammation was not clinically apparent and levels of IL-1beta were actually decreased. This is consistent with other reports of increased IRAP in photo-exposed skin sites. Nevertheless, other chemokines are capable of triggering an inflammatory infiltrate—i.e., increased macrophage inhibitory factor (MIF) and soluble stem cell factor (SCF)—as well as collagen and elastin fragments, which are also chemotactic. The mast cells and macrophages were found particularly at the sites of elastosis. Although Langerhans cells usually migrate out of the epidermis on UV stimulation (immunosuppression), increased dendritic cells were reported in this study, but these are thought to be of the "indeterminate type" as they had no Birbeck granules.

During UV-induced immunosuppression the skin has moved out of balance to a Th2 type of immune state, which seems to be driven by increased levels of IL-10, IL-4, TNF, PAF, and cis-urocanic acid. Urocanic acid can also cause degranulation of mast cells by binding to the histamine receptor releasing tumor necrosis factor-α (TNF-α) and further contributing to the immunosuppression. Proteases released by mast cell degranulation may then also degrade the extracellular matrix (36).

Morphology of a Wrinkle

By fixing the skin in vivo using superglue before a skin biopsy was taken, Green et al. (37) established that wrinkles are associated with thinning and compression of the epidermis at the wrinkle base with marked asymmetrical changes in matrix composition. The collagen network was aligned with the wrinkle with scarlike collagen under the wrinkle and a relatively photoprotected elastic network at the base of the wrinkle (Fig. 3). Thus reduced collagens I and III and an altered dermal matrix is present. Human skin is naturally under tension, but wrinkles appeared to be under compression in the upper walls of the wrinkle. Such tensional forces affect fibroblast alignment and collagen synthesis patterns. Underneath the wrinkle, the connective tissue showed distinctive evidence of an aligned matrix perpendicular across the wrinkle. The microscar extended

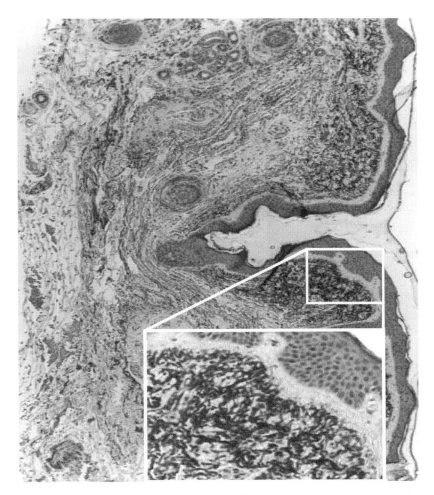

Figure 3 Stained wrinkle section perpendicular to the long axis of the wrinkle, displayed in the correct orientation for an upright adult. Aligned collagen can be seen at the base of the wrinkle whereas elastotic deposits are visible on the lower aspect of the wrinkle and absent from the base. *Source*: From Ref. 37

well beyond the visible wrinkle and may be involved in maintaining tension in the surrounding skin. Elastosis showed asymmetry with greater amounts in the lower face of the wrinkle, but the deep wrinkle had less. At the wrinkle base, collagen and biglycan was not being synthesized, but chondoitin-4-sulphate showed a slight increase. All of this indicates that significant remodeling of deeper collagen structures to reduce axial stiffness and new matrix production is needed to lead to wrinkle effacement.

(A) (B) (C)

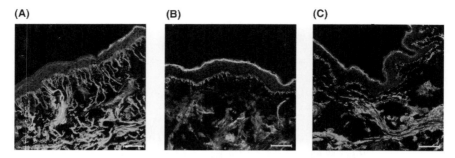

Figure 4 Oxytalan fibers. Comparison of elastic fibers aspect and distribution revealed by immunochemistry between non–sun-exposed skin (abdomen) (**A**), sun-exposed non-wrinkled skin of face (**B**) and sun-exposed, wrinkled skin of face (**C**). A distinct dimunition of oxytalan fibers can be seen in sun-exposed skin. *Source*: From Ref. 38.

In a recent study, Bosset et al. (38) also identified alterations in extracellular matrix components in the direct surroundings of skin wrinkles. The DEJ was modified by a decrease in the levels of collagen IV and VII combined with fewer oxytalan fibers under the wrinkles. Chrondriotin sulphate decreased, combined with an asymmetrical variation of GAGs on both sides of the wrinkles. A distinct dimunition of oxytalan elastic fibers and fibrillin can be seen in sun-exposed skin in Figures and 4B and C compared with non–sun-exposed skin (Fig. 4A).

WHAT WILL BIOTECHNOLOGY DELIVER IN TERMS OF TARGET IDENTIFICATION?

Biotechnological approaches have helped tremendously in deciphering the pathophysiology of aging. Without immunochemical approaches, we would not have the understanding of the molecular aberrations around a wrinkle. Other molecular approaches have been taken, such as serial analysis of gene expression (SAGE) of biopsies from skin of subjects with varying degrees of photodamage. SAGE has been used to identify mRNA profiles as a reflection of changes in global patterns of gene expression. Urschitz et al. (39) recently demonstrated with this method the changes in message levels for key epidermal proteins: keratin 1, macrophage inhibitory factor, and calmodulin-like skin protein. Many other genes were altered in the epidermis compared with the dermis, suggesting a major role of the epidermis in the pathomechanism of the changes associated with photoaging. Other approaches, such as proteomics and metabonomics, are also being applied in this area of research, and one will expect major advances in our understanding over the next decade.

SKIN ANTI-AGING TECHNOLOGIES

Nuclear Receptor Ligands

Gene expression is regulated through the interplay of specific DNA-binding transcription factors. On binding ligands, corepressors dissociate from the transcriptional machinery complex, and coactivators bind to initiate gene transcription. Nuclear hormone receptors are transcription factors that regulate many cellular functions. This superfamily of receptors has been segregated into four major subgroups. The class II subfamily consists of nuclear receptors that form heterodimers with the retinoid X receptor (RXR) (40) which, for example, include the retinoic acid receptor (RAR) and the peroxisome proliferator activated receptor (PPAR) (41). Stimulation of these receptors, in particular, regulates keratinocyte proliferation and differentiation, influences melanogenesis, and stimulates dermal matrix reconstruction.

Retinoid Receptors

Vitamin A is a recognized and well-established anti-aging active. Originally, used as an anti-acne treatment, retinoic acid is now used to treat the signs of aging. Retinoic acid mediates its effect via binding to its nuclear transcription factors. The RAR binds all *trans*-retinoic acid (RA) and its stereoisomer 9-*cis* RA; and the RXR binds 9-*cis* RA. A common feature of these receptors is that they bind to certain regions of DNA known as hormone response elements and thereby initiate ligand-dependent gene transcription. The retinoid transcription factors bind to a retinoic acid response element (RARE) in the promoter of genes, composed of a six base-pair sequence (AGGTCA) (Fig. 5). Similar base-pair sequences are shared by other members of this superfamily, which differ only by the insertion of additional base pairs. RARs and RXRs are known to contain at least three different subtypes: alpha, beta, and gamma, each of which have several isoforms. The RXRs predominate in human skin, especially RXRalpha. Of the RARs, 87% are RARgamma and 13% RARalpha. Only small amounts of RARbeta are found in dermal cells and melanocytes. Retinoic acid treatment results in major epidermal changes only weeks after treatment, but in the longer term, dermal effects are observed (angiogenesis, synthesis of new connective tissue components, and increases in the numbers of more active fibroblasts). Voorhees has also reported that 0.5% retinol (ROH) is as effective as 0.05% RA. However, this level of ROH cannot be used in cosmetic products, and even if it was allowed, the irritation levels are comparable between the two agents. Nevertheless, topical application of retinol can reverse the skin changes associated with aging by increasing fibroblast proliferation (Fig. 6), increasing skin collagen levels (Fig. 7), and decreasing MMP levels (Fig. 8) (42).

Although retinoic acid is the "gold standard" anti-aging treatment, it has its limitations, one being the retinoid resistance that usually occurs following

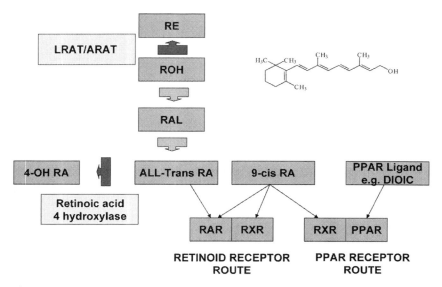

Figure 5 Simple schematic of retinol metabolism and interrelationships of RAR, RXR, and PPAR transcription factors. *Abbreviations*: RAR, retinoic acid receptor; RXR, retinoid X receptor; PPAR, peroxisome proliferator activated receptor.

treatment. Usually after approximately six months' application, no further benefit is accrued, which is thought to result from increased epidermal detoxifying enzymes that degrade retinoic acid to more polar metabolites (43). To circumvent these issues, azoles as cytochrome P450 inhibitors have been used to reduce the degradation of retinoic acid and increase its efficacy. For instance, Liarazole and Rambazole have been developed. Obviously these types of agents, which have been coined retinoic acid metabolism breakdown agents (RAMBAs) or retinomimetics, still have the potential to be used with ROH or RE if the ROH can be mainly directed to deliver RA (Fig. 5). Cosmetic azoles include climbazole, which is also known to inhibit the degradation of active vitamin D.

However, the effectiveness of RAMBAs will still not be optimal, as retinol esterification enzymes are present in the epidermis that will determine the ultimate flux of ROH to RA (Fig. 9) (44). Two enzyme activities that can catalyze retinyl ester synthesis from retinol are: acyl CoA retinol acyl transferase (ARAT) and lecithin retinol acyl transferase (LRAT). LRAT uses the acyl group at the sn-1 position of membrane phospholipids, whereas ARAT uses acyl-CoA. These are the first enzymes that need to be inhibited in the epidermis to ensure increases in RA bioavailability. Several agents have been identified to inhibit these enzymes, for instance, linoleoylmonoethanolamide (LAMEA) (45). Since then, a multitude of enzyme steps have been identified that are involved in retinol metabolism, and from this it is clear that activation and inhibition of several enzymes are needed to enhance retinoic acid bioavailability (46).

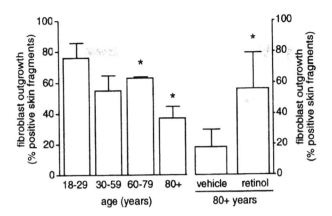

Figure 6 Fibroblast growth potential is reduced with increasing age and is increased with retinol treatment. Freshly obtained skin samples from persons of varying age were cut into small pieces (15–20 pieces/skin sample) and placed in culture to allow outgrowth of fibroblasts from the tissue. Skin from persons in the four age groups ($n = 12, 11, 12$, and 10, respectively) was analyzed. Data are presented as the percentage of skin pieces from which fibroblasts were isolated. *$p < 0.05$ versus 18- to 29-year-old group. Fibroblast outgrowth was also determined in skin samples from 17 persons 80+ years of age, who were treated with 1% retinol and its vehicle for 7 days. *$p < 0.05$ versus vehicle-treated skin. Values are mean ± SEM. *Source*: From Ref. 20.

"Retinoid boosters" have been identified by using keratinocyte assays that demonstrate synergy with retinol in cell proliferation and transglutaminases assays in particular. More sophisticated assays using fibroblast assays for the production of decorin and procollagen-1 have also been developed.

Peroxisome Proliferator Activated Receptors

Peroxisome proliferator activated receptors are a recently discovered family of nuclear transcription factors (41,47) and three PPAR receptor types, PPAR alpha, PPAR beta or delta, and PPAR gamma have been characterized. PPARs bind to the peroxisome proliferator response element within the promoter region of the DNA in the target gene in the form of homo- or heterodimers with the RXR (Fig. 5).

PPARs are activated by the fibrate hypolipidaemic drugs, fatty acids, eicosanoids, and prostanoids, but of these chemical types, the fatty acids are of the most interest for skin applications. The ability of saturated, monounsaturated, and polyunsaturated long chain fatty acids to bind and activate all three PPAR subtypes has been well documented. However, saturated fatty acids have very low activity as PPAR ligands, whereas monounsaturated fatty acids are substantially more active and polyunsaturated fatty acids are generally the most potent

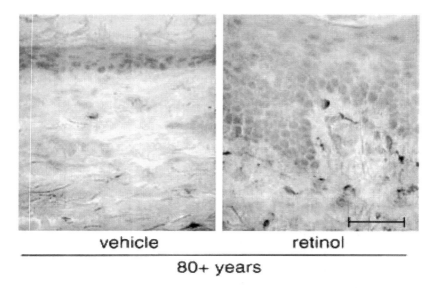

vehicle   retinol
80+ years

Figure 7   Retinol treatment increases type I procollagen expression in fibroblasts from aged skin. Representative immunohistologic staining of type I procollagen (α1 chain) in vehicle-treated (*left*) and retinol-treated (*right*) skin from an 86-year-old person. Tissue was frozen and stained by the immunoperoxidase method; scale bar: 100 μm. Data are representative of n = 6. *Source*: From Ref. 20.

with the optimum chain length required for activation being between C18 and C22. In terms of receptor subtype selectivity, the saturated and polyunsaturated fatty acids do not differentiate between PPARs, while in contrast the monounsaturated fatty acids appear to have a high affinity for PPAR alpha. Gamma-linoleic acid, myristic, and palmitic acids also show a greater affinity for PPAR alpha and PPAR delta compared with PPAR gamma, but their IC 50 values are still in the micromolar range (48).

PPARs were first identified in the epidermis in 1992. However, it was not until recently that the importance of PPARs in epidermal homeostasis has become apparent with the discovery that activation of PPAR alpha, with either lipids or the hypolipidaemic drug clofibrate, can accelerate epidermal barrier formation and induce epidermal differentiation. Rivier et al. (49) first reported that PPAR alpha ligands influence lipid biosynthesis in living skin equivalents. Keratinocyte serine palmitoyl transferase and glucocerebrosidase activities were increased in these studies, and there was a particular increase in ceramide biosynthesis particularly for ceramides 1, 2, and 3 (CER EOS, CER NS, and CER NP).

PPAR delta was recently observed to be the predominant PPAR subtype in human keratinocytes, whereas PPAR alpha and gamma were only induced during epidermal differentiation, suggesting nonredundant functions during

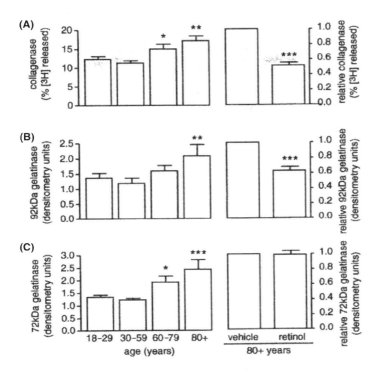

Figure 8 MMP levels are increased in skin with increasing age and partially reduced with retinol treatment. Skin samples of persons of varying age were analyzed for expression of three MMP: (**A**) MMP-1 (interstitial collagenase) (n = 10 persons per age group); (**B**) MMP-9 (92 kDa gelatinase); and (**C**) MMP-2 (72 kDa gelatinase) (n = 10, 11, 8, and 8 persons per age group). Values are mean ± SEM. *p < 0.05 versus 18–29 year old group. **p < 0.01 versus 18–29 year old age group. ***p < 0.001 versus 18–29 year old age group. Skin samples from 16 persons 80+ years of age who were treated with 1% retinol and vehicle for seven days were also analyzed for the three MMP. Values are mean ± SEM. Values for the vehicle-treated 80+ years old individuals were normalized to 1.0, and the other values expressed relative to the normalized values. ***p < 0.001, retinol versus vehicle-treated skin. *Abbreviation*: MMR, matrix metalloprotease. *Source*: From Ref. 20.

differentiation (50). PPAR delta ligands were found to be the most potent in inducing epidermal differentiation (tetrathioacetic acid) by increasing involucrin and transglutaminase while decreasing proliferation. This is consistent with PPAR delta deficient mice exhibiting an exacerbated epidermal hyperplastic response to TPO, in contrast to the minor abnormalities seen in PPAR alpha deficient mice.

Studies from scientists within my previous research group at Unilever have highlighted the benefits, particularly of petroselinic acid (51) and conjugated linoleic acid (52) as potent PPAR alpha activators improving epidermal

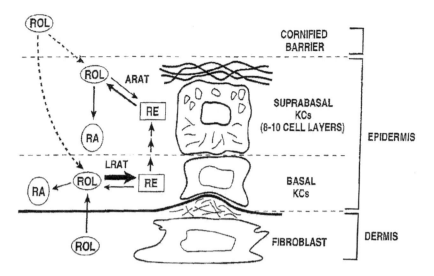

Figure 9   Model of all-*trans* retinol metabolism in human skin. All-*trans* retinol in blood
is supplied to skin through capillaries in the dermis (not shown). All-*trans* retinol is esterified by LRAT in basal keratinocytes. Retinyl esters (RE), formed in basal keratinocytes,
can be hydrolyzed to free all-*trans* retinol as basal keratinocytes differentiate and migrate
through cell layers. For simplicity, suprabasal layers, which are composed of 8 to 10 cell
layers, are depicted as a single cell layer. Exogenous all-*trans* retinol can be esterified
in suprabasal keratinocytes by ARAT, in addition to LRAT in basal keratinocytes. *Abbreviations*: ARAT, acyl coenzyme A retinol acyl transferase; LRAT, lecithin retinol acyl trans-
ferese. *Source*: From Ref. 44.

differentiation, reducing inflammation, increasing extracellular matrix components, and eliciting skin lightening. In vitro increases in levels of transglutaminase, involucrin, filaggrin, and corneocyte envelope formation were observed in
keratinocytes, whereas increased levels of pro-collagen 1 and decorin were
observed for fibroblasts. These effects were confirmed in vivo by short-term
patch testing studies over a three-week period, and increases in the levels of involucrin and filaggrin were also observed. These biochemical changes translated into
improvements in the signs of photodamage and skin tone in a 12-week clinical
study on forearm skin (53). There is further evidence that PPAR ligands can
also mitigate the pigmentation process and induce skin lightening, but the evidence, until now, has been fragmentary (54,55). Wiechers et al. (56) have reported
that octadecenedioic acid, a new nature-derived ingredient, evens Asian skin tone
(Fig. 10).

    Octadecenedioic acid cannot be made by traditional oxidative chemistry,
due to the presence of the double bond in the middle of the molecule. It is
derived via fermentation of oleic acid by naturally occurring yeast and consists

HOOC $\diagup\!\!\!\diagup\!\!\!\diagup\!\!\!\diagup\!\!\!\diagup\!\!\!\diagup\!\!=\!\!\diagup\!\!\!\diagup\!\!\!\diagup\!\!\!\diagup\!\!\!\diagup\!\!\!\diagdown$ COOH

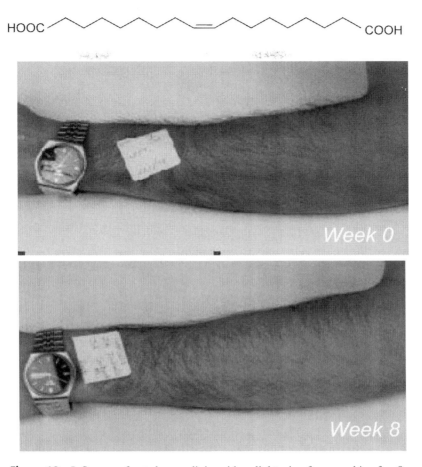

Figure 10 Influence of octadecene dioic acid on lightening forearm skin after 8 weeks. *Source*: From Ref. 56.

predominantly of $C_{18:1}$, $C_{18:2}$, and some C_{16} dicarboxylic acids. Normal yeasts rely on glucose and hydrocarbons, such as alkanes, fatty acids, and triglycerides for their energy consumption. The hydrocarbons are taken up into the microsomes within the cells and oxidized on one end to form a fatty acid, and then at the other end to form a dicarboxylic acid, generally known as dioic acid. These dioic acids are excreted from the microsome and taken up in the peroxisome where β-oxidation takes place, yielding acetyl-CoA. This acetyl-CoA is transferred to the mitochondria, where it is inserted into the tricarboxylic acid (TCA) cycle, yielding water, carbon dioxide, and energy in the form of adenosine triphosphate (ATP). A naturally occurring mutant of specific yeast was identified that follows the biological pathway described earlier, in which the peroxisome is inactive. This yeast will start the bioconversion of alkanes, fatty acids, and triglycerides, but cannot produce beyond the dicarboxylic acid phase. Such natural mutants can survive in nature because they can still obtain their energy via the conversion of glucose. When one feeds this natural mutant with only a very small amount of glucose to prevent it from dying and a relatively large amount of oleic acid as the fatty acid, it will convert oleic acid to *cis*-9-octadecenedioic acid (56).

In in vitro skin toning studies, the efficacy of octadecenedioic acid was compared to that of, among others, hydroquinone, kojic acid, and arbutin. In contrast to these molecules, octadecenedioic acid did not inhibit tyrosinase activity. However, most recently, in attempting to define its mechanism of action, Wiechers et al. (57) reported that octadenedioic acid was a pan PPAR agonist but with slightly greater affinity for the PPAR gamma transcription factor. Comparing it effects to pioglitazone (a specific PPAR gamma ligand) in melanoma cell lines demonstrated reduced cell proliferation and reduced melanogenesis. This was not due to the effects of octadecenedioic acid on tyrosinase enzyme itself but due to reduced levels of message and subsequently reduced total enzyme levels.

Octadecenedioic acid is thus a novel biotechnologically derived ingredient that binds to specific receptors that were first identified using molecular biological approaches. Due to its pan PPAR binding activities, it is expected to have a major influence on skin-aging processes. Clearly, however, it can also influence melanogenesis and melanocyte proliferation, which will contribute to the reduction in age-related increases in lentigines.

Anti-aging Peptides

The production of degradation fragments of collagen and elastin have previously only been considered to be the inert end products of the distruction of the dermal matrix. However, Francois Maquart proposed the name "matrikines" for peptides that are liberated by partial proteolysis of extracellular matrix macromolecules, that are able to regulate cell activities (57,58).

Elastin was reported to be an important source of matrikines. Alkaline hydrolysis of elastic fibers gives rise to a mixture of elastin peptides named Kappa-elastin (59), which possesses several activities typical of matrikines. For the purposes of this chapter, it inhibits elastase activity (60) and stimulates the proliferation of fibroblasts (61). VGPVG, a hydrophobic pentapeptide, is able to stimulate smooth muscle cells proliferation (62) and decrease their elastin production (63). This also stimulates gelatinase A/matrix metalloproteinase-2 (MMP-2) expression in human fibroblastic cells (64). The expression of the components of the MMP-2-activating complex and TIMP-2 was also increased. Further results demonstrated that VGVAPG also stimulates collagenase MMP-1 expression (65), which suggests that this peptide may play a major role in the regulation of connective tissue remodeling.

Several collagen-derived matrikines are also known. A typical matrikine is the tripeptide GHK. It is present in the a2(1) chain of type I collagen and in several other extracellular matrix macromolecules. GHK exhibits a high affinity for copper(II) ions, with which it forms a tripeptide–copper complex (GHK–Cu). GHK–Cu is chemotactic for monocytes/macrophages and mast cells (66,67), increases nerve tissue regeneration (68), and stimulates angiogenesis in vivo (69,70). GHK–Cu enhances extracellular matrix synthesis both in vitro (71,72) and in vivo (73,74). It was also shown to be able to modulate extracellular matrix remodeling by selectively increasing the expression and activation of gelatinase A/MMP-2 (75).

Pickart first studied the effects of GHK–Cu in vivo and found that the application of GHK–Cu-containing creams to human skin increased the thickness of the epidermis and dermis, increased skin elasticity, reduced wrinkles, and resulted in the removal of skin imperfections such as blotchiness and sun damage marks (76). More recently, Abulghani et al. (77) reported GHK–Cu was more effective in stimulating new collagen development than vitamin C, retinoic acid, or melatonin. Sigler et al. (78) also reported that in eight weeks, a GHK-containing liquid foundation improved epidermal thickness, increased skin elasticity, and improved skin appearance. Leyden et al. (79) equally found such creams to reduce visible signs of photodamage and increased skin density in eight weeks on facial skin (Fig. 11). Another placebo-controlled study found that a GHK–Cu-containing eye cream reduced wrinkles and fine lines and improved eye appearance (80). Clearly, this technology is effective on aged skin. Oddos et al. (81) demonstrated that the peptide–Cu complex was essential for activity.

Lys-Thr-Thr-Lys-Ser (KTTKS) is a fragment of procollagen I, that induces extracellular matrix (ECM) synthesis. KTTKS is the minimum sequence of collagen fragments that is necessary for the potent stimulation of collagen and fibronectin production in a variety of mesenchymal cells. To aid penetration through the stratum corneum, this peptide and other peptides have been acylated with palmitic acid. Recent clinical studies on the Pal–KTTKS peptide reveal spectacular

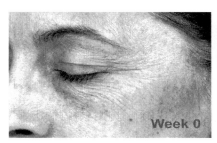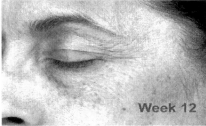

Figure 11 Photographic analysis of the effects of GHK–Cu cream versus placebo after 24 weeks. *Source*: Courtesy of Appa Y, Finkey M. Neutrogena.

results (82). One half-face study performed by Robinson et al. (83) included 92 panelists who used a basic moisturizer with (on one side of the face) and without (the other side) 3 ppm of Pal–KTTKS for three months (Fig. 12). Image analysis confirmed the wrinkle reducing efficacy of the peptide in comparison to the vehicle. Visual scoring of digital images demonstrated a significant skin improvement after only two months. In the second study, Chamberlin et al. (84) studied the effects of the same technology involving 60 volunteers, divided into two groups, one of which received a placebo cream, the other one the cream containing 5 ppm of peptide; two and four months' time points were determined, again by image analysis, photography, and assessment. Increased collagen IV and elastin levels were observed. It appears that the Pal–KTTKS peptide enhances elastin synthesis in the skin in significant amounts, whereas the placebo (vehicle) had no effect on this parameter.

A recent study also compared the effects of Pal–KTTKS in the same vehicle with retinol. A cream containing 3 ppm of lipopeptide was compared with that containing 700 ppm of retinol for two to four months on 16 volunteers. The volume of the wrinkle depth and length decreased similarly in the two actives. The scoring of the dermatologist also showed progressive improvement of the skin appearance with Pal–KTTKS and retinol. Results of echography studies show an approximately 9% increase in the skin thickness for both actives after four months, despite the fact that the effects of the peptide are more apparent after two months (85). Like GHK–Cu, Pal–KTTKS is an effective anti-aging ingredient.

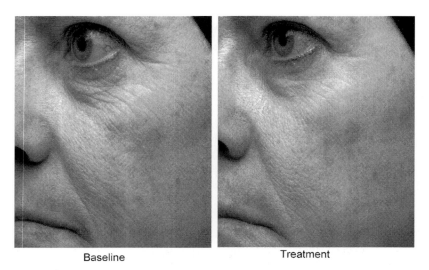

Baseline   Treatment

Figure 12 Photographic images of the effects of Pal–KTTS on photodamaged facial skin at baseline and after 12 weeks. *Source*: From Ref. 83.

Antioxidant Enzymes

As discussed earlier, exposure of human skin to solar UV irradiation is known to induce damage to cellular skin components such as lipids, proteins, and DNA, both directly and via the induction of reactive oxygen species (ROS). Oxidative stress plays a role in aging in general (86) and contributes to the photoaging of chronically exposed skin in particular (87–89). The long-term consequence of oxidative stress in the skin is determined by the balance between the amount of exposure to environmental sources of ROS, such as UV light, ozone, smoke, and air pollution, the individual's antioxidant defense capacity, and its ability to repair oxidative damage. Squalene is considered to be the first lipid at the skin surface to become oxidized upon UV exposure (90), forming squalene monohydroperoxide (sqOOH) isomers. More importantly, repeated topical application of sqOOH to hairless mice was reported to induce epidermal hyperplasia, collagen degradation, and skin wrinkling, suggesting that the formation of sqOOH at the skin surface might contribute to the induction of clinical features related to photoaging (91).

During the day, sqOOH accumulates at the surface of sun-exposed skin in summer and recovers back to baseline levels by the next morning. Topical treatment with an antioxidant mixture in the morning was shown to inhibit this increase and maintained sqOOH at baseline level during the entire day (92). The same formulation also inhibited lipid peroxidation at the skin surface upon exposure to cigarette smoke (93). To protect against oxidative damage, the skin is equipped with a network of enzymatic and nonenzymatic antioxidant defense systems (94). Even within the stratum corneum (SC) there is a redox gradient consisting of decreasing levels of vitamin E (95), vitamin C, and glutathione (96) toward the skin surface. In normal, healthy skin there is also a balance between the antioxidant enzymes superoxide dismutase (SOD) and catalase. SOD catalyzes the dismutation of the superoxide anion into O_2 and H_2O_2. Catalase neutralizes H_2O_2 to H_2O and O_2 and thereby prevents excessive H_2O_2 buildup. It has been reported that SOD and catalase activity decreases toward the skin surface, similar to the gradient described for nonenzymatic antioxidants. The endogenous protein levels of SOD and catalase were described to be lower in the SC and epidermis of photoaged skin (97). Use of topically applied SOD has been demonstrated to reduce skin-surface lipid peroxides (Fig. 13).

SPHINGOLIPIDS

Stratum Corneum Lipid Chemistry and Biophysics

The role of the stratum corneum barrier is to not only prevent excessive bodily water loss but also to be leaky enough to hydrate the outer layers of the stratum corneum in order to maintain its flexibility and to provide enough water to allow enzymes to facilitate stratum corneum maturation and desquamation. As a result, sharp phase separations between lipids should be minimized,

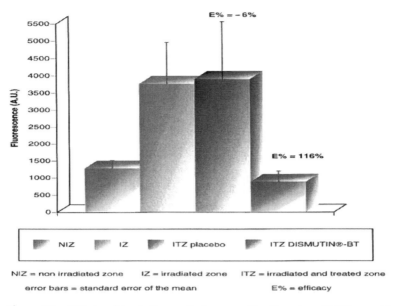

Figure 13 Effects of topically applied superoxide dismutase (SOD) on skin surface peroxides. *Source*: Courtesy of Dominik Imfeld, Pentapharm.

and from a functional point of view, the skin barrier should be as "homogeneous" as possible. As Norlen (98) has pointed out, this can only be achieved by hetero-geneity in stratum corneum lipid composition to broaden phase transition zones. Bouwstra et al. (99) have proved that ceramides are normally in a hexagonal lamellar state stabilized by cholesterol, and in the presence of long chain fatty acids the total lipid mixture is present as an orthorhombic lamellar gel state.

Ceramides constitute, on a weight basis, approximately 47%, cholesterol 24%, fatty acids 11%, and cholesterol esters 18%. Cholesterol has an important role to play in the lipid mixtures as it can increase the chain mobility of lipids in the gel state and decrease their mobility in the liquid crystalline state—a property likely to be important for barrier function during processing of glucosyl-ceramides to ceramides in the lower and upper regions of the stratum corneum. Ceramides are the most complex of stratum corneum (SC) lipids, and given this diversity, a nomenclature based on structure rather than as originally chroma-tographic migration characteristics, was proposed by Motta et al. (100). In this system, ceramides are classified in general as CER FB, where F is the type of fatty acid, and B indicates the type of base. When an ester-linked fatty acid is present, a prefix of E is used. Normal fatty acids (saturated or unsaturated), alpha hydroxy fatty acids and omega hydroxy fatty acids are N, A, O respect-ively, whereas sphingosines, phytosphingosines, and 6-hydroxysphingosines are indicated by S, P, and H, respectively (Fig. 14). Sphinganine not previously

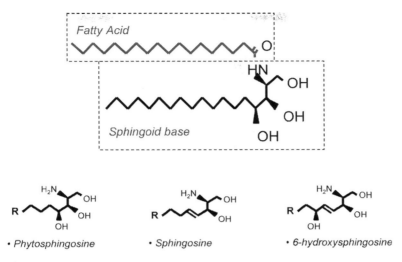

• *Phytosphingosine*   • *Sphingosine*   • *6-hydroxysphingosine*

Figure 14 Schematic of the ceramide nomenclature system.

classified is proposed to be SP in this nomenclature system. A novel long-chain ceramide containing branched-chain fatty acids is also found in vernix caseosa. Typical structures of human adult ceramides are given in Figure 15.

Lipids are also covalently attached to the corneocytes themselves and are esterified to involucrin on the corneocyte envelopes. These were originally

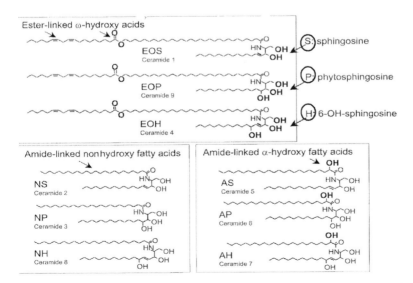

Figure 15 Typical structures of adult stratum corneum ceramides.

identified as ceramide A (sphingosine) and ceramide B (6-hydroxysphingosine) together with omega hydroxy fatty acids (101). Chopart et al. (102) recently identified covalently bound omega hydroxyl fatty acid containing sphinganine and phytosphingosine ceramides. All of these are believed to act as a template for lamellar lipid organization of the intercellular lipids. These covalently bound ceramides should now be named CER OS, CER OH, CER OSP, and CER OP. SP is proposed as a classification for sphinganine as given earlier.

All of the SC ceramides are synthesized from glucosylceramides, epidermosides, and sphingomyelin. Epidermosides are glycated precursors of omega hydroxyl-containing ceramides (103). The studies of Hamanaka et al. (104) have demonstrated that sphingomyelin provides some of CER NS and CER AS, whereas the glucosylceramides are precursors to ceramides, and epidermosides are precursors to the covalently bound ceramides together with CER EOS, CER EOH, and possibly CER EOP.

Examination of stratum corneum by transmission electron microscopy has revealed that the number of lipid lamellae between corneocytes varies, but in most regions there are multiples of three lamellae with a broad–narrow–broad spacing. When more lamellae are present, it is believed that CER EOS, EOH, and EOP play an essential role in formation of the additional lamellar arrangements. The repeated distances were found to be of 13 nm in dimension, composed of two units measuring approximately 5 nm each, and one unit measuring approximately 3 nm in thickness. These repeat lamellar patterns were also observed by X-ray diffraction studies and were named the long periodicity (LPP) and short periodicity (SPP) phases respectively.

Bouwstra et al. (99) recently proposed a new sandwich model consisting of two broad lipid layers with a crystalline structure separated by a narrow central lipid layer with fluid domains. Cholesterol and ceramides are important for the formation of the lamellar phase, whereas fatty acids play a greater role in the lateral packing of the lipids. Cholesterol is proposed to be located with the fatty acid tail of CER EOS in the fluid phase.

Lipids in vivo appear to exist as a balance between a solid crystalline state (orthorhombic packing) and gel (hexagonal packing) or liquid crystalline states. The orthorhombically packed lipids are the most tightly packed conformation and have the better barrier properties, and as shown by electron diffraction studies, these physical states change during migration of the corneocytes from the lower layers of the stratum corneum to the outer layers, where a greater proportion of hexagonally packed lipid conformations are observed (105). This is consistent with a weakening of the barrier toward the outer layers of the stratum corneum. It is believed that short-chain fatty acids from sebum contribute to the crystalline to gel transition in the upper stratum corneum layers (106).

Fatty acids also induce the formation of the short periodicity phase. pH has no effect on the lamellar ordering or lateral packing states of cholesterol and ceramide mixtures. However, when fatty acids are present, the LPP is observed at pH 7.4, whereas both the LPP and SPP are observed at pH 5 probably due to ionization of the fatty acids. This indicates that in addition to the lateral packing states, changes in the lamellar ordering might also occur toward the surface of the stratum corneum. In fact, the complexity of ordering is even further highlighted by the loss of the LPP at full hydration of the corneum (60% water) (107–109). However, Wiechers et al. (110) have reported that hydration of the stratum corneum does not affect the orthorhombic to hexagonal phase crystallization temperature.

In the absence of CER EOS, mostly hexagonal phases are also observed for total lipid mixtures. Nevertheless, the inclusion of CER EOS induces the formation of the LPP. Moreover, the importance of ceramide one or CER EOS in facilitating the formation of the long 13.4 nm LPP has been further elaborated by understanding the influence of the type of fatty acid esterified to the omega hydroxyl fatty acid (111). As a consequence, the LPP is seen mainly with linoleate-containing CER EOS, less with oleate-containing CER EOS, and is absent if only stearate-containing CER EOS is present in the lipid mixtures. These studies indicate that for formation of the LPP, a certain fraction of the lipids has to form a liquid phase. If the liquid phase is too high as with the oleate-containing CER EOS or too low as with stearate-containing CER EOS, the levels of the SPP increase at the expense of the LPP. It is important to remember that the fatty acid composition of CER EOS in vivo is highly complex but contains a large proportion of linoleic acid.

Changes to the composition of the SC lipids could, therefore, dramatically influence the condition of the skin. On the surface of the stratum corneum, cholesterol sulphate and CER EOS are hydrolyzed, leading to increased concentrations of short chain length fatty acids and decreased levels of pH and water. As a result, increased crystallization of cholesterol with simultaneous decrease in ceramide levels leading to perturbations to the lamellar ordering can be observed. In this respect, using electron microscopy of tape strippings from the outer layers of normal healthy skin, Rawlings et al. (112) reported complete loss of lamellar ordering in the outer layers of the stratum corneum.

The Management of Dry Skin

From the current understanding of the compositional changes in dry skin, five aspects of stratum corneum lipid biochemistry need to be corrected:

1. The lowered levels of lipids generally.
2. The reduced levels of phytosphingosine-containing ceramides.
3. The ceramide one linoleate (CEOS) insufficiency.
4. The lowered levels of covalently bound ceramides.
5. The chain length of the acyl groups in the ceramide sphingoid bases and free fatty acids.

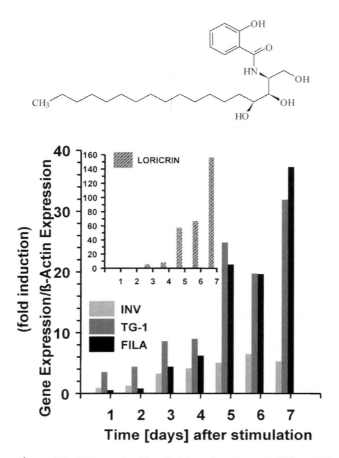

Figure 16 Effects of sphingolipids on keratinocyte differentiation. *Source*: Courtesy of Mike Farwick, Degussa.

Overall, however, the lipid lamellar architecture in the outer layers of the stratum corneum needs to be normalized in dry flaky skin conditions. Evidence also indicates that a reduction in long chain fatty acids also occurs in sodium lauryl sulphate (SLS)-induced dry skin. As these lipids are important for inducing an orthorhombic lateral packing state, these will also need to be supplied to the skin to more effectively correct barrier function. Equally, reduction in the levels of ceramides and especially linoleate-containing CER EOS can be found in aged skin (113).

The phytosphingosine ceramides are made through a combination of fermentation and chemistry. Tetracecetylphytosphingosine (TAPS) is produced by fermentation in the pichia ciferri yeast. After being recovered, the

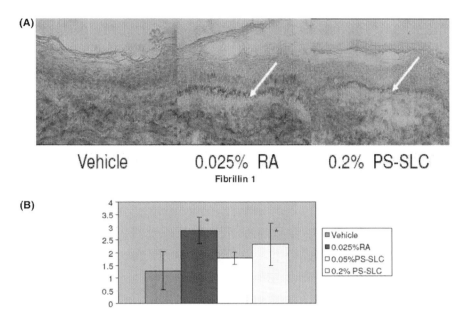

Figure 17 Fibrillin-1 immunohistochemistry: Application of all-*trans* retinoic acid produced deposition of fibrillin-1 proximal to the DEJ in volunteers. Application of 0.2% salicyoyl-phytosphingosine (PS-SLC) resulted in significantly increased fibrillin-1 deposition of 182% compared to the vehicle treated. (**A**) Typical images. The reappearance of the candelabra-type fibrillin fibers extending down from the DEJ can be seen following treatment with retinoic acid and salicyolyl-phytosphingosine (*white arrows*). (**B**) Histogram of results. *Source*: From Ref. 121.

phytosphingosine backbone is converted to different types of ceramides by chemically coupling different fatty acids to the phytosphingosine (114).

Several clinical studies evaluating the effects of ceramides have been conducted recently. However, it is important to remember that to derive the full benefits of ceramide technology, formulation into emulsions where other emollients dominant the formulation will be difficult to discern unless the ceramides are at a high enough concentration. Kucharekova et al. (115) found that the CER NP–containing cream significantly reduced TEWL, erythema, and epidermal proliferation compared with placebo cream. However, further improvements in efficacy were observed with complete lipid mixtures. De Paepe et al. (116) have demonstrated improvements in barrier functionality and stratum corneum hydration from a lipid mixture of CER NP (0.2%), CER AS (0.1%), and CER UP (0.2%) together with cholesterol (0.25%), linoleic acid (0.25%), and phytosphingosine (0.5%) compared with placebo lotions and a lotion containing only CER NP (0.6%) and CER UP (0.4%). Berardesca et al. (117) have also established that balanced lipid mixtures containing CER NP are effective in improving the

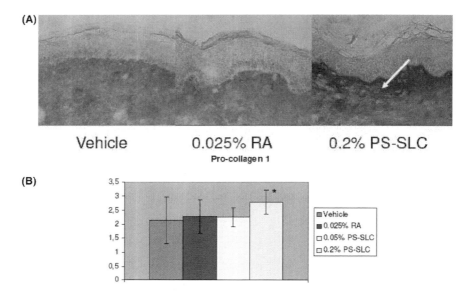

Figure 18 Pro-collagen I immunohistochemistry: Application of all-*trans* retinoic acid had little effect on the deposition of pro-collagen I proximal to the DEJ following 4-day occluded application (in agreement with previous short term studies but it is known to increase levels in the longer term). However, 0.2% salicyoyl-phytosphingosine (PS-SLC) significantly increased pro-collagen I to 130% of the level of the vehicle treated area content in the papillary dermis. Increased levels of pro-collagen-1 can be observed especially after treatment with salicyloyl-phytosphingosine (increased gray/black staining in the dermis *white arrows*). (**A**) Typical images. (**B**) Histogram of results. *Source*: From Ref. 121.

barrier properties and clinical condition of skin in subjects with contact dermatitis. Equally convincing are the studies of Chamlin et al. (118), showing that a ceramide dominant barrier repair lipid cream alleviates childhood atopic dermatitis. Over the six week treatment period, TEWL values decreased by 50%, and the number of D-squama tape-strippings required to break the barrier increased from approximately 12 to 22 strippings indicating a stronger stratum corneum barrier function.

The correct chirality is important for the optimal incorporation of ceramides in skin. Racaemic mixtures are incapable of producing the correct stratum corneum lamellar structure (119).

TAPS itself has also been shown to stimulate epidermal ceramide biosynthesis on its own and improve barrier function, especially when combined with juniperic acid and linoleic acid (120). Most recently Salicyloly-phytosphingosine has also been developed, and on analyzing its effects on keratinocyte gene expression, significant upregulation of differentiation marker genes has been observed (filaggrin, involucrin, loricrin, and transglutaminase; Fig. 16). Most recently this ingredient has been investigated in antiaging studies and it has been reported to increase fibrillin-1 and procollagen-1 levels (Fig 17 and 18) whereas decreased MMP's are reported (121).

CONCLUSIONS

Clearly, biotechnology has a role to play in the identification of technology for skin care. This is implicit in the identification of novel biological mechanisms and targets, such as the RAR/RXR and PPAR/RXR. Fermentation routes have developed to produce highly potent PPAR ligands that can inhibit skin lightening and potentially reverse the signs of age spots. Other PPAR ligands have also be shown to possess anti-aging properties like retinoids. Matrikines are useful peptide anti-aging ingredients. Antioxidant enzymes can reduce the levels of lipid peroxides that are thought to be involved in the aging process, and sphingolipids such as ceramides can repair the barrier and reverse some of the epidermal changes associated with the aging process. The future looks bright for the use of biotechnology in the development of anti-aging ingredients.

REFERENCES

1. Leyden JJ. Clinical features of ageing skin. Br J Dermatol 1990; 122 (suppl 33):1–3.
2. Ortonne JP, Marks R. Photodamaged Skin. London: Martin Dunitz Ltd, 1999: 1–149.
3. Chung JH. Photoaging in Asians. Photodermatol Photoimmunol Photomed 2003; 19(3):109–121.
4. Lock-Andersen J et al. Epidermal thickness, skin pigmentation and constitutive photosensitivity. Photoimmunol Photopigmentation & Constitutive Photosensitivity 1997; 13:153–158.
5. Sams WM et al. Mathematical morphological analysis of the aortic medial tissue. Anal Quant Cytol Histol 1993; 15:93–100.
6. Gilhar A et al. Aging of human epidermis, the role of apoptosis, fas and telomerase. Br J Dermatol 2004; 150:56–63.
7. Rawlings AV. Trends in stratum corneum research and the management of dry skin conditions. Int J Cosmet Sci 2003; 25:63–95.
8. Elias PM, Ghadially R. The aged permeability barrier: a basis for functional abnormalities. Clin Geriatr Med 2002; 18:103–120.
9. Gilchrest BA. Skin aging and photoaging: an overview. J Am Acad Dermatol 1989; 21: 610–613.
10. Anderson WK, Labadie R, Bhawan J. Histopathology of solar lentigines of the face: a quantitative study. J Am Acad Dermaol 1997; 36:444–447.
11. Fisher GJ, Kang S, Varani J, Bata-Csorgo Z, Wan Y, Datta S, Voorhees JJ. Mechanisms of photoaging and chronological skin aging. Arch Dermatol 2002; 138:1462–1470.
12. Welter JF, Eckert RL. Differential expression of the fos and jun family members c-fos, fosB, Fra-1, Fra-2, c-jun, junB and junD during human epidermal keratinocyte differentiation. Oncogene 1995; 11:2681–2687.

13. Manning MA, Davis RJ. Targeting JNK for therapeutic benefit: from junk to gold. Nature Rev 2003; 2:554–565.
14. Zingarelli B, Sheehan M, Wong HR. Nuclear factor-κB as a therapeutic target in critical care medicine. Crit Care Med 2003; 31.
15. Raza SL, Cornelius LA. Matrix metalloproteinases: pro- and anti-angiogenic activities. J Invest Dermatol Symp Proceed 2000; 5:47–54.
16. Chung JH, Seo Y, Choi HR, Lee MK, Youn CS, Rhie G, Cho KH, Kim KH, Park KC, Eun HC. Modulation of skin collagen metabolism in aged and photoaged human skin in vivo. J Invest Dermatol 2001; 117:1218–1224.
17. Quan T, He T, Kang S, Voorhees JJ, Fisher GJ. Ultraviolet irradiation alters transforming growth factor beta/smad pathway in human skin. J Invest Dermatol 2002; 119:499–506.
18. Quan T, He T, Voorhees JJ, Fisher GJ. Ultraviolet irradiation blocks cellular responses to transforming growth factor-beta by down-regulating its type-II receptor and inducing smad7. J Biol Chem 2001; 276(28):26349–26356.
19. Chung JH, Seo Y, Choi HR, Lee MK, Youn CS, Rhie G, Cho KH, Kim KH, Park KC, Eun HC. Modulation of skin collagen metabolism in aged and photoaged human skin in vivo. J Invest Dermatol 2001; 117:1218–1224.
20. Varani J, Perone P, Fligiel SEG, Fisher GJ, Voorhees JJ. Inhibition of type I procollagen production in photodamage: correlation between presence of high molecular weight collagen fragments and reduced procollagen synthesis. J Invest Dermatol 2002; 119:122–129.
21. El-Domyati M, Attia S, Saleh F, Brown D, Birk E, Gasparro F, Ahmad H, Uitto J. Intrinsic aging vs photoaging: a comparative histopathological, immunohistochemical, and ultrastructural study of skin. Exp Dermatol 2002; 11:398–405.
22. Seo JY, Lee S, Youn CS, Choi HR, Rhie G, Cho KH, Kim KH, Park HC, Eun C, Chung JH. Ultraviolet radiation increases tropoelastin mRNA expression in the epidermis of human skin in vivo. J Invest Dermatol 2001; 116:915–919.
23. Watson REB, Griffiths CEM, Craven NM, Shuttleworth CA, Kielty M. Fibrillin-rich microfibrils and reduced in photoaged skin. Distribution at the dermal-epidermal junction. J Invest Dermatol 1999; 112:782–787.
24. Watson REB, Craven NM, Kang S, Jones CJP, Kielty M, Griffiths CEM. A short-term screening protocol, using fibrillin-1 as a reporter molecule, for photoaging repair agents. J Invest Dermatol 2001; 116:672–678.
25. Tsukahara K, Takema Y, Moriwaki S, Tsuji N, Suzuki Y, Fujimura T, Imokawa G. Selective inhibition of skin fibroblast elastase elicits a concentration-dependent prevention of ultraviolet B-induced wrinkle formation. J Invest Dermatol 2001; 117:671–677.
26. Saarialho-Kere U, Kerkela E, Jeskanen L, Hasan T, Pierce R, Starcher B, Raudasoja R, Ranki A, Oikarinen A, Vaalamo M. Accumulation of matrilysin (MMP-7) and macrophage metalloelastase (MMP-12) in actinic damage. J Invest Dermatol 1999; 113:644–672.
27. Chung JH, Seo JY, Lee MK, Eun C, Le H, Kang S, Fisher J, Voorhees JJ. Ultraviolet modulation of human macrophage metalloelastase in human skin in vivo. J Invest Dermatol 2002; 119:507–512.
28. Cavarra E, Fimiani M, Lungarella G, Andreassi L, De SM, Mazzatenta C, Ciccoli L. UVA light stimulates the production of cathepsin G and elastase-like enzymes by

dermal fibroblasts: a possible contribution to the remodeling of elastotic areas in sun-damaged skin. Biol Chem 2002; 383(1):199–206.

29. Isnard N, Peterszegi G, Robert AM, Robert L. Regulation of elastase-type endopeptidase activity, MMP-2 and MMP-9 expression and activation in human dermal fibroblasts by fucose and a fucose-rich polysaccharide. Biomed Pharmacother 2002; 56:258–264.

30. Isnard N, Legeais JM, Renard G, Robert L. Effect of hyaluronan on MMP expression and activation. Cell Biol Int 2001; 25(8):735–739.

31. Varlet B, Chaudagne C, Saunois A, Barre P, Sauvage C, Berthouloux B, Meybeck, A, Dumas M, Bonte F. Age-related functional and structural changes in human dermo-epidermal junction components. J Invest Dermatol Symp Proceed 1998; 3: 172–179.

32. Amano S, Akutsu N, Matsunaga Y, Kadoya K, Nishiyama T, Champliaud MF, Burgeson RE, Adachi E. Importance of balance between extracellular matrix synthesis and degradation in basement membrane formation. Exp Cell Res 2001; 271:249–262.

33. Chung J, Yano K, Lee MK, Youn CS, Seo JY, Kim, Cho H, Eun HC, Detmar M. Differential effects of photoaging vs intrinsic aging on the vascularization of human skin. Arch Dermatol 2002; 138(11):1437–1442.

34. Huzaira M, Rius F, Rajadhyaksha M, Anderson RR, Gonzalez S. Topographical variations in normal skin as viewed by in vivo reflectance confocal microscopy. J Invest Dermatol 2001; 116:846–852.

35. Bosset S, Bonnet-Duquennoy M, Barre P, Chalon A, Kurfurst R, Bonte F, Schnebert S, Le Varlet B, Nicolas JF. Photoageing shows histological features of chronic skin inflammation without clinical and molecular abnormalities. Br J Dermatol 2003; 149:826–835.

36. Schwarz T. Photoimmunosuppression. Photodermatol Photoimmunol Photomed 2002; 18:141–145.

37. Green MR, Parish WE, Eastwood M, Wares J, Simon M, Siegel DM. The human periorbital wrinkle: immunohistology & computer modelling suggest key roles for directional collagen fibers and mechanical force in wrinkle maintenance. 22nd IFSCC Congress 2002, Edinburgh, Scotland; 1:1–6.

38. Contet-Audonneau JL, Jeanmaire C, Pauly G. A histological study of human wrinkle structures: comparison between sun-exposed area's of the face with or without wrinkles and sunprotected areas. Brit J Dermatol 1999; 140:1038–1047.

39. Urschitz J, Iobst S, Urban Z, Granda C, Souza KA, Lupp C, Schilling K, Scott I, Csiszar K, Boyd CD. A serial analysis of gene expression in sun-damaged human skin. J Invest Dermatol 2002; 119(1):3–13.

40. Griffiths CEM. Retinoids & vitamin D analogues: action on nuclear transcription. Hosp Med 1998; 59:12–16.

41. Wahli W. Peroxisome proliferator activated receptors: from metabolic control to epidermal wound healing. Swiss Med Wkly 2002; 132:83–91.

42. Varani J et al. Vitamin A antagonizes decreased cell growth and elevated collagen-degrading matrix metalloproteinases and stimulates collagen accumulation in naturally aged human skin. J Invest Dermatol 2000; 114:480–486.

43. Scott IR. Real performance in cosmetic antiaging products. 22nd IFSCC congress 2002, Edinburgh, Scotland; Volume 1.

44. Kurlandsky SB. Auto-regulation of retinoic acid biosynthesis through regulation of retinol esterfication in human keratinocytes. J Biol Chem 1996; 271:15, 346–15,352.

45. Granger S, Rawlings AV, Scott IR. Compositions containing retinol acyl transferase inhibitors-fatty acid amides. EP96302673 & US5599548, European & United States patents.

46. Iobst S, Feinberg C, Arce C, Carson R, Barratt M, Cardenas A, Matzke M, Santhanam U, Granger S, Rawlings AV, et al. Enhanced effects of vitamin A via manipulation of retinoid metabolism. 22nd IFSCC Congress Poster, 2002, Edinburgh, Scotland.

47. Wahli W. Peroxisome proliferator activated receptors: from metabolic control to epidermal wound healing. Swiss Med Wkly 2002; 132:83–91.

48. Rastinejad F. Retinoid X receptor and its partners in the nuclear receptor family. Curr Opin Struct Biol 2001; 11:33–38.

49. Rivier M et al. PPAR alpha enhances lipid metabolism in a skin equivalent model. J Invest Dermatol 2000; 114:681–687.

50. Westergaard M et al. Modulation of keratinocyte gene expression and differentiation by PPAR selective ligands & tetradecylthioacetic acid. J Invest Dermatol 2001; 116: 702–712.

51. Watkinson A, Lee RS, Paterson SE, Marti VJ, Rawlings AV, Ginger RS, Donovan M, Green MR, Mayes AE. PPAR alpha activators: petroselinic acid as a novel skin benefit agent for antiperspirants. 22nd IFSCC Congress Proceedings Oral Papers. Podium 11, 2002, Edinburgh, Scotland.

52. European & United states patents: US6423325, US6403064, US6287553, US6042841, WO0108650, WO0108652, WO0108649.

53. Mayes AE, Kealaher P, Watson LP, Donovan M, Green MR, Ginger RS, Barrett KE, Alaluf S, Rawlings AV, Brown M, et al. Antiaging and skin condition benefits from PPAR alpha activating molecules. 22nd IFSCC Congress Proceedings Poster, 2002, Edinburgh, Scotland.

54. Mossner R et al. Agonists of PPAR gamma inhibit cell growth in malignant melanoma. J Invest Dermatol 2002; 119:576–582.

55. Ando H et al. Linoleic and alpha linolenic acid lightens UV induced hyperpigmentation of the skin. Arch Dermatol Res 1998; 290: 375–381.

56. Wiechers JW, Groenhof FJ, Wortel VAL, Miller RM, Hindle NA, Drewitt-Barlow. Cosmet & Toilet 2002; 117:55–65.

57. Wiechers JW, Rawlings AV, Garcia C, Chesne C, Balaguer P, Nicolas JC, Corre S, Galibert MD. A possible new mechanism of action for skin whitening agents: Binding to the peroxisomal proliferator activated receptor. Int J Cosmetic Sci 2005; 27:123–132.

58. Maquart FX, Simeon A, Pasco S, Monboisse JC. Regulation de l' activite cellulaire par la matrice extracellulaire: le concept de matrikines. J Soc Biol 1999; 193:423–428.

59. Simeon A, Monier F, Emonard H, et al. Fibroblast-cytokineextracellular matrix interactions in wound repair. Curr Top Pathol 1999; 93:95–101.

60. Jacob MP, Hornebeck W. Isolation and characterization of insoluble and kappa-elastins. Front Matrix Biol 1985; 10:92–129.

61. Robert L, Tixier IM, Berenholc S, Levy O, Hornebeck W. Inhibition of elastase activity in human gingival extracts by elastin peptides. Pathol Biol (Paris) 1992; 40:879–882.
62. Kamoun A, Landeau IM, Godeau G, et al. Growth stimulation of human skin fibroblasts by elastin-derived peptides. Cell Adhes Commun 1995; 3:273–281.
63. Wachi H, Seyama Y, Yamashita S, et al. Stimulation of cell proliferation and auto-regulation of elastin expression by elastin peptide VPGVG in cultured chick vascular smooth muscle cells. FEBS Lett 1995; 368:215–219.
64. Tajima S, Wachi H, Seyama Y. Tropoelastin-derived degradation products down-regulate elastin expression in vascular smooth muscle cell in culture. Connect Tissue 1996; 28:231–235.
65. Brassart B, Randoux A, Hornebeck W, Emonard H. Regulation of matrix metallo-proteinase-2 (gelatinase A. MMP-2) membrane-type matrix metalloproteinase-I (MTI-MMP) and tissue inhibitor of metalloproteinases-2 (TIMP-2) expression in human HT-1080 fibrosarcoma cell line by elastin-derived peptides. Clin Exp Metast 1998; 16:489–500.
66. Brassart B, Fuchs P, Huet E, et al. Conformational dependence of collagenase (matrix metalloproteinase-1) up-regulation by elastin peptides in cultured fibroblasts. J Biol Chem 2001; 276:5222–5227.
67. Poole TJ, Zetter BR. Stimulation of rat peritoneal mast cells migration by tumor-derived peptides. Cancer Res 1983; 43:5857–5861.
68. Zetter BR, Rasmussen N, Brown L. An in vivo assay for chemoattractant activity. Lab Invest 1985; 53:362–368.
69. Grosse G, Lindner G. Experimental influence of phannacological agents on the regeneration of the nervous tissue in vitro. Folia Morphol (Praha) 1980; 28:345–347.
70. Lane TF, Iruela-Arispe ML, Johnson RS, Sage HE. SPARC is a source of copper-binding peptides that stimulate angiogenesis. J Cell Biol 1994; 125:929–943.
71. Raju KS, Alessandri G, Ziche M, Gullino PM. Ceruloplasmin, copper ions, and angiogenesis. J Natl Cancer Inst 1982; 69:1183–1188.
72. Maquart FX, Pickart L, Laurent M, et al. Stimulation of collagen synthesis in fibroblast cultures by the tripeptide-copper complex glycyl-L-histidyl-L-Iysine-Cu2+. FEBS Lett 1988; 238:343–346.
73. Wegrowski J, Maquart FX, Borel JP. Stimulation of sulphated glycosaminoglycan synthesis by the tripeptide–copper complex glycyl-L-histidyl-L-Iysine-Cu2+. Life Sci 1992; 51:1049–1056.
74. Maquart FX, Bellon G, Chaqour B, et al. In vivo stimulation of connective tissue accumulation by the tripeptide-copper complex glycyl-L-histidyl-L-Iysine-Cu2+. in rat experimental wounds. J Clin Invest 1993; 92:2368–2376.
75. Simeon A, Wegrowski Y, Bontemps Y, Maquart FX. Expression of glycosaminoglycans and small proteoglycans in wounds: modulation by the tripeptide-copper complex glycyl-L-histidyl-L-lysine-Cu. J Invest Dermatol 2000; 115:962–968.
76. Pickart L. Copperceuticals & the skin. Cosmet & Toilet 2003; 118:24–28.
77. Abulghani S, Morales-Tapia S, Solodkina, Robertson, Gottlieb. J Invest Dermatol 1998; 110:686.
78. Sigler ML, Stephens TJ, Barkovic S, Finkey MB, Barkovic S, Appa Y. A clinical evaluation of a copper-peptide-containing liquid foundation and cream concealer

designed for improving skin condition. Abstract P69. American Academy of Dermatology (AAD).

79. Leyden JJ, Grove G, Stephens TJ, Finkey MB, Barkovic S, Appa Y. Skin benefits of copper peptide containing facial cream. Abstract P67. AAD meeting 2002. American Academy of Dermatology (AAD).

80. Leyden JJ, Grove G, Stephens TJ, Finkey MB, Barkovic S, Appa Y. Skin benefits of copper peptide containing eyecreams. Abstract P68. AAD meeting 2002. American Academy of Dermatology (AAD).

81. Oddos T, Jurmeau-Lafond A, Ries G. Requirement of copper tripeptide GHK complex formation for collagen synthesis activity in normal human fibroblasts. Abstract P66. AAD meeting 2002. American Academy of Dermatology (AAD).

82. Lintner K, Peschard O. Biologically active peptides: from a laboratory bench curiosity to a functional skin care product. Int J Cosmet Sci 2000; 22:207–218.

83. Robinson LR, Fitzgerald NC, Doughty DG, Dawes NC, Berge CA, Bissett DL. Palmitoyl-pentapeptide offers improvement in human photoaged facial skin. Poster Proc 20th World Congress Of Dermatology 2002.

84. Mas-Chamberlain C, Lintner K, Basset L, Adoute H, Revuz J. Relevance of antiwrinkle treatment with a peptide: 4 months clinical double blind study vs. excipient. Poster Proc 20th World Congress Of Dermatology 2002.

85. Mas-Chamberlain C, Lintner K. Penta-peptide facilitates matrix regeneration in photoaged skin. Poster Proc 20th World Congress Of Dermatology 2002.

86. Golden TR, Hinerfeld DA, Melov S. Oxidative stress & aging: beyond correlation. Aging Cell 2002; 1:117–123.

87. Giacomoni PU, Declercq L, Hellemans L, Maes D. Aging of human skin: review of a mechanistic model and first experimental data. IUBMB Life 2000; 49:259–263.

88. Nishigori C, Hattori Y, Arima Y, Miyachi Y. Photoaging & oxidative stress. Exp Dermatol 2003; 12 (suppl 2):18–21.

89. Ohido M, Yoshino K, Matsuo I. Lipid peroxide of human skin. Curr Probl Dermatol 1980; 10:269–278.

90. Ekanayake Mudiyanselage S, Hamburger M, Elsner P, Thiele JJ. UV A induces generation of squalene monoperoxide isomers in human sebum and skin surface lipids in vitro and in vivo. J Invest Dermatol 2003; 120:915–922.

91. Chiba K, Kawakami K, Sone T, Onoue M. Characteristics of skin wrinkling and dermal changes induced by repeated application od squalene monohydroperoxide to hairless mouse skin. Appl Skin Physiol 2000; 16:242–251.

92. Maes D, Mammone T, McKeever MA. Non invasive techniques for measuring oxidation products on the surface of human skin. Methods Enzymol 2000; 319:612–622.

93. Pelle E, Miranada EP, Fthenakis C. Cigarette smoke-induced lipid peroxidation in human skin & its inhibition by topically applied antioxidants. Skin Pharmacol Appl Skin Physiol 2001; 15:63–68.

94. Thiele JJ, Schoeter C, Hsieh SN, Podda M, Packer L. The antioxidant network of the stratum corneum. Oxidants & antioxidants in cutaneous biology 2001; 29:26–42.

95. Thiele JJ, Traber MG, Packer L. Depletion of human stratum corneum vitamin E: an early and sensitive in vivo marker of UV induced photo-oxidation. J Invest Dermatol 1988; 110:756–761.

96. Weber SU, Thiele JJ, Cross CE, Packer L. Vitamin C, uric acid and glutathione gradients in murine stratum corneum and their susceptibility to ozone exposure. J Invest Dermatol 1999; 113:1128–1132.

97. Lu CY, Lee HC, Fahn HJ, Wei YH. Oxidative damage elicited by imbalance of free radical scavenging enzymes is associated with large scale mtDNA deletions in aging human skin. Mutant Res 1999; 423:11–21.

98. Norlen. Skin barrier structure and function: The single gel phase model. J Invest. Dermatol 2001; 117:830–836.

99. Bouwstra J, Pilgram G, Gooris G, Koerten H, Ponec M. New aspects of the skin barrier organization. Skin Pharm Appl Skin Physiol 2001; 14:52–62.

100. Motta SM, Monti M, Sesana S, et al. Ceramide composition of psoriatic scale. Biochim Biophys Acta 1993; 1182:147–151.

101. Downing DT, Stewart ME. Epidermal composition. In: Loden M, Maibach HI, eds. Dry Skin and Moisturizers Chemistry and Function. 2000:13–26.

102. Chopart M, Castiel-Higounenc I, Arbey E, Schmidt R. A new type of covalently bound ceramide in human epithelium. Stratum corneum III 2001, poster. Stratum Corneum III, Basel, Switzerland.

103. Hamanaka S, Asagami C, Suzuki M, Inagaki F, Suzuki A. Stucture determination of glucosyl beta1-n-{omega-O-Linoleoyl}-acylsphingosines of human epidermis. J Biochem 1989; 105:684–690.

104. Hamanaka S, Hara M, Nishio H, Otsuka F, Suzuki A, Uchida Y. Human epidermal glucosylceramides are major precursors of stratum corneum ceramides. J Invest Dermatol 2002; 119:416–423.

105. Pilgram GSK, Engelsma-van Pelt AM, Bouwstra JA, Koerten HK. Electron diffraction provides new information on human stratum corneum lipid organisation studied in relation to depth and temperature. J Invest Dermatol 1999; 113: 403–409.

106. Brancaleon L, Bamberg MP, Sakamaki T, Kollias N. Attenuated total reflection-fourier transform infrared spectroscopy as a possible method to investigate biophysical parameters of stratum corneum in vivo. J Invest Dermatol 2001; 116: 380–386.

107. Bouwstra JA, Gooris GS, Dubbelaar FR, Ponec M. Phase behaviour of lipid mixtures based on human ceramides: coexistence of crystalline and liquid phases. J Lipid Res 2001; 42:759–1770.

108. Bouwstra J, Gooris GS, Cheng K, et al. Phase behaviour of isolated skin lipids. J Lipid Res 1996; 37:999–1011.

109. Bouwstra JA, Gooris GS, Salomons E, et al. Structure of human stratum corneum as a function of temperature and hydration. Int J Pharm 1992; 8:205–216.

110. Weichers JW, Bouwstra JA, Burgess A, et al. A multifaceted approach to elucidating skin moisturization & elasticity. 22nd IFSCC Congress, Edinburgh 2002; P133.

111. Bouwstra J, Gooris GS, Dubbelaar FR, Ponec M. Phase behaviour of stratum corneum lipid mixtures based on human ceramides: The role of natural and synthetic ceramide 1. J Invest Dermatol 2002; 118:606–617.

112. Rawlings AV, Watkinson A, Rogers J, et al. Abnormalities in stratum corneum structure lipid composition and desmosome degradation in soap-induced winter xerosis. J Soc Cosmet Chem 1994; 45:203–220.

113. Rogers J, Harding C, Mayo A, Banks J, Rawlings A. Stratum corneum lipids: the effect of ageing and the seasons. Arch Dermatol Res 1996 Nov; 288(12):765–770.

114. Lambers JWJ, Barendse RCM, Overwater AJ, van der Berg H, Keuig W. Yeast-derived ceramides. Proceedings Biocosmetics—Skin Aging. 1993; II:348–353.

115. Kucharekova M, Schalkwijk J, Van De Kerkhof PC, Van De Valk PG. Effect of a lipid-rich emollient. Contact Dermatitis 2002; 46:331–338.

116. De Paepe K, Roseeuw D, Rogiers V. Repair of acetone- and sodium lauryl sulphate-damaged human skin barrier function using topically applied emulsions containing barrier lipids. JEADV 2002; 16:587–594.

117. Berardesca E, Barbareschi M, Veraldi S, Pimpinelli N. Evaluation of efficacy of a skin lipid mixture in patients with irritant contact dermatitis, allergic contact dermatitis or atopic dermatitis: a multicenter study. Contact Dermatitis 2001; 45:280–285.

118. Chamlin SL, Kao J, Frieden IJ, Sheu MY, Fowler AJ, Fluhr JW, Williams ML, Elias PM. Ceramide-dominant barrier repair lipids alleviate childhood atopic dermatitis: changes in barrier function provide a sensitive indicator of disease activity. J Am Aca Dermatol 2002; 47:198–208.

119. Wollenberger U, Korevaar K, Rawlings AV, Schick. Application of a skin-identical lipid concentrate for enhanced skin moisturization and protection. SOFW J 2004; 130:12–18.

120. Davies A, Verdejo P, Feinberg C, Rawlings AV. Increased stratum corneum ceramide levels and improved barrier function following topical treatment with tetraacetylphytosphingosine. Annual Meeting Of Society For Investigative Dermatology, Washington, USA. J Invest Dermatol 1996; 106(abstract 678):918.

121. Farwick M, Watson REB, Rawlings AV, Lersch P, Griffiths CEM. Salicyoyl-phytosphingosine: A novel agent for the repair of photodamaged skin. In Press, 2006.

8

Biotechnology in Skin Care (IV): Skin Pigmentation, Lightening, and Darkening

Miri Seiberg

*Skin Research Center, Johnson & Johnson CPPW,
Skillman, New Jersey, U.S.A.*

SKIN COLOR, LIGHTENING, AND DARKENING

Skin color has always been of concern to human beings, and both men and women often desire to alter skin color for medical or cosmetic reasons. In certain cultures, general body whitening and "porcelain white" skin are desired, whereas in certain geographic areas of the world, it is the "tanned look" that is preferred. Interestingly, the need to remove hyperpigmentation and to reduce the visibility of age spots, freckles, or uneven skin color is universal, resulting in a worldwide need for safe and effective pigment-modulating agents. Concerns of changes in skin color are also frequently raised for medical reasons. Pigmentary disorders can be inherited (e.g., vitiligo, Waardenburg syndrome), acquired (e.g., post-inflammatory pityriasis alba, idiophatic guttate hypomelanosis, melasma), medication related (minocycline, bleomycin, busulfan, zidovudine), or transmitted through infection (e.g., tinea versicolor), (reviewed in 1). Many methods have been proposed to alter skin color. For example, tyrosinase inhibitors, hydroquinones, retinoids, and melanocyte cytotoxic agents are all used for depigmentation. However, the currently available topical agents that are based on these mechanisms are sometimes disappointing, and there is a need for more effective, safer, and less irritating depigmenting technologies (reviewed in 2). Skin darkening could be obtained through natural UV exposure or artificial tanning devices. These, however, result in accelerated skin aging and in increased incidence of skin cancer (e.g., 3–5). Alternative methods for "sunless tanning" have evolved, such as the use of dihydroxyacetone or topical synthetic melanins (e.g., reviewed in 6). Unfortunately, such products might produce a "nonnatural" skin color, they only minimally protect the user from UV irradiation (7), and they are ineffective when skin hydration is high (8). Thus, products are needed that could enhance the natural pigment content of the skin, leading to a desired skin color and to enhanced photoprotection, without the need of UV exposure.

Pigment Production and Distribution

During the development process, melanoblasts migrate from the embryonal neural crest into the skin. Within the epidermis, the melanoblasts mature into melanocytes, the pigment producing cells (Fig. 1A), which produce melanin in secretory granules called melanosomes. The melanocytes reside within the epidermal–melanin unit, a functional unit that produces and distributes melanin and is composed of one melanocyte and approximately 36 neighboring keratinocytes (reviewed in 9,10). Melanogenesis occurs within the melanosome, and the produced pigment is later distributed to keratinocytes by the melanocyte dendrites (Fig. 1A). Melanosomes containing newly synthesized pigment molecules translocate from their site of origin in the perinuclear cytoplasm toward the melanocyte dendrite tips (Fig. 1A) using microtubule-based and actin-based motor proteins (11–13). They are then transferred into the recipient keratinocytes, producing "cap" structures over the keratinocytes' nuclei (Figs. 1B, 2), to provide the keratinocyte genetic material with UV protection (reviewed

(A)   **(B)**

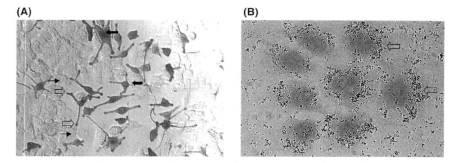

Figure 1   (**A**) A coculture of keratinocytes and melanocytes. Melanocytes (*dark arrow*) are stained with DOPA, the substrate of tyrosinase, demonstrating active melanogenesis. Melanocyte dendrites are extended from their cell bodies. The dendrite tips (*open arrow*) are ready to interact with the neighboring keratinocytes (line arrow, not stained) to transfer pigment-containing melanosomes. (**B**) Melanosome ingestion and cap formation in culture. Cultured keratinocytes (nuclei shown in *gray*) were provided with melanosomes (Fontana–Mason staining, black, documents pigment deposition), previously isolated from B16 cells. The keratinocytes ingest the melanosomes, and arrange them in a cap-like structure (*open arrows*) around their nuclei.

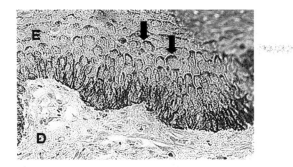

Figure 2 A histological section of a hyperpigmented human skin. D is the upper part of the dermis; E is the lower part of the epidermis. Fontana-Mason staining documents pigment deposition. Melanin caps over the nuclei of epidermal keratinocytes (*arrows*) protect the genetic material within the keratinocytes nuclei from UV damage.

in 14). As the epidermal keratinocytes mature, they move with their melanin content upward in the epidermis (reviewed in 15). It is the pigment content within the epidermis, and in particular within the stratum corneum, the uppermost layer of the epidermis, that results in visible skin color; the pigment within the melanocytes is not visible to the naked eye.

The chemical and enzymatic basis of melanogenesis is heavily documented (reviewed in 9,10,16–21). The key enzyme in melanogenesis is tyrosinase, which is the only enzyme absolutely essential for melanin formation in mammals. Tyrosinase initiates a cascade of reactions that convert the amino acid tyrosine to the biopolymer melanin. During the first reaction in the melanin biosynthesis process, tyrosinase catalyzes the hydroxylation of tyrosine, to create 3,4-dihydroxyphenylalanine (DOPA). Once DOPA is formed, it could either spontaneously, or with the aid of tyrosinase, be oxidized to dopaquinone, or, in the presence of sulfhydryl groups (e.g., Glutathione, or the amino acid cysteine), form cystenyldopa. Following a series of decarboxylation and oxidation reactions, a heterogeneous mixture of melanins is produced, consisting of two types of melanins, eumelanin (insoluble black, brown) and pheomelanin (somewhat soluble red, yellow) (reviewed in 17,22). Two tyrosinase-related proteins, TRP-1 (which is the most abundant glycoprotein in melanocytes) and TRP-2 (Dopachrome tautomerase), share about 40% homology with tyrosinase and have both catalytic activities and regulatory roles during melanogenesis (reviewed 17,22). Although these enzymes are not rate limiting in melanogenesis, the ratio of TRP-1: TRP-2 affects the ratio of very black, insoluble eumelanins to brown, more soluble eumelanins, therefore affecting skin color. Moreover, TRP-1 stabilizes the tyrosinase protein (e.g., 23–25), therefore the downregulation of TRP-1 should result in reduced tyrosinase half-life and consequently in reduced pigment production. Although TRP-1 has not been documented as a target for lightening agents, the indirect downregulation of TRP-1 mRNA expression was shown to correlate with depigmentation (26).

In Search for Tyrosinase Inhibitors

Based on the detailed biochemical knowledge of the melanogenic process, depigmenting agents were designed to inhibit the enzymatic activity of tyrosinase. Mushroom tyrosinase has been, and is still, used in the evaluation of tyrosinase activity (e.g., 27), and earlier industrial efforts for the search of tyrosinase inhibitors were heavily relied on mushroom-derived tyrosinase in a test-tube enzymatic assay. Obviously, the mushroom tyrosinase is not identical to the human one, resulting in inhibitory agents that were only partially active against the human enzyme. Unfortunately, the use of biochemically purified human tyrosinase (e.g., 28) was found to be too costly and could not be used for routine industrial screenings. As a result, many skin-lightening products that are based on mushroom tyrosinase inhibition are not as effective as desired. More recently, the use of human melanocyte lysate-based assays has provided tyrosinase-inhibition data that are more relevant to human skin depigmentation. However, before efficient cell-based pigmentation screenings were developed (e.g., 29), such lysates were also too costly and were used primarily for basic research (e.g., 30). Advances in biotechnology enabled the cloning of the human tyrosinase (31) and the expression of this enzyme in bacteria (e.g., 32). Efforts for the expression of tyrosinase in mammalian systems were first geared toward therapeutic goals, in particular in the area of melanoma research (e.g., 33), and not toward cosmetic applications. Although not documented in peer-reviewed publications, it is clear that the overexpression of the human tyrosinase in melanocytes or in other permissive cell types, and the production of lysates of tyrosinase that overexpressing cells, could be easily achieved with today's technologies. This could provide an alternative test method for tyrosinase-inhibitory agents, which is commercially feasible and is highly related to the human enzyme. Interestingly, the cloning and expression of the human tyrosinase did not lead to a breakthrough in the identification of skin lightening or darkening agents. In particular, no reports are available describing screens for potential darkening agents that act to stabilize the enzyme, to increase its half-life, or to enhance its efficiency. Similarly, no commercial products are available that are based on the direct induction of tyrosinase gene expression.

BIOTECHNOLOGY-GENERATED RESEARCH TOOLS FOR PIGMENTATION STUDIES

With the increased availability of biotechnology research tools, knowledge of the chemistry of melanogenesis was enhanced, and the understanding of the integration of these chemical and enzymatic activities and their regulation at the cellular level was dramatically increased. To an unusual extent, most of these advances stemmed from molecular approaches, resulting in the in vitro reconstruction and modulation of the overall chemical activity of melanocytes. Furthermore, these studies led to the identification of regulatory factors other than tyrosinase, which could be used as targets for the discovery of new pigment modulating agents. The increase in molecular knowledge of pigment-related genes (reviewed in 34,35) had expanded the traditional concept of melanogenesis inhibition. New concepts were further enhanced by recombinant DNA technologies and by the engineering of cells that overexpress or null express various pigmentary proteins, not only tyrosinase. With the additional molecular learning gained from the mechanistic understanding of different pigmentary mutant animals and cells (reviewed in 34,35), a whole new plethora of gene products and factors, and in particular of membrane-bound receptors, were found to affect pigment production.

At the cellular level, the understanding of cell–cell interactions and their importance in the regulation of pigment production resulted in the development of complex in vitro cellular systems. Keratinocyte–melanocyte cocultures and pigmented epidermal equivalents were developed to enable epidermal differentiation and cell–cell contact in vitro, making these research tools more representative of in vivo skin pigmentation (e.g., 36,37). The development of tissue-engineered skin (also called "skin substitutes," or "epidermal/dermal equivalents") was first geared toward therapeutic targets and resulted first in products for improving wound healing. Apligraf, an engineered bilayered skin equivalent, has been approved by the FDA for the treatment of venous ulcers (38). Such sophisticated in vitro systems were proven crucial for the discovery of new pathways involved in melanosome transfer and in pigment distribution, as well as in the regulation of pigment production (e.g., 26). Pigmented epidermal equivalents are now commercially available and are routinely used as a research and screening tool for pigment-modulating agents, enabling the identification of agents that affect both keratinocytes and melanocytes and their interactions. Efforts in the area of "designed in vitro equivalents" were initiated toward studies of melanoma development. Models consisting of epidermal keratinocytes plated onto fibroblast-contracted collagen gels and supplemented with normal melanocytes or melanoma-derived cell lines are continuously evaluated for growth and migration of the melanoma cells in the dermal component, as well as for tumorigenicity in vivo (39). The ability to genetically modify cells and then create these 3D in vitro epidermal structures is not yet fully exploited. It is expected that "designer equivalents" with gene knockouts or overexpressed genes will be soon used for pigmentary studies and for drug or cosmetic agent discovery.

The introduction of genetic material into the germ line of mammals resulted in major advances in pigment cell research and its applications. The ability to modulate pigmentary gene expression in vivo resulted in numerous applications for basic and applied research. The testing of designed mutants in the form of transgenic mice was proven a powerful and a valuable tool in the correlation of pigmentary phenotypes with patterns of gene expression (e.g., 40). Transgenic animal studies had extended our knowledge of the regulation of pigment production and distribution, and pigmentary mutants led to the identification of numerous new molecular targets for the modulation of pigment production. However, it is important to note that the mouse skin has no, or very few, (specifically localized) epidermal melanocytes, and, therefore, the mouse skin is not pigmented. Most transgenic rodents with a pigmentary phenotype demonstrate only hair color changes and not epidermal (skin) pigmentation. Interpretation of data generated from these genetically engineered animals for skin color modulation should be, therefore, carefully analyzed. Mutant mice of enhanced epidermal pigmentation have been created using chemical mutagenesis (e.g., 41), but transgenic mice with engineered enhancement of epidermal pigmentation are yet to be created.

SKIN COLOR MODULATION—MORE THAN TYROSINASE INHIBITION

This chapter will not discuss the technologies of tyrosinase inhibition or selective melanocyte cytotoxicity. It will rather concentrate on newer approaches, mainly of biotechnology nature, that enable the modulation of skin color. Although the chemical synthesis of melanin is well documented, the regulation of pigment production and the processes involved in pigment distribution at the cellular level are only partially understood. Therefore, until recently, most topical depigmenting agents available in cosmetic products were either tyrosinase inhibitors or melanocyte cytotoxic agents, whereas available darkening agents consisted mainly of dihydroxyacetone and topically applied melanins. Using the most recent understanding of pigment biology, it is now possible not only to inhibit pigment production, but also to enhance skin color. New, yet incomplete understanding of different pathways and regulatory molecules is currently evaluated, and novel pigment-modulating agents are expected to be developed.

Molecules involved in the regulation of pigmentation, rather than in the biogenesis of melanin, were identified as targets for pigment-altering agents. Examples of the experimental use of such targets for the modulation of skin color are described later. These targets were identified using molecular and cellular technologies, and the proof of concept studies for the ability to alter skin color via these targets were performed with the aid of biotechnology. Many of these targets are membrane-bound receptors, which are considered as ideal targets for intervention. Cellular receptors control and modulate numerous cellular functions, including developmental processes, cell–cell communication, and metabolic pathways, by inducing a signal transduction cascade. Membrane-bound receptors are desired pharmacological targets, because they are relatively accessible. Moreover, agonist and antagonist molecules could be designed to affect these receptor-controlled processes, based on the nucleic acid sequence of the desired receptor. "Designer peptide" agonists and antagonists have been created based on the structures of receptors and their ligands, and they have been employed in the modulation of numerous tissue functions (reviewed in 42). Some examples of the use of receptor agonists and/or antagonists in skin color modulation as well as the use of novel, regulatory molecules as target for pigment alteration are described later. This chapter will focus on proteins and peptides and will not discuss nucleic-acid-based products. Using such technologies as Ribozymes, silencing RNA and antisense was shown to specifically reduce or inhibit desired biological activities. However, these technologies are yet immature even for medical use, and their industrial production, stability, and delivery have not been fully investigated.

The Melanocortin-1 Receptor and Its Ligands

The melanocortin-1 receptor (MC1-R) plays a key role in determining the type of melanin (eumelanin vs. pheomelanin) that is produced within melanocytes. Binding of the proopiomelanocortin (POMC)-derived peptides melanocyte stimulating hormone (MSH) and adrenocorticotropic hormone (ACTH) to the MC1-R increases tyrosinase activity and eumelanin production, resulting in skin darkening (43,44). MC1-R is also involved in UV-induced melanogenesis (tanning). Mutations of the MC1-R gene are associated with variation in hair and skin color. Loss-of-function MC1-R mutations result in a "red hair" phenotype in humans and are associated with fair skin and with the decreased ability to tan (45). Five melanocortin receptors (MC1 through MC5) have been identified, which are expressed in numerous tissues and share ligand bindings, resulting in complex physiological responses. The melanocortin receptors were most studied for their physiological actions in the brain (e.g., 46). MC-R agonists and antagonists are constantly being synthesized and evaluated, and MSH analogs have been extensively used in many of these studies (e.g., 47–49). Although these efforts target primarily the MC4-R, for such indications as weight loss and management, anxiety control, or depression (e.g., 50–53), agents useful for the study and modulation of all other melanocortin receptors were created via these studies. As in many other situations, agents, that are created first using new technologies aim for a therapeutic need. Such agents are later used for "lighter" indications, sometimes following modifications that reduce their potency or alter their specificity. Similarly, agents targeting the MC-Rs were later evaluated for their potential to alter skin color. The melanocortin receptors are activated by MSH and ACTH and are antagonized by Agouti and Agouti-related protein. Indeed, the peptides MSH and ACTH induce pigment production, whereas the Agouti protein inhibits pigment production in rodent experimental systems (e.g., 54).

In humans, enhancement of the melanin content of the skin was achieved using either MSH, or synthetic MSH analogs (e.g., the "super-potent" analogs Melanotan-1 and -2, reviewed in 6). Melanotan-1, a synthetic MSH-like peptide that is a nonselective melanocortin receptor agonist, was found to induce skin darkening upon injection or when used in an implant. Melanotan-1 is promoted to protect fair-skinned individuals from sunburn; however, the most at-risk population, namely individuals with MC1-R loss-of-function mutations, cannot benefit from such an agent. Moreover, because the darkening effect of MSH is enhanced upon UV exposure, MSH-like products encourage sun exposure and therefore do not reduce the risk of skin cancer development. The side effects of systemic MSH treatment include not only flushing upon injection, but also, in some men, an erectile response. These systemic side effects produced by the MSH-like peptide treatment were found to be of high commercial value, and Melanotan-2, the second-generation cyclic peptide, is currently evaluated in animals for decreased food uptake (e.g., 55) and in human subjects with erectile dysfunction (e.g., 56).

Interestingly, the POMC peptides (POMC is the precursor of the MC-Rs ligands) are produced in skin not only by melanocytes, but also by keratinocytes (e.g., 57–59, for a detailed review, see 60). This suggests that local modulation of MSH or ACTH production within the epidermis, as well as the use of topical agents with agonist or antagonist activity toward the MC1-R, could be effective in modulating skin color with no systemic undesired effects. MSH-like peptides with either agonist or antagonist activity were already designed and could be further improved and produced using simple and available biotechnology systems. Although topical skin delivery of peptides is still inefficient, progress in the field has been made. Liposomal delivery vehicles, peptide modifications, and energy-enhanced delivery (e.g., iontophoresis) were all used to enhance peptide penetration through the stratum corneum, and efforts for the topical delivery of melanotropic peptides for skin darkening in vivo were initiated (e.g., 61). A cost-efficient process for peptide production, and better understanding of peptide delivery through the stratum corneum, would enable the creation of topical treatments that could, theoretically, avoid most of the side effects produced by the systemic delivery and provide safe and effective skin color altering agents.

The c-Kit Receptor and Its Ligand

c-Kit is a membrane receptor with tyrosine kinase activity, which is expressed in human melanocytes. The c-kit receptor and its ligand, the growth factor Stem Cell Factor (SCF) are essential for melanocyte differentiation and survival, and are known to induce pigment production (e.g., 62,63). In experimental systems, blocking the c-kit receptor with injection of antibodies inhibits UVB-induced pigmentation (64), suggesting that c-kit could serve as a target for pigment modulating agents. Mutations in c-kit or in its ligand result in a failure of melanocytes to reach the skin during embryogenesis (65). These developmental effects might suggest that modulation of the c-kit pathway after birth would happen "too late" to affect pigmentation. However, incubation of melanocytes with SCF led to a transient increase of tyrosinase activity at two to four hours post-incubation (66). This early response of tyrosinase activation is possibly mediated by modifications of the tyrosinase protein like phosphorylation, suggesting that the kinase activity of c-kit could be targeted for skin color modulation. SCF is synthesized as both soluble (S) and membrane-associated (MA) proteins, but the physiologic role(s) of these two isoforms is not yet understood. In transgenic mice that overexpress the MA isoform of human SCF (hSCF), an antagonist effect was identified. Mice expressing the hSCF transgene have coat color deficiency and display a pronounced forehead blaze, white spots over the cervical region, and a large white belly spot (67). It might be possible, therefore, to design an SCF-like agonist or a c-kit antagonist that would modulate skin color. Although the technology for the design and production of such agents is available, the overall biological effects of c-kit modulating agents are not yet completely understood. More basic research is required before c-kit agonists and antagonists could be safely used to modulate skin color.

The Endothelin-1 Receptor Pathway

The vasoconstrictive peptide endothelin-1 (ET-1) is expressed in human keratinocytes, and the ET-1 receptor (ET-1R) is found on melanocytes. UVB irradiation results in ET-1 secretion from keratinocytes (68). The addition of ET-1 to cultured human melanocytes resulted in elevated levels of tyrosinase and tyrosinase-related protein-1 expression, an increase in tyrosinase activity, and, consequently, in an increase in pigment production (69). Extracts of M. Chamomilla act as an antagonist for ET-receptor mediated signaling but have no inhibitory effect on tyrosinase activity in culture. These extracts inhibited UVB-induced pigmentation in vivo when applied daily to human skin, immediately after UVB exposure (70). This suggests that agent(s) within this plant extract could act as ET-R1 antagonists. Alternatively, ET-1R agonists and antagonists could be engineered and evaluated for their effect on skin pigmentation.

The membrane-bound metalloproteinase, endothelin-converting enzyme (ECE-1), specifically cleaves the inactive precursor of ET-1 to produce the mature, active ET-1 peptide, which is then secreted. Like ET-1, ECE-1 is also expressed in human keratinocytes, and its expression is increased following Interleukin-1 alpha treatment (71). This suggests that ECE-1 could play a role in the processing and in the UVB-inducible secretion of ET-1 by human keratinocytes, leading to the stimulation of pigment production in the epidermis (71). Cloning and expression of ECE-1 could be used to identify molecules that enhance, prolong, or inhibit its activation, resulting in novel darkening or lightening agents that affect the ET-1 pathway. Assuming that the specificity of ECE-1 is indeed restricted, antisense or small interfering RNA molecules against ECE-1 could be used for proof of concept studies, and possibly even as bioengineered depigmenting molecules.

Microphthalmia

The microphthalmia-associated transcription factor (MITF) is involved in the differentiation, growth, and survival of pigment cells (e.g., 72,73). Many growth factor signaling pathways regulate MITF at both the protein and the promoter levels. The c-kit signaling pathway is linked to phosphorylation of MITF at Ser73 and Ser409 through activation of MAP kinase and RSK-1, respectively (74,75). Phosphorylation of MITF is also conducted at Ser298 through GSK3beta, although the signaling pathway for this event still remains to be understood. Both the WNT and the MSH signaling pathways regulate MITF at the promoter level, and endothelins may regulate MITF at the protein and promoter levels (e.g., 72,73). MITF has four isoforms, one of which (M) is melanocyte specific. This MITF isoform is a major transcriptional regulator of the melanogenic genes. MITF binds to the promoters of tyrosinase and tyrosinase-related protein-1 and -2 and transactivates their expression. The MITF promoter contains a cAMP response element (CRE) that may mediate cAMP-induced melanogenesis and differentiation of melanocytes. (For a review of the role of cAMP in melanogenesis, see e.g., 76). Homozygous mutations at the mouse microphthalmia (Mi) locus lead to a complete loss of pigmentation, and mutation in the human MITF gene results in abnormal pigmentation, as observed in Waardenburg Syndrome type II (e.g., 75,77,78).

The central role of MITF in the regulation of melanocyte development and melanogenesis makes it an ideal target for the modulation of skin pigmentation. Using bioengineered nucleic acid constructs that express a reporter gene from the MITF promoter, agents were identified that modulate MITF expression (79). A natural extract (TCM-1) that enhances MITF expression in vitro was identified and was found to enhance pigment deposition in culture. Lipoic acid and dihydrolipoic acid, which were found to reduce MITF promoter activity, were shown to inhibit pigment deposition both in vitro and in vivo (79). These data demonstrate the potential of a biotechnology-based screening procedure, in combination with pigmentation genomics data, to provide novel agents for altering skin color.

Protein Kinase C Beta

The beta isoform of the Protein Kinase C (PKC) can regulate melanogenesis in vitro through tyrosinase activation via the MSH pathway (80,81). A diacylglycerol analog was found to increase the melanin content of cultured human melanocytes. This increase was completely blocked by the PKC inhibitors H-7 and sphingosine (82). Activation of PKC by phorbol dibutyrate increased tyrosinase activity in cultured melanocytes. Depletion of PKC resulted in reduction in tyrosinase activity, and reintroduction of the PKC activity induced the recovery of tyrosinase activity. Transient transfection with PKC-beta cDNA increased tyrosinase activity, suggesting that PKC-beta could serve as a target for pigment modulating agents (80). However, in vivo data for the direct effect of PKC beta on tyrosinase are not yet available, and no isoform-selective PKC inhibitors are available, which could affect tyrosinase phosphorylation only. Moreover, data also suggest that PKC regulates melanogenesis by controlling the constitutive expression of tyrosinase and, to a lesser extent, of TRP-1, and that B16 clones overexpressing PKC alpha have increased tyrosinase activity as well (83). Clearly, more basic research is required before applications for skin pigmentation could be created. The cloning and expression of the desired isozymes in bacteria, yeast, or baculovirus could aid in a search for PKC isoform-specific inhibitors and in comparing their binding profile to those of the other PKC isozymes expressed in skin. Identified agents could be evaluated in monolayer cocultures or in pigmented equivalents, for their possible pigment modulating activities, as well as for their undesired effects on other PKC isoforms.

The PAR-2 Pathway

The regulation of keratinocyte–melanocyte interactions and the mechanism of melanosome transfer into keratinocytes are not yet completely understood. This chapter describes the identification of a pathway involved in melanosome transfer, the application of this knowledge to the discovery of new targets, and the development of new products for the modulation of skin pigmentation. The direct and indirect contributions of biotechnology and recombinant DNA technologies, and their impact on the identification of the PAR-2 pathway and its role in pigmentation, are detailed later.

Melanosome Transfer

Pigment-loaded melanosomes are transferred from the melanocyte dendrite tips into the recipient keratinocytes (Fig. 1A). Numerous mechanisms for melanosome transfer have been suggested, such as endocytosis, direct inoculation ("injection"), keratinocyte–melanocyte membrane fusion and phagocytosis (reviewed in 12). Phagocytosis is a receptor-mediated process, resulting in the ingestion of 0.5 to 1 micron size particles (e.g., 84–86). This process is associated with macrophages, neutrophils, and monocytes (reviewed in 82), but epidermal keratinocytes were also shown to have phagocytic ability (87). The mechanism and regulation of keratinocyte phagocytosis and its role in epidermal homeostasis are not yet completely understood. The Protease-activated receptor-2 (PAR-2) (88) is a seven transmembrane G-protein-coupled receptor that is activated by a serine protease cleavage at the extracellular domain. PAR-2 cleavage by trypsin or mast cell tryptase exposes a new N-terminus, which then acts as a tethered ligand (88). PAR-2 could also be specifically activated using synthetic peptides such as SLIGRL, which correspond to the new N-terminus of the naturally activated receptor. PAR-2 is expressed in keratinocytes (89,90), but not in melanocytes (26), and its activation results in Ca^{++} mobilization and IP_3 hydrolysis (reviewed in 91,92). Interestingly, PAR-2 was found to regulate pigmentation by affecting keratinocyte phagocytosis (26,93–95). PAR-2 activation increases the ability of keratinocytes to ingest melanosomes, resulting in skin darkening, and inhibition of PAR-2 activation by serine protease inhibitors reduces pigment transfer and leads to depigmentation. Moreover, the inhibition of PAR-2 activation prevents UVB-induced pigmentation and reduces tanning (95, reviewed in 96).

Research Tools Essential to the Identification of the PAR-2 Pathway

Because PAR-2 is expressed on keratinocytes, but not on melanocytes (26), PAR-2 was not evaluated earlier as a target for pigment modulation. It is the use of biotechnology tools, and in particular the ability to coculture keratinocytes and melanocytes under specific growth conditions, that enabled the identification of this pathway and its role in pigmentation. The coculturing of keratinocytes and melanocytes requires a well-defined growth medium, with measurable quantities of numerous growth factors, instead of the classic use of nondefined mixtures such as bovine serum. It is the use of recombinant DNA technology that enabled the mass production of specific growth factors in a cost-effective manner and, therefore, enabled the creation of controlled cell culture conditions. Indirectly, therefore, it is the recombinant DNA technology that enabled the identification of the PAR-2 pathway. In order to identify the role of PAR-2 in the regulation of pigmentation, the signaling of the keratinocyte to the melanocyte had to be preserved in the experimental systems. Without the ability to produce bioengineered growth factors and to control tissue culture conditions, the role of PAR-2 in pigmentation would not be identified. Melanocyte-only cultures are not responsive to PAR-2 signaling modulation, since melanocytes do not express PAR-2 (14,26). The PAR-2 pigmentary effect was observed only in keratinocytes–melanocytes cocultures that enabled physical contact between the two cell types (26, reviewed in 14). It is the ability to maintain complex coculture systems that led to a new paradigm in the identification of pigment-regulating agents.

In order to study the role of PAR-2 in pigmentation, research tools were required to activate PAR-2 and to inhibit its activation. PAR-2 activating peptides like SLIGRL could be easily synthesized. However, since no PAR-2 antagonists were available, only the inhibition of the PAR-2-activating proteases was possible. Serine protease inhibitors were used as research tools during the earlier studies of PAR-2 in pigmentation. These inhibitors were designed based on a structure–function analysis of the PAR-2 cleavage site, and the amino acid sequence of the receptor (97). These agents were extremely useful in the elucidation of the pathway and could be developed into prescription-drug type lightening agents. However, these small serine protease inhibitors could not be used as cosmetic skin-lightening agents. Once the role of the PAR-2 pathway was understood, agents of natural source were sought and evaluated for their ability to inhibit PAR-2 activation and to induce skin lightening. STI, a soybean-derived serine protease inhibitor, was found to inhibit PAR-2 activation in vitro, and was used in proof-of-principle studies in vivo (Fig. 3) (95). Similarly, the

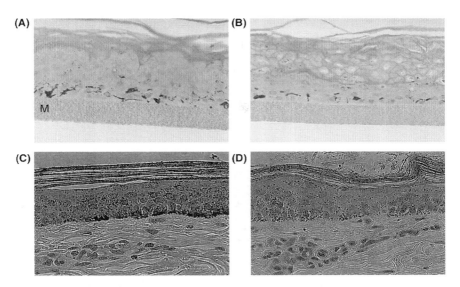

Figure 3 STI reduces pigment deposition in pigmented epidermal equivalents and in vivo. Pigmented equivalents grown on membranes (M) were treated daily, for three days, with STI (**B**) or vehicle (**A**), and formalin fixed by the fourth day. Histological sections were stained with Fontana–Mason to document melanin deposition, which is reduced following the STI treatment (**B**). Dark-skinned Yucatan swine were treated daily, for eight weeks, with STI, in liposomes. Fontana–Mason staining of skin sections demonstrates reduced pigment deposition following STI (**D**) treatment, relative to the vehicle treated site (**C**).

PAR-2 activating peptide SLIGRL was shown to induced pigment deposition in culture and in vivo (Fig. 4), (94).

Knowledge Results in Simplified Research Systems

Once the PAR-2 pathway was identified, the complex and costly systems of keratinocyte–melanocyte cocultures and pigmented epidermal equivalents, used for the search of pigment-modulating agents, could be used for secondary evaluations only. PAR-2 was found to be a phagocytic receptor (93), involved in melanosome ingestion. Studies of melanosome ingestion by keratinocytes were used as a proof of concept (93) (Fig. 1B) but were later replaced with the ingestion of fluorescently labeled microspheres, which was easier to detect (93). Cell-based assays for macrophage phagocytosis using fluorescently labeled *E. coli* particles were later adapted to keratinocytes. This led to the creation of a 96-well plate assay that was used for screening of agents with pigment modulation potential, by evaluating their effects on keratinocyte phagocytosis (93). Because PAR-2 is activated by trypsin, agents with trypsin

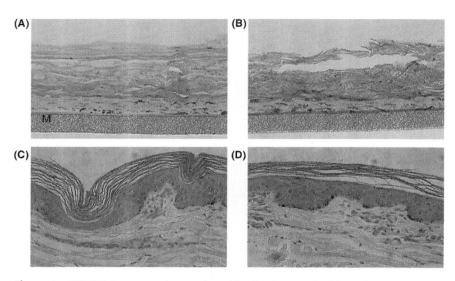

Figure 4 SLIGRL increases pigment deposition in pigmented epidermal equivalents and in vivo. Pigmented equivalents grown on membranes (M) were treated daily, for three days, with SLIGRL (**B**) or vehicle (**A**), and formalin fixed by the fourth day. Histological sections were stained with Fontana–Mason to document melanin deposition, which is increased following the SLIGRL treatment (**B**). Lightly pigmented Yucatan swine were treated daily, for eight weeks, with SLIGRL. Fontana–Mason staining of skin sections demonstrates increased pigment deposition following SLIGRL (**D**) treatment, relative to the vehicle treated site (**C**).

inhibitory activity could potentially reduce pigment production. Trypsin inhibition assays were set as screening tools for potential depigmenting agents. A peptide with a serine protease cleavage site, which fluoresces upon cleavage, was commercially available, and was used as a first line screen. Recombinant trypsin was used to cleave this peptide and to create a fluorescence signal. Agents that were able to inhibit trypsin activity in this system were further evaluated (95). A more specific assay was then created to evaluate the inhibition of trypsin in cleaving the PAR-2 specific sequence (26,96). Agents that were able to inhibit the cleavage of a peptide comprising the PAR-2 cleavage site in a dose-dependent manner were identified and were further evaluated in the phagocytosis assay. The pigment modulating activity of promising agents was later verified in pigmented equivalents. These enzymatic and phagocytosis inhibition, 96-well plate assays, were proven most useful during the development of PAR-2-based depigmenting products. Different formulations could be efficiently evaluated for their efficacy, and each ingredient could be evaluated for incompatibility with the active agents. Efficacy evaluations were incorporated into long-term stability studies, to ensure the creation of effective depigmenting products.

Modulation of the PAR-2 Pathway Alters Skin Color

The soybean-derived proteins Soybean trypsin inhibitor (STI) and Bowman–Birk inhibitor (BBI) inhibit the enzymatic activity of trypsin. Therefore, they were considered as natural candidates for cosmetic skin lightening by inhibition of the PAR-2 pathway. These proteins were positive in the assays described earlier and were later shown to reduce pigment deposition in epidermal equivalents (Fig. 3B, compare to 3A) (95). The PAR-2 activating peptide SLIGRL was positive in the phagocytosis assay and was shown to enhance pigment deposition in vitro (Fig. 4B, compare to 4A). The modulation of pigmentation by SLIGRL and STI was then evaluated in vivo to verify their activity in a physiological environment. The species of choice for this evaluation was the pigmented Yucatan swine, because mice have minimal or no epidermal pigmentation. STI treatment of dark-skinned Yucatan swine induced a dose-dependent visible skin lightening, which was confirmed histologically (Fig. 3D, compare to 3C) (95). Topical treatment of light-skinned Yucatan swine with SLIGRL led to increased pigment deposition within the epidermis (Fig. 4D, compare to 4C), (94, reviewed in 14).

To further examine the modulation of pigmentation by SLIGRL and STI, human skins transplanted onto severe combined immunodeficiency (SCID) mice were used. SCID is a lymphoid deficiency disease, which impairs the differentiation of both T- and B-lymphocytes, creating an immuno-suppressed status that enables xeno grafting with no rejection (98). The immune deficiency of these mice has provided an animal model to examine the in vivo function and the therapeutic intervention of many transplanted human tissues. The use of SCID mice in medical research and biotechnology is constantly increasing, enabling the evaluation of drug responses of a whole human tissue, within a real human physiological environment (reviewed in 99,100). Using the SCID mouse system for pigmentation studies provided the final proof that PAR-2 can regulate pigmentation. Human Caucasian skin transplanted onto SCID mice showed a visible increase in pigmentation following SLIGRL treatment, relative to a vehicle-treated transplant from the same donor. An increase in pigment deposition was documented histologically (94,14). A hyperpigmented human skin transplanted onto SCID mice, which was treated with STI, showed reduced pigment deposition, which was confirmed histologically (14,94). No other changes were observed in the SLIGRL or STI-treated human skins; skin architecture was normal and intact, and no inflammatory infiltrate was detected histologically. These data suggest that SLIGRL and STI could be used to modulate pigmentation of human skin (14).

PAR-2 in Human Skin

The PAR-2 mediated pigmentary effects are reversible, indicating no permanent damage to the pigmentary system. For example, four weeks after termination of STI treatment, the STI-depigmented site was no longer visible. Histological analysis revealed a gradual increase in pigment production and distribution even before the visual observation of repigmentation (e.g., 94). Human studies with STI-containing soy extracts that were performed at a later stage induced significant skin lightening with no side effects, demonstrating that the inhibition of PAR-2 is a novel approach to human skin depigmentation (101). The inhibition of PAR-2 activation also prevented UVB-induced pigmentation in vitro (26,95). Therefore, the possibility that PAR-2 is involved in UV-mediated tanning was examined. Increasing doses of UVB irradiation of keratinocyte cultures induced the secretion of a protease activity, which was able to cleave a peptide comprising the PAR-2 cleavage site in a dose-dependent manner (93,14). In vivo, this UVB-induced PAR-2 cleaving activity could be inhibited with STI-containing compositions (95,14), which led to reduced or eliminated UVB-induced tanning. Yucatan swine that were minimally UVB irradiated produced visible tanning, but daily treatments with STI prevented this tanning (95). PAR-2 was found to be upregulated in UVB-irradiated human skin (100), and the distribution of the PAR-2 protein within the epidermis was found to change following UVB exposure (102). Ethnic skin studies revealed an increase in PAR-2 and trypsin (the PAR-2 activator) expression in darker skins (103). Similarly, the distribution of the PAR-2 protein within the epidermis was found to correlate with the level of pigment deposition (103). Genomic studies (gene chips) confirmed this observation, and activity analyses documented that the PAR-2 pathway is more active in darker-skinned individuals (103). These studies further confirmed that PAR-2 modulation is a promising approach for affecting skin color.

Combining Science and Technology with Nature

Combining the mechanistic understanding of the PAR-2 pathway with the consumer desire for a safe and effective "natural" depigmenting agent might sound contradictory, if not impossible. Based on the depigmenting activity of STI and BBI, nondenatured soybean extracts were developed and were found to induce human skin lightening (101). When used for the proof of concept studies, STI and BBI were combined with liposomes (e.g., 104), to enable protein delivery through the stratum corneum (95). To verify protein delivery, new molecular techniques were employed. In one case, the STI protein was tagged with a fluorescent marker and was later visualized in histological sections. In another study, treated skin extracts were processed for Western blotting analysis, and STI was detected in the swine skin extract using anti-STI antibodies. The presence of the liposome-delivered STI protein in skin was not only verified, but was also found to correlate with skin lightening in a dose-dependent manner. Similar studies were performed to verify that formulated, nondenatured soybean extracts could deliver STI through the stratum corneum, into the epidermis. Nondenatured soy extracts led to skin lightening and were shown to contain intact STI protein by Western blotting. Soybean extracts that were denatured experimentally, or commercially available denatured soy extracts (e.g., soymilk for nutritional consumption), failed to induce skin lightening (95). These nutritional extracts were found to contain no intact or active STI, as determined by Western blotting and by trypsin inhibition assays. During the course of product development, product formulation, and stability evaluation, the presence of intact and active STI was verified, and trypsin inhibitory activity was followed throughout these processes. All skin-care products that are based on nondenatured soybean extracts must demonstrate the ability to inhibit PAR-2 activation, as an integral part of their quality-control process. The application of PAR-2 knowledge into product development systems resulted in the incorporation of molecular and biotechnology research tools into the processes of product development and analytical evaluation.

The production of a natural extract containing nondenatured and active proteins required the application of protein biochemistry knowledge into the industrial process. In order to keep proteins in their native form, the use of standard raw material processing procedures—such as heat, detergents, organic solvents, or pH modification—was eliminated. Novel processes needed to be developed to enable extraction of soybeans without affecting the compositions, ratios, and activities found in the raw beans. Formulation ingredients were individually evaluated for possible interference with protein activity, and many commonly used, inactive cosmetic ingredients were found incompatible with STI activity. From thickening agents to preservatives and to scents, every ingredient was analyzed in combination with the actives to ensure that STI and BBI activities are preserved. These demands result in a major challenge to the aesthetics of the product, and novel approaches and materials were developed to obtain aesthetic products containing nondenatured, active proteins. Microorganism control of a natural product is usually achieved using standard sterilization techniques. However, since these involve heat and pressure, protein denaturation is unavoidable. Similar to the sterility issues of cell-based products for transplantation, systems were developed to enable microorganism control while keeping STI and BBI intact and active in the nondenatured soy extracts. With the application of new molecular technologies in the product development processes, analytical assays, and sterilization procedures, the cost of the final product was kept within the accepted range of the skin-care industry. Since the nondenatured soy products were developed in a research and technology-based program, the results were novel, safe, efficacious, and cost-effective products. Advertising of these products, therefore, emphasizes the mechanism of action, demonstrating that the understanding of biological processes, combined with the ability to use biotechnology research tools could be translated into new concepts in skin care products.

The PAR-2 pathway is not the only pathway involved in melanosome transfer. Over the past few years, significant advance has been made toward the understanding of melanosome transfer. Ongoing studies aim not only for a comprehensive understanding of PAR-2-induced events, but also of other pathways involved in melanosome transfer. Future studies of the mechanism of melanosome transfer are likely to focus on the identification of key molecules involved in the dendrite–keratinocyte interaction, the "glue" molecules that enable keratinocyte phagocytosis, and their regulation. These studies should yield new targets, all remain to be elucidated, and future products would modulate skin pigmentation by interacting with these molecules.

PROTEINS AND PEPTIDES IN PIGMENT-ALTERING PRODUCTS: THE CHALLENGES

Many of the pathways described in this chapter were identified using biotechnology, and proofs of concept for lightening and darkening were obtained with similar strategies. However, these studies resulted in very few biotechnology-produced pigment-modulating agents that are commercially available. More interestingly, although the general use of biotechnology-derived recombinant proteins and chemically synthesized peptides as therapeutic agents is increasing, peptides and proteins are not yet available even for the treatment of pigmentary disorders. Possible key issues affecting the development of pigmentary products are mentioned later.

Proteins and Peptides in Pigment-Altering Products: Challenges Beyond the Proof of Principle

The use of proteins and peptides for skin care is facing challenges at three functional levels. The first level has the same issues found in all protein products used to treat humans: The stability and activity of the protein, its safety and immunological profile, and the cost-effective production of the product, all need to be optimized. The second level is skin-specific and is directly related to the expectation and to the desire to treat skin topically and to avoid systemic side effects. At this level, the ability to deliver the active agent across the stratum corneum is a major challenge. Moreover, when pigmentary changes are desired, the active agent might need not only to cross the skin barrier, but also to travel deep into the epidermis, to reach the surface of the melanocytes, or sometimes to enter the melanosomes. A third cycle of challenges is related to the creation of consumer products, which are used and stored in a less controlled manner relative to therapeutic agents, resulting in higher demands on protein stability and activity.

For a pigment-altering cosmetic product, which contains proteins as their active agents, several major issues remain to be solved. Protein delivery through the stratum corneum is clearly a key issue. Previous efforts in the area of protein delivery were dedicated primarily to the transdermal delivery of proteins, namely to the ability to deliver an agent like insulin, systemically, through the skin. For a pigment-altering protein, the desired delivery system should target the epidermis only, while avoiding the deeper skin layers where the agent could lead to systemic effects. Liposomal delivery vehicles and instrument-enhanced localized delivery systems (e.g., patches, iontophoresis) have been evaluated, but they are still far from being optimized. For a protein-containing skin-care product, another important factor is maintaining protein stability and activity within the formulated product during storage, not only within the skin following application. Unlike drugs, skin-care products are stored at varied room temperatures, are not expected to be reconstituted or hydrated only at the time of use, and are not consumed immediately as their container is opened. Therefore, skin-care products are exposed to numerous environmental insults that would result in protein oxidation, degradation, or change in structure. Proteins need to be correctly folded to enable their activity, as little modifications in their three-dimensional structure will render them inactive. The proper folding of proteins, as well as their post-translational modifications must remain intact within the product. Protein stability of a skin care product must be significantly enhanced to retain activity over long periods of storage under less than optimal conditions. A cost-effective process to obtain such stable proteins is highly desired.

Current trends of consumer expectations desire the use of "natural" products, which are conceived as safe and effective. However, natural extracts contain numerous "unknown" ingredients that could, sometimes, reduce the safety or the efficacy of such products. Purified proteins, expressed in bioengineered systems, could provide higher efficacy and reduced side effects. Bacteria, plants, and mammalian cells as well as live animals are already used to express desired proteins, which, following required modifications, are demonstrated to be active in numerous biological systems. In the area of skin pigmentation, cloned, expressed, and purified STI, for example, could be used as a depigmenting agent. This cloned protein could also be genetically modified to enhance its specificity and to decrease its undesired activities. Similarly, trypsin could be used to enhance skin color, and a "super-trypsin" could be engineered with a selectivity and high specificity for PAR-2 cleavage only. A "super-tyrosinase," although as easy to construct recombinantly, might be more challenging to use, because it would require the specific delivery into the melanosome.

Using peptides in pigment-altering consumer products has some advantages relative to proteins. Being smaller, peptides might be less sensitive to proteolytic degradation, and theoretically they should be easier to penetrate the stratum corneum. Some simple modifications, such as the addition of a fatty acid side chain or a short poly-Arginine peptide, as well as the use of liposomes or iontophoresis were shown to enhance peptide delivery into human skin. In many cases, the desired peptide activity was not impaired following the use of such strategies. Most peptides are too small to acquire a precise folding structure and are more "flexible" than proteins. Usually they do not require post-translational modifications; therefore their production should be less expensive relative to protein expression and modification. Peptides that act as receptor agonists or antagonists do not need to enter into the cells or into certain subcellular organelles like the melanosome, so they should reach their targets more efficiently. However, skin delivery of small peptides is far from being optimized, and more research is needed in the area of peptide delivery. Moreover, the industrial production of small peptides is not yet cost-effective; therefore, up till now, peptides were not a major component of consumer products. Regardless, peptide-based skin-care products are increasingly appearing in the market. Conversely, peptide-containing lightening or darkening products for topical use are not readily available. Such products are within the reach of the industry. For example, mimetic MSH peptides with higher activity were already designed, and could be further optimized for their specificity, but their delivery had not been optimized to eliminate systemic side effects. Studies for the optimization of topical peptide delivery, and in particular targeting the epidermis only, would lead to a major advance in the field of skin-pigmentation products. Following the optimization of peptide delivery, immunogenicity and safety parameters should be evaluated for each peptide and protein.

A shift in consumer perception is required before resources will be allocated to solve these problems and to create bioengineered, biotechnology-designed proteins for pigment-modulating skin-care products. Consumers currently accept the use of engineered, and even "enhanced" proteins, in only very few "end user" areas (e.g., in laundry detergents) but not yet in skin care. Interestingly, there are no negative misconceptions associated with peptides in skin-care use, and products containing "active peptides" for skin care have recently emerged.

Proteins and Peptides in Pigment-Altering Products: Summary

1. Advances in science and biotechnology resulted in novel understanding of the regulation of pigmentation. Novel molecular targets for pigment modulation were identified. Proof of concept studies in experimental systems demonstrated the ability to modulate pigmentation via numerous biological pathways, not only by directly affecting tyrosinase. Recent advances in pigment cell research and current developments in biotechnology have made it possible to design and produce specific skin pigmentation modifiers, which have the potential for greater effectiveness and fewer side effects relative to currently available products.

2. Although protein expression and purification systems are the hallmark of the biotechnology industry, proteins that regulate skin color are not yet available in skin-care products. Pigment-altering proteins and peptides need to be produced in a cost-efficient manner. The three-dimensional structure and post-translational modifications of proteins must remain stable under storage-and-use conditions, and protein and peptide delivery systems need to be optimized. The safety and the possible immune reaction of such agents need to be examined under physiological conditions, before such agents could be commercialized.

3. A shift in consumer opinion is required in order to allocate resources for the creation of protein-based products and for demonstrating their long-term safety of efficacy.

4. Biotechnology has been extensively used in the research and development of pigment-altering products. The commercial success of biotechnology-produced proteins in altering skin pigmentation is yet to be demonstrated.

REFERENCES

1. Hacker SM. Common disorders of pigmentation: when are more that cosmetic cover-ups required? Postgrad Med 1996; 6:177–186.
2. Jimbow K, Jimbow M. Chemical, pharmacologic and physical agents causing hypo-melanoses. In: Nordlund JJ, Boissy RE, HearingVJ, King RA, Ortonne J-P, eds. The Pigmentary System. New York: Oxford University Press, 1998:621–627.
3. de Gruijl FR. Skin cancer and solar UV radiation. Eur J Cancer 1999; 35(14):2003–2009.
4. Armstrong BK, Kricker A. The epidemiology of UV induced skin cancer. J Photo-chem Photobiol B 2001; 63(1–3):8–18.
5. Karagas MR, Stannard VA, Mott LA, Slattery MJ, Spencer SK, Weinstock MA. Use of tanning devices and risk of basal cell and squamous cell skin cancers. J Natl Cancer Inst 2002; 94(3):224–226.
6. Pawelek JM. Approaches to increasing skin melanin with MSH analogs and synthetic melanins. Pigment Cell Res 2001; 14(3):155–160.
7. Draelos ZD. Self-tanning lotions: are they a healthy way to achieve a tan? Am J Clin Dermatol 2002; 3(5):317–408.
8. Nguyen BC, Kochevar IE. Influence of hydration on dihydroxyacetone-induced pigmentation of stratum corneum. J Invest Dermatol 2003; 120(4):655–661.
9. Jimbow K. Current update and trends in melanin pigmentation and melanin biology. Keio J Med 1995; 44(1):9–18.
10. Hadley ME, Quevedo WC Jr. Vertebrate epidermal melanin unit. Nature, 1966; 209(30):1334–1335.
11. Lambert J, Vancoillie G, Naeyaert JM. Molecular motors and their role in pigmenta-tion. Cell Mol Biol (Noisy-le-grand)1999; 45:905–918.
12. Jimbow K, Sugiyama S. Melanosomal translocation and transfer. In: Nordlund JJ, Boissy RE, Hearing VJ, King RA, Ortonne J-P, eds. The Pigmentary System. New York: Oxford University Press, 1998:107–114.
13. Wu X, Hammer JA. Making sense of melanosome dynamics in mouse melanocytes. Pigment Cell Res 2000;13:241–247.
14. Seiberg M. Keratinocyte-melanocyte interactions during melanosome transfer. Pigment Cell Res 2001; 14(4):236–242.
15. Fuchs E. Epidermal differentiation: the bare essentials. J Cell Biol 1990; 111(6):2807–2814.
16. Urabe K, Aroca P, Hearing VJ. From gene to protein: determination of melanin synthesis. Pigment Cell Res 1993; 6:186–192.
17. Hearing VJ, King RA. Determinants of skin color: melanocytes and melanization. In: Levine N, ed. Pigmentation and Pigmentary Disorders. Boca Raton, FL: CRC Press, 1993:3–33.
18. Winder A, Kobayashi T, Tsukamoto K,Urabe K, Aroca P, Kameyama K, Hearing V. The tyrosinase gene family—interactions of melanogenic proteins to regulate melanogenesis. Cell Mol Biol Res 1994; 40(7–8):613–626.
19. Sanchez-Ferrer A, Rodrigez-Lopez JN, Garcia-Canovas F, Garcia-Carmona. Tyrosinase: a comprehensive review of its mechanism. Biochem Biophys Acta 1995; 1247(1):1–11.
20. Barsh GS. The genetics of pigmentation: from fancy genes to complex traits. Trends Genet 1996; 12(8):299–305.
21. del Marmol V, Beermann. Tyrosinase and related proteins in mammalian pigmen-tation. FEBS Lett 1996; s381:165–168.

22. Pawelek JM, Chakraborty AK. The enzymology of melanogenesis. In: Nordlund JJ, Boissy RE, Hearing VJ, King RA, Ortonne J-P, eds. The Pigmentary System. New York: Oxford University Press, 1998:399–400.
23. Hearing VJ, Tsukamoto K, Urabe K, Kameyama K, Montague PM, Jackson. Functional properties of cloned melanogenic proteins. I J Pig Cell Res 1992; 5:264–270.
24. Orlow SJ, Zhou BK, Chakraborty AK, Drucker M, Orlow SJ, Pawelek JM, Pifko-Hirst S. High molecular weight forms of tyrosinase and thetyrosinase-related proteins: evidence for a melanogenic complex. J Invest Dermatol 1994; 103:196–201.
25. Winder A, Kobayashi T, Tsukamoto K,Urabe K, Aroca P, Kameyama K, Hearing V. The tyrosinase gene family—interactions of melanogenic proteins to regulate melanogenesis. Cell Mol Biol Res 1994; 40(7–8):613–626.
26. Seiberg M, Paine C, Sharlow E, Costanzo M, Andrade-Gordon P, Eisinger M, Shapiro SS. The protease-activated receptor-2 regulates pigmentation via keratinocyte–melanocyte interactions. Exp Cell Res 2000; 254(1):25–32.
27. No JK, Soung DY, Kim YJ, Shim KH, Jun YS, Rhee SH, Yokozawa T, Chung HY. Inhibition of color red tyrosinase by green tea components. Life Sci 1999; 65(21):241–246.
28. Vijayan E, Husain I, Ramaiah A, Madan NC. Purification of human skin tyrosinase and its protein inhibitor: properties of the enzyme and the mechanism of inhibition by protein. Arch Biochem Biophys 1982; 217(2):738–747.
29. Dooley TP, Gadwood RC, Kilgore K, Thomasco LM. Development of an in vitro primary screen for skin depigmentation and antimelanoma agents. Skin Pharmacol 1994; 7(4):188–200.
30. Lemic-Stojcevic L, Nias AH, Breathnach AS. Effect of azelaic acid on melanoma cells in culture. Exp Dermatol April 1995; 4(2):79–81.
31. Kwon BS, Haq AK, Kim GS, Pomerantz SH, Halaban R. Cloning and characterization of a human tyrosinase cDNA. Prog Clin Biol Res 1988; 256:273–282.
32. Kong KH, Park SY, Hong MP, Cho SH. Expression and characterization of human tyrosinase from a bacterial expression system. Comp Biochem Physiol B Biochem Mol Biol 2000; 125(4):563–569.
33. Li J, Holmes LM, Franek KJ, Wagner TE, Wei Y. Murine tyrosinase expressed by a T7 vector in bone marrow-derived dendritic progenitors effectively prevents and eradicates melanoma tumors in mice. Cancer Gene Ther 2000; 7(11):1448–1455.
34. Oetting B, King RA. Molecular approaches to the study of pigment cells. In: Nordlund JJ, Boissy RE, Hearing VJ, King RA, Ortonne J-P, eds. The Pigmentary System. New York: Oxford University Press, 1998:199–206.
35. Shibahara S. Genetic regulation of the pigment cell. In: Nordlund JJ, Boissy RE, Hearing J, King RA, Ortonne J-P, eds. The Pigmentary System. New York: Oxford University Press, 1998:251–274.
36. Bessou S, Pain C, Taieb A. Use of human skin reconstructs in the study of pigment modifiers. Arch Dermatol 1997; 133(3):331–336.
37. Nakazawa K, Kalassy M, Sahuc F, Collombel C, Damour O. Pigmented human skin equivalent—as a model of the mechanisms of control of cell–cell and cell–matrix interactions. Med Biol Eng Comput 1998; 36(6):813–820.
38. Kirsner RS. The use of Apligraf in acute wounds. J Dermatol Dec 1998; 25(12):805–811.

39. Meier F, Nesbit M, Hsu MY, Martin B, Van Belle P, Elder DE, Schaumburg-Lever G, Garbe C, Walz TM, Donatien P, et al. Human melanoma progression in skin reconstructs: biological significance of bFGF. Am J Pathol 2000; 156(1):193–200.

40. Beermann F. Advances in transgenic animal models. In: Nordlund JJ, Boissy RE, Hearing VJ, King RA, Ortonne J-P, eds. The Pigmentary System. New York: Oxford University Press, 1998:275–282.

41. Fitch KR, McGowan KA, van Raamsdonk CD, Fuchs H, Lee D, Puech A, Herault Y, Threadgill DW, Hrabe de Angelis M, Barsh GS. Genetics of dark skin in mice. Genes Dev 2003; 17(2):214–228.

42. Hruby VJ. Designing peptide receptor agonists and antagonists. Nat Rev Drug Discov 2002; 1:847–858.

43. McLeod SD, Smith C, Mason RS. Stimulation of tyrosinase in human melanocytes by pro-opiomelanocortin-derived peptides. J Endocrinol 1995; 146(3):439–447.

44. Tsatmali M, Ancans J, Thody AJ. Melanocyte function and its control by melanocortin peptides. J Histochem Cytochem 2002; 50(2):125–133.

45. Schaffer JV, Bolognia JL. The melanocortin-1 receptor: red hair and beyond. Arch Dermatol 2001; 137(11):1477–1485.

46. Adan RA, Cone RD, Burbach JP, Gispen WH. Differential effects of melanocortin peptides on neural melanocortin receptors. Mol Pharmacol Dec 1994; 46(6):1182–1190.

47. Hunt G, Todd C, Cresswell JE, Thody AJ. Alpha-melanocyte stimulating hormone and its analogue Nle4DPhe7 alpha-MSH affect morphology, tyrosinase activity and melanogenesis in cultured human melanocytes. J Cell Sci Jan 1994; 107(1):205–211.

48. Yang Y, Dickinson C, Haskell-Luevano C, Gantz I. Molecular basis for the interaction of [Nle4,D-Phe7]melanocyte stimulating hormone with the human melanocortin-1 receptor. J Biol Chem Sept 1997; 272(37):23000–23010.

49. Prusis P, Muceniece R, Mutule I, Mutulis F, Wikberg JE. Design of new small cyclic melanocortin receptor-binding peptides using molecular modelling: role of the his residue in the melanocortin peptide core. Eur J Med Chem 2001; 36(2):137–146.

50. Hruby VJ, Lu D, Sharma SD, Castrucci AL, Kesterson RA, al-Obeidi FA, Hadley ME. Cone RD cyclic lactam alpha-melanotropin analogues of Ac-Nle4-cyclo[Asp5, D-Phe7,Lys10] alpha-melanocyte-stimulating hormone-(4–10)-NH2 with bulky aromatic amino acids at position 7 show high antagonist potency and selectivity at specific melanocortin receptors. J Med Chem 1995; 38(18):3454–3461.

51. Han G, Quillan JM, Carlson K, Sadee W, Hruby VJ, Design of novel chimeric melanotropin–deltorphin analogues. Discovery of the first potent human melanocortin 1 receptor antagonist. J Med Chem 2003; 46(5):810–909.

52. Thirumoorthy R, Holder JR, Bauzo RM, Richards NG, Edison AS, Haskell-Luevano C. Novel Agouti-related-protein-based melanocortin-1 receptor antagonist. J Med Chem 2001; 44(24):4114–4124.

53. Holder JR, Haskell-Luevano C. Melanocortin tetrapeptides modified at the N-terminus, His, Phe, Arg, and Trp positions. Ann NY Acad Sci 2003; 994:36–48.

54. Graham A, Wakamatsu K, Hunt G, Ito S, Thody AJ. Agouti protein inhibits the production of eumelanin and phaeomelanin in the presence and absence of alpha-melanocyte stimulating hormone. Pigment Cell Res 1997; 10(5):298–303.

55. Schuhler S, Horan TL, Hastings MH, Mercer JG, Morgan PJ, Ebling FJ. Decrease of food intake by MC4-R agonist MTII in Siberian hamsters in long and short photoperiods. Am J Physiol Regul Integr Comp Physiol 284, 2003; 1:R227–232.

56. Wessells H, Levine N, Hadley ME, Dorr R, Hruby V. Melanocortin receptor agonists, penile erection, and sexual motivation: human studies with Melanotan II. Int J Impot Res 2002; 12(Suppl 4):S74–S79.

57. Zubair A, Lakshmi MS, Sherbet GV. Expression of alpha-melanocyte stimulating hormone and the invasive ability of the B16 murine melanoma. Anticancer Res 1992; 12(2):399–402.

58. Schauer E, Trautinger F, Kock A, Schwarz A, Bhardwaj R, Simon M, Ansel JC, Schwarz T, Luger TA. Proopiomelanocortin-derived peptides are synthesized and released by human keratinocytes. J Clin Invest 1994; 93(5):2258–2262.

59. Bhardwaj RS, Luger TA, Proopiomelanocortin production by epidermal cells: evidence for an immune neuroendocrine network in the epidermis. Arch Dermatol Res 1994; 287(1):85–90.

60. Luger TA, Paus R, Lipton JM, Slominski AT. Cutaneous Neuroimmunomodulation, the Poroopiomelanocortin System. New York: The New York Academy of Sciences, 1999.

61. Hadley ME, Wood SH, Lemus-Wilson AM, Dawson BV, Levine N, Dorr RT, Hruby VJ. Topical application of a melanotropic peptide induces systemic follicular melanogenesis. Life Sci 1987; 40(19):1889–1895.

62. Wehrle-Haller B, Weston JA. Altered cell-surface targeting of stem cell factor causes loss of melanocyte precursors in Steel17H mutant mice. Dev Biol 1999; 210(1):71–86.

63. Kunisada T, Yoshida H, Yamazaki H, Miyamoto A, Hemmi H, Nishimura E, Shultz LD, Nishikawa S, Hayashi S. Transgene expression of steel factor in the basal layer of epidermis promotes survival, proliferation, differentiation and migration of melanocyte precursors. Dev 1998; 125(15):2915–2923.

64. Hachiya A, Kobayashi A, Ohuchi A, Takema Y, Imokawa G. The paracrine role of stem cell factor/c-kit signaling in the activation of human melanocytes in ultraviolet-B-induced pigmentation. J Invest Dermatol 1996; 116(4):578–586.

65. Halaban R, Moellmann G. White mutants in mice shedding light on humans. J Invest Dermatol 1993; 100(2 suppl):176S–185S.

66. Luo D, Chen H, Searles G, Jimbow K. Coordinated mRNA expression of c-kit with tyrosinase and TRP-1 in melanin pigmentation of normal and malignant human melanocytes and transient activation of tyrosinase by Kit/SCF-R. Melanoma Res 1995; 5(5):303–309.

67. Kapur R, Everett ET, Uffman J, McAndrews-Hill M, Cooper R, Ryder J, Vik T, Williams DA. Overexpression of human stem cell factor impairs melanocyte, mast cell, and thymocyte development: a role for receptor tyrosine kinase-mediated mitogen activated protein kinase activation in cell differentiation. Blood 1997; 90(8):3018–3026.

68. Yohn JJ, Morelli JG, Walchak SJ, Rundell KB, Norris DA, Zamora MR. Cultured human keratinocytes synthesize and secrete endothelin-1. J Invest Dermatol 1993; 100(1):23–26.

69. Imokawa G, Miyagishi M, Yada Y. Endothelin-1 as a new melanogen: coordinated expression of its gene and the tyrosinase gene in UVB-exposed human epidermis. J Invest Dermatol 1995; 105(1):32–37.

70. Imokawa G, Kobayashi T, Miyagishi M, Higashi K, Yada Y. The role of endothelin-1 in epidermal hyperpigmentation and signaling mechanisms of mitogenesis and melanogenesis. Pigment Cell Res 1997; 10(4):218–228.

71. Hachiya A, Kobayashi T, Takema Y, Imokawa G. Biochemical characterization of endothelin-converting enzyme-1alpha in cultured skin-derived cells and its postulated role in the stimulation of melanogenesis in human epidermis. J Biol Chem 2002; 277(7):5395–5403.

72. Tachibana M. MITF: a stream flowing for pigment cells. Pigment Cell Res 2004; 13(4):230–240.

73. Yasumoto K, Yokoyama K, Shibata K, Tomita Y, Shibahara S. Microphthalmia-associated transcription factor as a regulator for melanocyte-specific transcription of the human tyrosinase gene. Mol Cell Bio 1994; 114:8058–8070.

74. Hemesath TJ, Price ER, Takemoto C, Badalian T, Fisher DE. MAP kinase links the transcription factor Microphthalmia to c-kit signalling in melanocytes. Nature 1998; 391:298–301, 6664.

75. Price ER, Ding HF, Badalian T, Bhattacharya S, Takemoto C, Yao TP, Hemesath TJ, Fisher DE: Lineage-specific signaling in melanocytes. C-kit stimulation recruits p300/CBP to microphthalmia. J Biol Chem 1998; 273:17983–17986.

76. Busca R, Ballotti R. Cyclic AMP a key messenger in the regulation of skin pigmentation. Pigment Cell Res 2002; 13(2):60–69.

77. Hemesath TJ, Steingrimsson E, McGill G, Hansen MJ, Vaught J, Hodgkinson CA, Arnheiter H, Copeland NG, Jenkins NA, Fisher DE. Microphthalmia, a critical factor in melanocyte development, defines a discrete transcription factor family. Genes Dev 1994; 8:2770–2780.

78. Silvers WK. Microphthalmia and other considerations. In: The Coat Colors of Mice. New York: Springer-Verlag, 1979:268–332.

79. Lin BZ, Babiarz L, Liebel F, Roydon Price E, Fisher D, Gendimenico G, Seiberg M. Modulation of microphthalmia-associated transcription factor gene expression alters skin pigmentation. J Invest Dermatol 2002; 119(6):1330–1340.

80. Park HY, Russakovsky V, Ohno S, Gilchrest BA. The beta isoform of protein kinase C stimulates human melanogenesis by activating tyrosinase in pigment cells. J Biol Chem 1993; 268(16):11742–11749.

81. Park HY, Russakovsky V, Ao Y, Fernandez E, Gilchrest BA. Alpha-melanocyte stimulating hormone-induced pigmentation is blocked by depletion of protein kinase C. Exp Cell Res 1996; 227(1):70–79.

82. Gordon PR, Gilchrest BA, Human melanogenesis is stimulated by diacylglycerol. J Invest Dermatol 1989; 93(5):700–702.

83. Mahalingam H, Vaughn J, Novotny J, Gruber JR, Niles RM. Regulation of melanogenesis in B16 mouse melanoma cells by protein kinase C. J Cell Physiol 1996; 168(3):549–558.

84. Brown EJ. Phagocytosis. BioEssays 1995; 17:109–117.

85. Kwiatkowski K, Sobota A. Signaling pathways in phagocytosis. BioEssays 1999; 21:422–431.

86. Allen LA, Aderem A. Mechanisms in phagocytosis. Curr Opin Immunol 1996; 8:36–40.

87. Wolff K, Konrad K: Phagocytosis of latex beads by epidermal keratinocytes in vivo. J Ultrastructural Res 1972; 39:262–280.

88. Nystedt S, Emilsson K, Larsson AK, Strombeck B, Sundelin J. Molecular cloning and functional expression of the gene encoding the human proteinase-activated receptor 2. Eur J Biochem 1995; 232:84–89.

89. Marthinuss J, Andrade-Gordon P, Seiberg M. A secreted serine protease can induce apoptosis in pam12 keratinocytes. Cell Grow Differ 1995; 6:807–816.

90. Santulli RJ, Derian CK, Darrow AL, Tomko KA, Eckardt AJ, Seiberg M, Scarborough RM, Andrade-Gordon P. Evidence for the presence of a protease-activated receptor distinct from the thrombin receptor in human keratinocytes. Proc Natl Acad Sci USA 1995; 92:9151–9155.

91. Dery O, Corvera CU, Steinhoff M, Bunnett NW. Proteinase-activated receptors: novel mechanisms of signaling by serine proteases. Am J Physiol 1998; 247: C1429–C1452.

92. Macfarlane SR, Seatter MJ, Kanke T, Hunter GD, Plevin R. Proteinase-activated receptors. Pharmacol Rev 2001; 53:245–282.

93. Sharlow E, Paine C, Eisinger M, Shapiro S, Seiberg M. The protease-activated receptor-2 upregulates keratinocyte phagocytosis. J Cell Sci 2000; 113:3093–3101.

94. Seiberg M, Paine C, Sharlow, Costanzo M, Andrade-Gordon P, Eisinger M, Shapiro S. Inhibition of melanosome transfer results in skin lightening. J Invest Dermatol 2000; 115(2):162–167.

95. Paine C, Sharlow E, Liebel F, Eisinger, M, Shapiro S, Seiberg M. An alternative approach to depigmentation by Soybean extracts via inhibition of the PAR-2 pathway. J Invest Dermatol 2001; 116(4):587–595.

96. Seiberg M. PAR-2 regulates pigmentation via melanosome phagocytosis. In: Ortonne JP, Balotti R, eds. Mechanisms of Tanning. London: Martin Dunitz. 2002:215–228.

97. Costanzo MJ, Maryanoff BE, Hecker LR, Schott MR, Yabut SC, Zhang H-C, Andrade-Gordon P, Kauffman JA, Lewis JM, Krishnan R, et al. A potent thrombin inhibitors that probe the S1 subsite: tripeptide transition state analogues based on a heterocycle-activated carbonyl group. J Med Chem 1996; 39:3039–3043.

98. Bosma GC, Custer RP, Bosma MJ. A severe combined immunodeficiency mutation in the mouse. Nature 1983; 301:527–530, 5900.

99. Sandhu JS, Boynton E, Gorczynski R, Hozumi N. The use of SCID mice in biotechnology and as a model for human disease. Crit Rev Biotechnol 1996; 16(1):95–118.

100. Nonoyama S, Ochs HD. Immune deficiency in SCID mice. Int Rev Immunol 1996; 13(4):289–300.

101. Hermanns JF, Petit L, Martalo O, Pierard-Franchimont C, Cauwenbergh G, Pierard GE. Unraveling the patterns of subclinical pheomelanin-enriched facial hyperpigmentation: effect of depigmenting agents. Dermatol 2000; 201(2):118–122.

102. Scott G, Deng AC, Rodriguez-Burford C, Seiberg M, Han RJ, Babiarz L, Grizzle W, Bell W, Pentland A. Protease-activated receptor-2 (PAR-2), a receptor involved in melanosome transfer, is upregulated in human skin by UV irradiation. J Invest Dermatol 2001; 117(6):1412–1420.

103. Babiarz-Magee L, Chen N, Seiberg M, Lin CB. The Expression and Activation of PAR-2 Correlate with Skin Color. Pigment Cell Res 2004; 17:241–251.

104. Niemiec SM, Ramachandran C, Weiner N. Influence of nonionic liposomal composition on topical delivery of peptide drugs into pilosebaceous units: an in vivo study using the hamster ear model. Pharm Res 1995; 12(8):1184–1188.

9

Biotechnology in Skin Care (V): UV and Sun Protection

Yasuhiro Matsumura

*Department of Immunology, The University of Texas,
M.D. Anderson Cancer Center, Houston, Texas, U.S.A.,
and Department of Dermatology, Kansai Medical University, Osaka, Japan*

Honnavara N. Ananthaswamy

*Department of Immunology, The University of Texas,
M.D. Anderson Cancer Center, Houston, Texas, U.S.A.*

INTRODUCTION

Sunlight is composed of a continuous spectrum of electromagnetic radiation that is divided into three main regions of wavelengths (Fig. 1): ultraviolet (UV), visible, and infrared. UV radiation comprises the wavelengths from 200 to 400 nm, the span of wavelengths just shorter than those of visible light (400–700 nm). UV radiation is further divided into three sections, each of which has distinct biological effects: UVA (320–400 nm), UVB (280–320 nm), and UVC (200–280 nm). UVC is effectively blocked from reaching the earth's surface by the stratospheric ozone layer. UVA and UVB radiation both reach the earth's surface in amounts sufficient to have important biological consequences to the skin and eyes. Wavelengths in the UVB region of the solar spectrum are absorbed into the skin, producing erythema, burns, and, eventually, skin cancer. Although UVA is the predominant component of solar UV radiation to which we are exposed, it is supposed to be weakly carcinogenic and to cause aging and wrinkling of the skin. In addition, the important role of UVA radiation in the induction of systemic immunosuppression is becoming a major concern.

The incidence of skin cancer has been increasing at an astonishing rate over the past several decades, and it is estimated that more than one million new cases

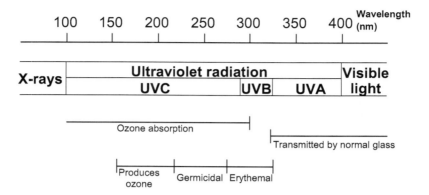

Figure 1 UV radiation spectrum and the chemical, physical, and biological effects.

of nonmelanoma skin cancer (NMSC) occur each year in the United States (1). The relevance of sunlight exposure to NMSC epidemic is well known (2). The skin responds to sun exposure by tanning and skin thickening, which provides some protection from further damage by UV irradiation. The degree of pigmentation in the skin and the ability to tan are important risk factors in skin cancer development, and the risk of NMSC is highest in people who sunburn easily and suntan poorly (1). Recent developments in molecular biology and research using laboratory animals have clarified the central role of UV radiation in NMNC carcinogenesis. UV radiation induces skin cancers by damaging the ability of keratinocytes to control cell proliferation; the cell has mechanisms to counteract this damage before cancer can develop, including DNA repair, apoptosis, and immune surveillance.

Sunscreens are the most effective and widely available intervention for sun damage that is currently available, other than sun avoidance or the use of protective clothing (3). Data from experimental studies in animals and human volunteers have clearly established that sunscreens reduce photoaging and other harmful effects of UV (4). However, sunscreens vary widely in their relative ability to screen various UV waveband components, and their testing has been applied variable to outcomes other than for erythema to determine sunburn protective factors (SPF), a measure primarily of UVB filtration only (3). SPF is defined as the ratio of the time of UV exposure necessary to produce minimally detectable erythema in sunscreen-protected skin to that for unprotected skin. Although this is a convenient endpoint for such an assessment, it is nonetheless a crude indicator of UV-induced damage. The purpose of this article is to provide an overview of recent advances in molecular mechanism of photocarcinogenesis and UV-induced immunosuppression, to assess the effectiveness and problems of sunscreens that are presently used, and to mention novel indexes and methods of photoprotection.

SHORT-TERM UV EFFECTS ON SKIN

The clinical aspects of human skin after acute UV irradiation include sunburn and immunomodulation (Fig. 2). Acute UV irradiation (a single exposure) induces DNA lesions such as pyrimidine dimers and photoproducts (4–6), which could lead to DNA mutations if they are not repaired. To prevent DNA mutations, cells are equipped with DNA repair mechanisms.

UV-induced DNA Lesions and the Repair Mechanisms

UV irradiation from 245 to 290 nm is absorbed maximally by DNA (5). UV irradiation is able to induce mutagenic photoproducts or lesions in DNA between adjacent pyrimidines in the form of dimers (6). These dimers are of two main types: cyclobutane dimers (CPDs) between adjacent thymine (T) or cytosine (C) residues and pyrimidine (4–6) photoproducts between adjacent pyrimidine residues. CPDs are formed between the C-4 and C-5 carbon atoms of any two adjacent pyrimidines; the double bonds become saturated to produce a four-membered ring (7). Similarly, (4–6) photoproducts are formed between the 5-prime 6 position and the 3-prime 4 position of two adjacent pyrimidines, most often between TC and CC residues (5). CPDs are produced three times as often overall as (4–6) photoproducts (5). Both lesions occur most frequently in areas of tandem pyrimidine residues, which are known as "hot spots" of UV-induced mutations (7). Although both lesions are potentially mutagenic, CPDs are supposed to be the major contributor to mutations in mammals (5).

All mammalian cells are equipped with several DNA repair systems, which are able to protect the cell from the effects of DNA-damaging compounds by removing DNA lesions (8). Depending upon the primary DNA lesion, one or more repair pathways become active, such as direct repair, base excision repair, mismatch repair, double-stranded break repair, and nucleotide excision

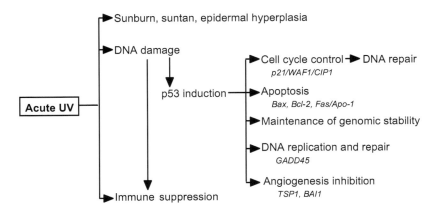

Figure 2 Effects of acute UV irradiation on the skin.

repair (NER). CPD and (4–6) photoproducts generated by UV irradiation are primarily repaired by NER, which removes bulky DNA damage (9).

If not repaired, UV-induced DNA lesions can lead to mutations in the DNA sequences. These mutations are in the form of C to T and CC to TT transitions, known as UV "signature" mutations. The "A rule" has been proposed to explain how UV signature mutations arise from DNA lesions (10). According to the A rule, DNA polymerase-eta inserts adenine (A) residues by default opposite lesions that it cannot interpret. A mutation is then created upon DNA replication of the strands containing base-pair changes. The TT cyclobutane dimers do not result in mutations because A normally is paired with T, and no mutation would result from the insertion of A residues by default opposite the dimer. However, with CC CPDs, a CC to TT transition occurs because two A residues are placed opposite the dimer by default in the place of two guanine (G) residues. In (4–6) photoproducts between a pyrimidine and a C residue, the 5-prime residue base-pairs correctly, but the 3-prime C residue resembles a noninstructional site (7). A C to T mutation occurs because an A residue is placed opposite the C residue by default.

p53 Protein, Cell Cycle Arrest, and Apoptosis

Despite the ability of human cells to repair UV-induced DNA damage, some damage will remain. The cells of the skin contain mechanisms to prevent such DNA damage from leading to skin carcinogenesis. One of these mechanisms is growth arrest followed by DNA repair, and the other is cell death by apoptosis (11). Both of these mechanisms prevent the transmission of mutations to daughter cells that can lead to transformation and carcinogenesis. The *p53* protein is important in both these mechanisms.

Upon DNA damage by acute UV irradiation, *p53* transcription is upregulated, and the *p53* protein is activated by phosphorylation of Serin 15 and Serin 20 (12). The accumulation of activated *p53* protein induces a cell cycle arrest at the G1 phase, which allows the repair of DNA damage before its replication in the S phase (13). In this pathway, *p21/WAF1/CIP1* was discovered as an inhibitor of cyclin-dependent kinase (CDK), whose induction is associated with the expression of *p53* (14). *p21/WAF1/CIP1* inactivates the CDK–cyclin complex by competitively forming a complex with CDK, thus leading the cell into G1 arrest.

If the DNA damage caused by UV irradiation is too severe and cannot be repaired, apoptotic pathways are activated to eliminate damaged cells. *p53* also plays a leading role in the apoptotic pathways. As a transactivator of transcription, *p53* protein can induce apoptosis by upregulating the expression of apoptosis-promoting genes, such as *Bax, Fas/Apo-1*, or by downregulating the expression of apoptosis-suppressing genes, such as *Bcl-2* (15). In addition, wild-type *p53* protein can activate the *Fas* gene by binding to the transcriptional activation site within the *Fas* gene as well as to its promoter region (16). Recent studies have shown that Fas/Fas-L interactions are essential for the induction of sunburnt cells in UV-irradiated mouse skin (17).

p53 also contributes to the maintenance of genomic stability (18), promotes proper DNA replication and repair via *GADD45* gene (19), and inhibits angiogenesis via *TSP1* and *BAI1* genes, which is a critical factor in the progression to malignancy (20,21). In this way, *p53* plays a pivotal role in the protection of genome, cells, and skin tissue from UV irradiation.

Immunological Responses

The skin contains Langerhans cells (LCs) that serve as antigen-presenting cells (APCs) and are capable of communicating with T, and probably non-T, lymphocytes. In addition, keratinocytes produce several cytokines that might also participate in immune recognition in the skin. These cells, together with the regional draining lymph nodes that serve them, have been labeled "skin-associated lymphoid tissues" (SALT) (22). UV irradiation induces immunosuppression by affecting this system, including suppressing contact hypersensitivity (CHS) (23) and delayed-type hypersensitivity (DTH) (24).

DNA damage is proposed to initiate UV-induced immunosuppression by the following evidence: (*i*) UV-induced suppression of CHS in American opossum, whose DNA damage is repaired by visible light-activated photoreactivating enzyme, was completely prevented by exposing opossum skin to visible light immediately after UVB irradiation (25), (*ii*) topical application of T4N5 (bacteriophage T4 endonuclease V, an excision repair enzyme for CPDs in DNA) to UVB-irradiated mouse skin prevented UVB-induced suppression of DTH and CHS responses and the induction of suppressor T cells (26), and (*iii*) IL-10, which is shown to be responsible for systemic immune suppression, is produced by cultured keratinocytes after UV irradiation but not by keratinocytes pretreated with T4N5, suggesting that UV-induced DNA damage may trigger the production of soluble immunosuppressive mediators, such as IL-10, from keratinocytes (27).

The involvement of the immune system in human skin carcinogenesis is suggested by the increased risk of malignancy in patients undergoing immunosuppressive therapies. The increased risk of skin cancer in renal transplant patients is approximately sevenfold (28), and patients treated with immunosuppressive chemotherapeutic agents also appear to be at an increased risk for the development of skin cancer (29). By analogy, the immunosuppressive state caused by UV irradiation could lead to an increased risk of skin cancers.

LONG-TERM UV EFFECTS ON SKIN

Long-term and recurrent exposure to sunlight causes the gradual deterioration of cutaneous structure and function. It apparently occurs as a result of cumulative DNA damage resulting from recurrent, acute DNA injury and from the effects

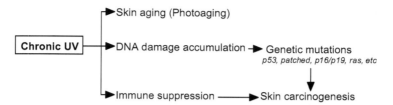

Figure 3   Effects of chronic UV irradiation on the skin.

of chronic inflammation. Those actinic damages could ultimately lead to the development of skin cancers, which is a multistep process involving induction of mutations and escape from immune surveillance (Fig. 3).

Skin Carcinogenesis

Among NMSCs, actinic keratosis (AK) is a precancerous tumor that is commonly observed on the face, the dorsa of the hands, and the bald portion of the scalp in persons who had been exposed to excessive sunlight over many years without adequate protection against it (30). When left untreated, it has been estimated that in 20% of patients with solar keratoses, squamous cell carcinoma (SCC) develops in one or more of the lesions (31). SCC is a malignant skin tumor that is derived from keratinocytes in the epidermis. The most frequent cause of SCC is AKs, and next is the scars from burns and stasis ulcers (32). The incidence of metastasis amounts to 2–3%, with death resulting in about three quarters of the patients with metastases (32). Basal cell carcinoma (BCC) is another skin cancer that is derived from basal cells of the epidermis. BCCs are observed almost exclusively on sun-exposed sites, especially on the face (33). Unlike SCCs, BCCs almost never metastasize. Multiple development of AKs, SCCs, and BCCs are often observed in xeroderma pigmentosum (XP) patients who are inherently defective in repairing UV-induced DNA damage, suggesting that UV irradiation plays the key role in NMSC tumorigenesis.

Carcinogenesis is usually thought of as a multistep process involving initiation, promotion, and progression. UV irradiation causes mutations and increases cellular proliferation; it is therefore able to cause skin cancer without additional initiators or promoters being present and is thus termed a "complete carcinogen." Carcinogenesis by UV radiation often involves the inactivation of one or more tumor-suppressor genes or the overactivation of growth-stimulatory proto-oncogenes. Tumor-suppressor genes are negative growth regulators and usually are recessive in that they require both copies of the gene to be inactivated before loss of control of cell growth occurs. Accumulation of proteins that bind to and sequester tumor-suppressor proteins can also make the cell more susceptible to further mutations. Activation of oncogenes is dominant in that a change in only one copy of the gene is required to have an effect. Proto-oncogenes, the normal versions of oncogenes, act to control cell proliferation and differentiation and are divided into three groups: growth factors and growth factor receptors, signal transduction proteins, and nuclear factors (7). Carcinogenesis can result either from the expression of a mutant or altered gene product. Several genes have been extensively studied that have important roles in skin carcinogenesis, including *p53, patched, p19,* and *ras* genes (11).

The *p53* gene is the most frequent target of genetic alteration identified so far in human cancers including NMSC (33). Loss or mutation of *p53* has been demonstrated in approximately 50% of all human cancers examined, although the frequency of mutations varies, greatly depending on the type of cancer. The basic function of *p53* protein is to maintain a cell in normal status against various extracellular stress including UV irradiation or to lead the cell into apoptosis when its DNA is severely damaged in order to prevent the carcinogenesis procedure. A number of investigators have detected *p53* gene mutations in a large proportion of human SCCs, BCCs, and AKs (11). Ziegler et al. (34) reported that *p53* gene mutations in NMSCs were detected at a high frequency (about 50–90%) compared with those of internal malignancy, and the predominant alterations are C to T and CC to TT transitions at dipyrimidine sites. One report compared multiple SCCs with and without *p53* mutations that had developed in the same patient and found that the former tended to exhibit more rapidly growing and/or histologically immature clinical features, suggesting that *p53* gene mutations would bring more malignant characteristics to UV-induced skin cancers (35).

Malignant Melanoma and UV Irradiation

Malignant melanoma incidence and mortality rates are increasing in most countries throughout the world where they are being recorded (36). The likelihood of melanoma occurring in any individual is a combination of inherited or constitutional predisposition and exposure to environmental factors relevant to tumorigenesis. The major constitutional risk factor for melanoma is skin color and skin reaction against sunlight exposure; fair-skinned people who only burn and never tan after exposure of sunlight have relatively higher incidence of melanoma (37). The only environmental risk factor that has been shown relevant to the development of melanoma is exposure to sunlight. A history of exposure to large doses of sunlight sufficient to cause sunburn in childhood is particularly important in the formation of melanoma, which could occur many years later (38). Some studies also suggest that recreational activity leading to sunburn in adulthood is also associated with the risk of melanoma (38,39).

A great advance has been seen in the analyses of the molecular mechanisms of melanoma carcinogenesis in the recent decade. Linkage analysis of familial melanoma suggested the presence of a melanoma susceptibility gene on chromosome 9p21 (40,41), and, a few years later, *p16* or *CDKN2A* gene at the locus was identified as a melanoma susceptibility gene (42,43). The germline mutations in *p16/CDKN2A* gene have been identified in familial melanomas (44,45). To date, it is estimated that approximately 20% of melanoma families worldwide are linked to *p16* mutations (46,47). Alternatively, *p16* may still be involved with gene methylation, mutations in the promoter region of the gene, which may explain the lack of *p16* mutations in 9p21-linked families (48). Melanoma has also been linked to chromosome 1p36 by linkage and loss of heterozygosity (LOH) studies, and this locus has been implicated in other cancers, which suggests the presence of a new tumor-suppressor gene in that locus (49). The intragenic mutations of *p16* gene in human sporadic melanomas were detected at frequencies of 0–26% (11). UV signature mutations occupy approximately half of the whole mutations, implying that the causal role of UV in *p16* gene mutation is not as clear-cut as in the case of *p53* gene mutations in NMSC.

PHOTOPROTECTIVE MECHANISMS OF TOPICAL SUNSCREENS

Historical Aspect

In the early twenteeth century, zinc cream was applied to the nose, lips, and cheeks for outdoor activities to prevent sunburn, with no thought of preventing skin cancer, in Western countries (50). The first documented use of sunscreen occurred in 1928 with the introduction of an emulsion composed of benzyl salicylate and benzyl cinnamate in the United States, followed by the use of a protective agent containing 10% phenyl salicylate in Australia (51). By 1935, protective lotions containing quinine oleate and quinine bisulfate had appeared in the United States (52). The first commercially available sunscreen product was introduced by L'Oreal in 1936 (53). In the 1940s, dermatologists began prescribing 2–5% *p*-aminobenzoic acid (PABA) in aqueous cream or in 70% alcohol (50). Patented in 1943, PABA led the way for the development of numerous derivatives (52). Continuing into the 1950s and 1960s, dermatologists regularly prescribed sunscreens containing PABA or its derivatives, and most of these early sunscreens were directed toward UVB. In the early 1970s, the FDA began to consider the value of sunscreens. In 1972, the FDA reclassified sunscreens from cosmetics to over-the-counter (OTC) drugs, and applied more stringent labeling requirements. In 1978, a Federal Register published the established guidelines for the formulation and evaluation of sunscreens marketed in the United States (54). These guidelines were re-evaluated in 1988 and further revised in 1993 and in 1999 (55,56). By the late 1970s, the FDA declared sunscreens as safe and effective in helping to prevent skin cancer, alleviate premature aging of the skin, and prevent sunburn (57). Dermatologists educated people on the proper use of sunscreen and of the long-term consequences of early childhood sunburn correlated to the development of skin cancer (58). Beginning in the 1990s, the sunscreen industry offered products that provided protection against UVB plus UVA radiation. Foundation makeup with sunscreen offered full-spectrum UVA protection, achieved through high pigment content and inorganic particulates. The first PABA-free sunscreen formulation with the UVA blocker

Parsol 1789 was introduced in the United States in 1993. In 1999, the FDA published the Final Sunscreen Monograph (56). Currently available products offer excellent protection from both UVB and UVA radiation. The particulate sunscreens have gained popularity over the last decade due to their low toxicity potential and effectiveness.

Current Sunscreen Filters

The increased awareness of protection against skin cancer has led to a worldwide rise in the usage of topically applied chemical sunscreen agents (59). Sunscreen agents (i.e., UV filters) are widely incorporated into skin products designed for daily use in the form of emulsions, gels, oils, and lipsticks with an adequate sun protection factor. Modern sun protection products contain a variety of UV filters to (*i*) broaden the sun protection range, (*ii*) increase the SPF, and (*iii*) reduce the concentration of particular UV filters with regard to their toxicological risk. There are two categories of sunscreen agents: Chemical (organic) filters absorb UVB/UVA radiation, and physical (inorganic) filters block UVB/UVA radiation mainly through reflection and scattering (60). Chemical filters are classified into seven groups and subdivided into either UVB or UVA filters (Table 1). Chemical filters have been the mainstay of sunscreen formulations for decades and are still used in the majority of products. However, the

Table 1 Chemical Sunscreen Filters, Their Active Agents, and Their Commercial Names

	Active agents	Commercial names
UVB filters		
p-Aminobenzoate derivatives (PABA)	2-ethylhexyl-4-dimethylaminobenzoate amyl-4-dimethylaminobenzoate	Padimate-O, Octyl Dmimethyl PABA, Escalol 507 Padimate-A, Escalol 506
Camphor derivatives	terephthalydene dicamphor sulfonic acid 4-methylbenzylidine caphor	Mexoryl SX
Cinnamate derivatives	octyl methoxycinnamate (OMC)	
Salycylate derivatives	octyl salicylate trolamine salicylate	
UVA filters		
Anthranilate derivatives	methyl anthranilate	
Benzophenone derivatives	4,4'-bis(dimethylamino) benzophenone	Michler's ketone
Dibenzoylmethane derivatives	butyl-methoxy dibenzoylmethane	Parsol 1789, Parsol A

concern regarding potential adverse health effects of chemical sunscreens have led to a reconsideration of the safety of these products (see Chap. 3–4). In response to this health concern, physical filters are used with increasing frequency because of their safety and effectiveness, particularly in blocking UVA (59). The most commonly used physical filters are titanium dioxide (TiO_2) and zinc monoxide (ZnO). Inorganic sunscreens are generally viewed as harmless substances that cannot penetrate into the skin and are not altered by light energy, unlike organic sunscreens that can be modified by sunlight (59).

The Assessment of the Effectiveness of Sunscreens

The use of cancer induction as an endpoint for assessing the effectiveness of sunscreen compounds in experimental animals is a labor-intensive, time-consuming, long-term endpoint. In addition, tumor induction cannot be studied readily in humans because of ethical considerations and the length of time involved. It is therefore important to develop other earlier endpoints that might be more accurate than erythema formation in predicting the effectiveness of sunscreens in preventing skin cancer. As mentioned in chapter 2, analyses of human skin cancers and UV-induced mouse skin cancers for *p53* gene mutations have provided new insights into the molecular mechanisms by which UV radiation induces skin cancer. The mutant *p53*-positive clusters are detected well before the appearance of skin cancers in UVB-irradiated mouse skin (61), and *p53* gene mutations are considered to be causally related to skin cancer development (62). Ananthaswamy et al. (63) investigated if sunscreen application would block the induction of *p53* gene mutations with using a UVB-absorbing sunscreen and a sunscreen that absorbed both UVB and UVA (both had a human SPF of 15) in mouse models chronically irradiated with FS-40 sunlamps. They found that both sunscreens significantly blocked the induction of *p53* gene mutations in irradiated skin. Compared with the UV + vehicle-treated control, they noted an 88% reduction in mutation frequency when the UVB-absorbing sunscreen was applied, and noted a 92% reduction when the UVB- and UVA-absorbing sunscreen was applied. They repeated the studies with an UV solar simulator, and the results were identical to those described above (64). In order to test the hypothesis that blocking sunlight-induced p53 mutations should interfere with the development of skin cancer, they irradiated groups of mice with UV solar stimulator without or with sunscreen application (64). The results indicated that 100% of mice that received a cumulative dose of $1000 \, kJ/m^2$ of UVB only, or vehicle +UVB, developed skin tumors, whereas the probability of tumor development in all the mice treated with the sunscreens $+1000 \, kJ/m^2$ of UVB was 2%, and those two sunscreens were almost equally effective in preventing skin tumor development (Fig. 4). They concluded that the mutagenic and carcinogenic effect of solar-simulator radiation is caused mainly by UVB and not UVA wavelengths.

UV-induced immunosuppression is another harmful influence as well as DNA damage; however, the action spectrum on immunosuppression has not

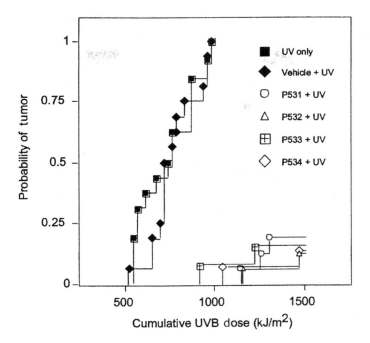

Figure 4 Sunscreen application prevents UV-induced skin cancer induction in mouse models. Sunscreen preparations containing only UVB absorbers (P531 and P532) or both UVB and UVA absorbers (P533 and P534) were applied to the dorsal skin of mice 30 minutes before each UV exposure. Both types of sunscreens were effective to the same extent in preventing skin cancer formation. *Source*: Ref. Adapted from 64.

been clarified, especially in the case of human skin (65). Nghiem et al. (66) compared the immunosuppressive effects of UVA I (340–400 nm) only, UVA only, and UVA + UVB radiation in the solar-simulated radiation in mouse models. As a result, dose-response curves for immune suppression observed in mice exposed to UVA + UVB, or UVA only, were identical. On the other hand, no immune suppression was noted when the mice were irradiated with UVA I only, indicating that UVA II (320–340 nm) present in the solar-simulated radiation was responsible for suppressing established immune reactions. In addition, they confirmed the finding by using two sunscreens: P532 that only absorbs in the UVB region of the spectrum and P533 that absorbs both UVB and UVA (66). Both sunscreens had a human SPF of 15. No immune protection was observed when P532 was applied to the mice prior to UV exposure. When P533 was applied 30 minutes prior to UV exposure, no immune suppression was observed, which implies that UVA radiation is the critical wavelength for suppressing established immune reactions and that UVA protection is indispensable for preventing UV-induced immunosuppression. Because UVA is more immunosuppressive than it is erythromogenic (65), SPF would not be sufficient to predict the ability of sunscreens to protect from UV-induced immune suppression. Considering different photobiological mechanisms are involved in suppressing the induction of immunity (UVB) and the elicitation of immunity (UVAII), complete immune protection requires a sunscreen that absorbs both UVB and UVA radiation.

Problems of Present Sunscreens

PABA, which filters out some but not all the UVB radiation, has been widely used for many years, although harmful side effects of sensitizing the formation of pyrimidine dimers were reported (67,68). One of PABA derivatives, 2-ethylhexyl-4-dimethylaminobenzoate, is assumed to produce very reactive oxygen species upon illumination and thus to be mutagenic (69). Another PABA derivative, amyl-4-dimethylaminobenzoate, is known to cause photoallergies and other skin problems (69). TiO_2 is also reported to be genotoxic to human skin (70). Ultrafine sunscreen-grade TiO_2 irradiated with simulated sunlight is photocatalytically active and is harmful to supercoiled plasmid DNA, causing single- and double-strand breaks (71). Photoexcited TiO_2 specimens were shown to inflict similar DNA damage in the nuclei of human skin cells (71).

The potential permeation of the UV filters through skin and the subsequent toxic effects should not be neglected. Up to 2% of an applied dose of benzophenone and its metabolites were found to be excreted in the urine in humans (72). 2-ethylhexyl-4-dimethylaminobenzoate is absorbed through human skin and is 32–36% metabolized, the rest remaining unaffected (73).

Since most commercial formulations employ a combination of chemical and physical filters to provide broadband protection over the UVB and UVA regions, the combination might affect the UV protective ability of each ingredient. The combination of octyl methoxycinnamate (OMC) and butyl-methoxy dibenzoylmethane, for example, is not recommended, because photoadducts are formed between OMC and photogenerated fragments of butyl-methoxy dibenzoylmethane and lead to its photoinstability (60).

NEW MEASURES OF PHOTOPROTECTION

Novel Indexes of Sun Protection

Rouabhia et al. (74) evaluated the effect of physical sunscreen on CPDs and (4–6) photoproducts formation using engineered human skin (EHS) exposed to increasing doses of simulated sunlight (SSL). They determined the degree of sunscreen protection against DNA damage accordingly and defined a DNA damage protection factor (DNA-PF). Because CPDs and (4–6) photoproducts formation is closely relevant to UV-induced carcinogenesis, DNA-PF could be a novel index of sunscreen efficacy against skin cancer by further tumorigenesis studies using animal models and DNA damage determinations in human skin in vivo. From a carcinogenesis point of view, however, protection against endpoints that are associated with chronic UV effects are preferable to endpoints that are associated with acute UV effects. In that sense, the measurement of mutant *p53*-positve clusters after four to eight weeks of UV-irradiated mouse skin with or without topical application of sunscreen compounds could be more appropriate biological endpoint (62).

Determination of an immune protection factor (IPF) has been proposed as an alternative or adjunctive measure to SPF, and recent studies show that IPF can indeed detect added in vivo functionality of sunscreens, such as high levels of UVA protection that SPF cannot (3). IPF is measured using various in vivo outcome factors, such as contact sensitivity induction, contact sensitivity elicitation, delayed-type hypersensitivity elicitation, antigen-presenting cell function or numbers, and cytokine modification including IL-10. However, the universal definition of IPF has not been determined yet. Development of IPF standards for regulatory or product claim purposes would allow the integration of both UVB and non-UVB (UVA, blue, and infrared) solar waveband effect-reversals, would be applied to other ingredients with protective function, such as antioxidants and retinoids, and would spur development of more advanced and complete protection products.

Perspectives on Sun Protection and Skin Cancer Prevention

The desirable site of action of the UV filters is restricted to the skin surface or to the uppermost part of the stratum corneum. However, it has been demonstrated that penetration into skin, permeation through skin, and retention of UV filters in the skin from topical products can differ significantly between formulations used (75). It is evident that future vehicle development is aimed at formulating vehicles that support penetration of the UV filters only into the uppermost part of the stratum corneum. At the same time, the UV filters should be retained at this location and permeation through the skin should be prevented. In addition, each ingredient in a cosmetic (or OTC) product should ideally exert no photosensitizing effect, should be photochemically stable and nontoxic to human skin and DNA, and should not unfavorably affect another. Several sunscreens containing new chemicals or specimens that have more stable and less harmful characteristics are currently under investigation.

Because UV-induced DNA damage, *p53* mutation, proliferation, and immunosuppression are key events in skin cancer development, inhibition of one or more of these events may protect against skin cancer development (Fig. 5). Use of sunscreens alone may not be sufficient to prevent skin cancer because they are limited by cases of noncompliance and, when they are used, must be applied before each exposure to sunlight and reapplied every few hours or after coming into contact with water. Because of these limitations, it may be difficult to completely prevent such events as DNA damage and *p53* mutation. Thus, in addition to the lotions containing sunscreens that are

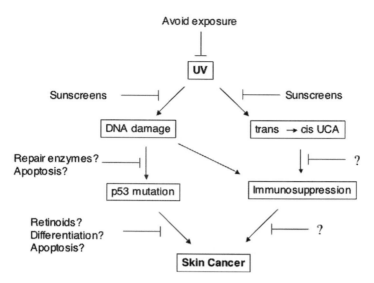

Figure 5 A model for key events in UV-induced skin damage and skin cancer and potential intervention points.

applied before exposure, the use of creams containing agents that enhance the repair of UV-induced DNA damage after sun exposure may abrogate key events in photocarcinogenesis. In fact, recent studies have shown that the treatment of UV-irradiated mouse skin with liposomes containing T4N5 endonuclease or DNA photolyase enhanced the DNA repair of UV-induced pyrimidine dimers and abrogated UV-induced suppression of CHS (76) and IL-10 release from keratinocytes (77). Recently, Yarosh et al. reported the effectiveness of topically applied T4N5 liposome lotion in preventing skin cancer development in XP patients without significant adverse effects (78). In addition, comprehensive skin cancer prevention plans should also include intervention strategies that are directed at later stages of UV-induced carcinogenesis, such as preventing cells containing *p53* mutations from progressing into a tumor or preventing secondary skin tumors. The development and use of new drugs that can scavenge free radicals, or can induce differentiation or apoptosis of premalignant cells, may provide a novel intervention. To date, retinoids (derivatives of vitamin A) (79), green tea polyphenols, silymarin (80), butyrated hydroxytoluene, and carotenoids (81) have been reported to be effective in reducing the incidence of UV-induced skin cancers. Among them, retinoids may be most applicable or effective in reducing the number and severity of new skin cancers in high-risk patients who present with single or multiple primary skin cancers (82). Further study should lead to a greater understanding of the genetic and immune suppression pathways in UV-induced carcinogenesis and, as a result, to more effective protective measures and/or restorative treatment.

SUMMARY

UV irradiation generally causes "more harm than good" in normal human skin and could ultimately result in skin cancer development. According to the recommendations to prevent skin cancer development by International Agency for Research on Cancer (IARC), the most effective way to protect against solar UV irradiation is staying indoors in the midday and wearing adequate clothing (83). In addition, the use of sunscreens is also recommended as a means of accomplishing this purpose. The development of skin tumors is a multistep process involving induction of mutations and escape from immune surveillance. DNA photoproducts induced by UV irradiation may be repaired, lead to cell death, or result in a mutation. Mutations may occur in the repair genes themselves or in oncogenes and tumor-suppressor genes. Impairment of immunologic containment of outgrowth of the transformed cell may be initiated via DNA damage, photoisomerization of urocanic acid, cell membrane damage, or cytokine release. Topical application of sunscreens can block both of the pathways, thus protecting skin cancer development. The continuing studies will result in a greater understanding of the genetic and immune suppression pathways mentioned in this review, and the development of more efficient protective measures of skin cancers as well as actual repair of pre-existing photodamage to skin.

ACKNOWLEDGMENT

This study was supported by NIH grant R01-CA-46523 to H.N.A.

REFERENCES

1. Gloster HM, Brodland DG. The epidemiology of skin cancer. Dermatol Surg 1996; 22:217–226.
2. Strom S. Epidemiology of basal and squamous cell carcinomas of the skin. In: Weber R, Miller M, Goepfert H, eds. Basal and Squamous Cell Skin Cancers of the Head and Neck. Baltimore, MD: Williams and Wilkins, 1996:1–7.
3. Cooper KD, Baron ED, LeVee G, Stevens SR. Protection against UV-induced suppression of contact hypersensitivity responses by sunscreens in humans. Exp Dermatol 2002; 11(suppl 1):20–27.
4. Hawk JLM. Cutaneous photoprotection. Arch Dermatol 2003; 139:527–530.
5. Tornaletti S, Pfeifer GP. UV damage and repair mechanisms in mammalian cells. BioEssays 1996; 18:221–228.
6. Ananthaswamy HN. Ultraviolet light as a carcinogen. In: Bowden GT, Fischer SM, eds. Comprehensive Toxicology, Vol. 12. Chemical Carcinogens and Anticarcinogens. Oxford: Pergamon, 1997:255–279.
7. Kanjilal S, Ananthaswamy HN. Molecular biology of skin carcinomas. In: Weber R, Miller M, Goepfert H, eds. Basal and Squamous Cell Skin Cancers of the Head and Neck. Baltimore, MD: Williams and Wilkins, 1996:25–26.
8. Wood RD. DNA repair in eukaryotes. Ann Rev Biochem 1996; 65:135–167.
9. Lehmann AR. Nucleotide excision repair and the link with transcription. Trends Biochem Sci 1995; 20:402–405.

10. Tessman I, Liu SK, Kennedy MA. Mechanism of SOS mutagenesis of UV-irradiated DNA: mostly error-free processing of deaminated cytosine. Proc Natl Acad Sci USA 1992; 89:1159–1163.

11. Matsumura Y, Ananthaswamy HN. Molecular mechanisms of photocarcinogenesis. Front Biosci 2002; 7:D765–783.

12. Prives C, Hall PA. The p53 pathway. J Pathol 1999; 187:112–126.

13. Huang LC, Clarkin KC, Wahl GM. Sensitivity and selectivity of the DNA damage sensor responsible for activating p53-dependent G1 arrest. Proc Natl Acad Sci USA 1996; 93:4827–4832.

14. Harper JW, Adami GR, Wei N, Keyomarsi K, Elledge SJ. The p21 cdk-interacting protein Cip1 is a potent inhibitor of G1 cyclin-dependent kinases. Cell 1993; 75:805–816.

15. Mullauer L, Gruber P, Sebinger D, Buch J, Wohlfart S, Chott A. Mutations in apoptosis genes: a pathogenetic factor for human disease. Mutat Res 2001; 488:211–231.

16. Muller M, Wilder D, Bannasch D, Israeli K, Lehibach M, Li-Weber SL. p53 activates the CD95 (APO1/Fas) gene in response to DNA damage by anticancer drugs. J Exp Med 1998; 188:2033–2045.

17. Hill LL, Ouhtit A, Loughlin SM, Kripke ML, Ananthaswamy HN, Owen-Schaub LB. Fas ligand: a sensor for DNA damage critical in skin cancer etiology. Science 1999; 285:898–900.

18. Lane DP. p53, guardian of the genome. Nature 1992; 358:15–16.

19. Kastan MB, Zhan Q, El-Deiry WS, Carrier F, Jacks T, Walsh WV, Plunkett BS, Vogelstein B, Fornace AJ Jr. A mammalian cell cycle checkpoint pathway utilizing p53 and GADD45 is defective in ataxia-telangiectasia. Cell 1992; 71:587–597.

20. Dameron KM, Volpert OV, Tainsky MA, Bouck N. Control of angiogenesis in fibroblasts by p53 regulation of thrombospondin-1. Science 1994; 265:1582–1584.

21. Nishimori H, Shiratsuchi T, Urano T, Kimura Y, Kiyono K, Tatsumi K, Yoshida S, Ono M, Kuwano M, Nakamura Y, Tokino T. A novel brain-specific p53-target gene, BAI1, containing thrombospondin type 1 repeats inhibits experimental angiogenesis. Oncogene 1997; 15:2145–2150.

22. Streilein JW, Tigelaar RE. SALT: Skin-associated lymphoid tissue. In: Parrish JA, ed. Photoimmunology. New York: Plenum, 1983:95–103.

23. Noonan FP, Kripke ML, Pedersen GM, Greene MI. Suppression of contact hypersensitivity in mice by ultraviolet irradiation is associated with defective antigen presentation. Immunology 1981; 43:527–533.

24. Molendijk A, van Gurp RJ, Donselaar IG, Benner R. Suppression of delayed-type hypersensitivity to histocompatibility antigens by ultraviolet radiation. Immunology 1987; 62:299–305.

25. Applegate LA, Ley RD, Alcalay J, Kripke ML. Identification of the molecular target for the suppression of contact hypersensitivity by UV radiation. J Exp Med 1989; 170:1117–1131.

26. Kripke ML, Alas LG, Yarosh DB. Pyrimidine dimers in DNA initiate systemic immunosuppression in UV-irradiated mice. Proc Natl Acad Sci USA 1992; 89:7516–7520.

27. Nishigori C, Yarosh DB, Ullrich SE, Vink AA, Bucana CD, Roza L, Kripke ML. Evidence that DNA damage triggers interleukin 10 cytokine production in UV-irradiated murine keratinocytes. Proc Natl Acad Sci USA 1996; 93:10354–10359.

28. Hoxtell EO, Mandel JS, Murray SS, Schuman LM, Goltz RW. Incidence of skin carcinoma after renal transplantation. Arch Dermatol 1977; 113:436–438.

29. Hill BHR. Immunosuppressive drug therapy potentiator of skin tumors in five patients with lymphoma. Aust J Dermatol 1976; 17:46–52.

30. Lever WF, Schaumburg-Lever G. Histopathology of the skin. 7th ed. Philadelphia, PA: J.B. Lippincott, 1990:542–546.

31. Lever WF, Schaumburg-Lever G. Histopathology of the skin. 7th ed. Philadelphia, PA: J.B. Lippincott, 1990:552–563.

32. Lever WF, Schaumburg-Lever G. Histopathology of the skin. 7th ed. Philadelphia, PA: J.B. Lippincott, 1990:622–634.

33. Hollstein M, Sidransky D, Vogelstein B, Harris CC. *p53* mutation in human cancers. Science 1991; 253:49–53.

34. Ziegler A, Jonason AS, Leffell DJ, Simon JA, Sharma HW, Kimmelmann J, Remington L, Jacks T, Brash DE. Sunburn and p53 in the onset of skin cancer. Nature 1994; 372:773–776.

35. Matsumura Y, Sato M, Nishigori C, Zghal M, Yagi T, Imamura S, Takebe H. High prevalence of mutations in the p53 gene in poorly differentiated squamous cell carcinomas in xeroderma pigmentosum patients. J Invest Dermatol 1995; 105:399–401.

36. Marks R. Epidemiology of melanoma. Clin Exp Dermatol 2001; 25:459–463.

37. Evans RD, Kopf AW, Lew RA, Rigel DS, Bart RS, Friedman RJ, Rivers LK. Risk factors for the development of malignant melanoma I. Review of case-control studies. J Dermatol Surg Oncol 1988; 14:393–406.

38. Whiteman DC, Whiteman CA, Green AC. Childhood sun exposure as a risk factor for melanoma: a systematic review of epidemiologic studies. Cancer Causes Cont 2001; 12:69–82.

39. Elwood M, Jopson J. Melanoma and sun exposure: an overview of published studies. Int J Cancer 1997; 73:198–203.

40. Cannon-Albright LA, Goldgar DE, Meyer LJ, Lewis CM, Anderson DE, Fountain JW, Hagi ME, Wiseman RW, Kwiatkowski DJ, Piepkorn MW, et al. Assignment of a locus for familial melanoma, MLM, to chromosome 9p13-p22. Science 1992; 258:1148–1152.

41. Fountain JW, Karayiorgon M, Ernstoff MS, Kirkwood JM, Vlock DR, Titus-Ernstoff L, Bouchard B, Vijayasaradhi S, Houghton AN, Lahti J, et al. Homozygous deletions within human chromosome band 9p21 in melanoma. Proc Natl Acad Sci USA 1992; 89:10557–10561.

42. Kamb A, Gruis NA, Weaver-Feldhaus J, Liu Q, Harshman K, Tavtigian SV, Stockert E, Day RS, Johnson BE, Skolnick MH. A cell cycle regulator potentially involved in genesis of many tumor types. Science 1994; 264:436–440.

43. Nobori T, Miura K, Wu DJ, Lois A, Takabayashi K, Carson DA. Deletions of the cyclin-dependent kinase-4 inhibitor gene in multiple human cancers. Nature 1994; 368:753–756.

44. Hussussian CJ, Struewing JP, Goldstein AM, Higgins PA, Ally DA, Sheahan MD. Germline mutations in familial melanoma. Nat Genet 1994; 8:15–21.

45. Gruis NA, van der Velden PA, Sandkuijl LA, Prins DE, Weaver-Feldhaus J, Kamb A, Bergman W, Frants RR. Homozygotes for CDKN2 (p16) germline mutation in Dutch familial melanoma kindreds. Nat Genet 1995; 10:351–353.

46. Foulkes WD, Flanders TY, Ploock PM, Hayward NK. The CDKN2 (p16) gene and human cancer. Mol Med 1997; 3:5–20.

47. Greene MH. The genetics of hereditary melanoma and naevi 1998 update. Cancer 1999; 86:2464–2477.

48. Harland M, Holland EA, Ghiorzo P, Mantelli M, Bianchi-Scarra G, Goldstein AM, Tucker MA, Ponder BA, Mann GJ, Bishop DT, et al. Mutation screening of the CDKN2A promoter in melanoma families. Genes Chromosomes Cancer 2000; 28:45–57.
49. Smedley D, Sidhar S, Birdall S, Bennett D, Herlyn M, Cooper C, Shipley J. Characterization of chromosome 1 abnormalities in malignant melanomas. Genes Chromosomes Cancer 2000; 28:121–125.
50. Mackie BS, Mackie LE. The PABA story. Austral J Dermatol 1999; 40:51–53.
51. Groves G. The sunscreen industry in Australia; past, present, and future. In: Lowe NJ, Shaath NA, eds. Sunscreen. New York: Marcel Dekker, 1997.
52. Safer and more successful suntanning. Consumers Guide. New York: Wallaby Pocketbooks, 1979:1–33.
53. Rebut D. The sunscreen industry in Europe; past, present, and future. In: Lowe NJ, Shaath NA, eds. Sunscreen. New York: Marcel Dekker, 1997.
54. Sunscreen products for over-the-counter use. Federal Register 43. 1978:28269.
55. Sunscreen drug products for over-the-counter human use: tentative final monograph: proposed rule. Federal Register 58. 1993:28194–28302.
56. Sunscreen drug products for over-the-counter human use: final monograph: final rule. Federal Register 64. U.S. Food and Drug Administration, 1999:27666–27693.
57. Sikes R. The history of suntanning; a love/hate affair. J Aesthet Sci 1998; 1:6–7.
58. Gasparro FP. Sunscreens, skin photobiology, and skin cancer: the need for UVA protection and evaluation of efficiency. Environ Health Perspect 2000; 108:71–78.
59. Gasparro FP, Mitchnick M, Nash JF. A review of sunscreen safety and efficacy. Photochem Photobiol 1998; 68:243–256.
60. Sunscreen drug products for over-the-counter human use: Final Monograph, Federal Register 64. Rockville, MD: U.S. Food and Drug Administration, 2000:27666.
61. Berg RJ, van Kranen HJ, Rebel HG, de Vries A, van Vloten WA, van Kreijl CF, van der Leun JC, de Gruijl FR. Early p53 alterations in mouse skin carcinogenesis by UVB radiation: immunohistochemical detection of mutant p53 protein in clusters of preneoplastic epidermal cells. Proc Natl Acad Sci USA 1996; 93:274–278.
62. Ananthaswamy HN, Ullrich SE, Kripke ML. Inhibition of UV-induced p53 mutations and skin cancers by sunscreens: implication for skin cancer prevention. Exp Dermatol 2002; 11(suppl 1):40–43.
63. Ananthaswamy HN, Loughlin SM, Cox P, Evans RL, Ullrich SE, Kripke ML. Sunlight and skin cancer: inhibition of p53 mutations in UV-irradiated mouse skin by sunscreens. Nat Med 1997; 3:510–514.
64. Ananthaswamy HN, Ullrich SE, Mascotto RE, Fourtanier A, Loughlin SM, Khaskina P, Bucana CD, Kripke ML. Inhibition of solar simulator-induced p53 mutations and protection against skin cancer development in mice by sunscreens. J Invest Dermatol 1999; 112:763–768.
65. Young AR, Walker SL. Effects of solar simulated radiation on the human immune system: influence of phototypes and wavebands. Exp Dermatol 2002; 11(suppl 1): 17–19.
66. Nghiem DX, Kazimi N, Clydesdale G, Ananthaswamy HN, Kripke ML, Ullrich SE. Ultraviolet A radiation suppresses an established immune response: implications for sunscreen design. J Invest Dermatol 2001; 117:1193–1199.
67. Sutherland BM. p-Aminobenzoic acid-sunlamp sensitization of pyrimidine dimer formation and transformation in human cells. Photochem Photobiol 1982; 36:95–97.

68. Sutherland C, Griffin KP. p-Aminobenzoic acid can sensitize the formation of pyrimidine dimers in DNA: direct chemical evidence. Photochem Photobiol 1984; 40:391–394.
69. Serpone N, Salinaro A, Emeline AV, Horikoshi S, Hidaka H, Zhao J. An in vitro systematic spectroscopic examination of the photostabilities of a random set of commercial sunscreen lotions and their chemical UVB/UVA active agents. Photochem Photobiol Sci 2002; 1:970–981.
70. Nagakawa Y, Wakuri S, Sakamoto K, Tanaka N. The photogenoxicity of titanium dioxide particles. Mutat Res 1997; 394:125–132.
71. Dunford R, Salinaro A, Cai L, Serpone N, Horikoshi S, Hidaka H, Knowland J. Chemical oxidation and DNA damage catalyzed by inorganic sunscreen ingredients. FEBS Lett 1997; 418:87–90.
72. Hayden CG, Roberts MS, Benson HA. Systemic absorption of sunscreen after topical application. Lancet 1997; 350:863–864.
73. Kenney GE, Sakr A, Lichtin JL, Chou H, Bronangh RL. In vitro skin absorption and metabolism of Padimate-O and a nitrosamine formed in Padimate-O-containing cosmetic products. J Soc Cosmet Chem 1995; 46:117–127.
74. Rouabhia M, Mitchell DL, Rhainds M, Claveau J, Drouin R. A physical sunscreen protects engineered human skin against artificial solar ultraviolet radiation-induced tissue and DNA damage. Photochem Photobiol Sci 2002; 1:471–477.
75. Chatelain E, Gabard B, Surber C. Skin penetration and sun protection factor of five UV filters: effect of the vehicle. Skin Pharmacol Appl Skin Physiol 2003; 16:28–35.
76. Vink AA, Yarosh DB, Kripke ML. Chromophore for UV-induced immunosuppression: DNA. Photochem Photobiol 1996; 63:383–386.
77. Nishigori C, Yarosh DB, Ullrich SE, Vink AA, Bucana CD, Roza L, Kripke ML. Evidence that DNA damage triggers interleukin 10 cytokine production in UV-irradiated murine keratinocytes. Proc Natl Acad Sci USA 1996; 93:10354–10359.
78. Yarosh D, Klein J, O'Connor A, Hawk J, Rafal E, Wolf P. Effect of topically applied T4 endonuclease V in liposomes on skin cancer in xeroderma pigmentosum: a randomised study. Lancet 2001; 357:926–929.
79. Moon TE, Levine N, Cartmel B, Bangert JL. Retinoids in prevention of skin cancer. Cancer Lett 1997; 114:203–205.
80. Agarwal R, Mukhtar H, Cancer chemoprevention by polyphenols in green tea and artichoke. Adv Exp Med Biol 1996; 401:35–50.
81. Black HS, Mathews-Roth MM. Protective role of butylated hydroxytoluene and certain carotenoids in photocarcinogenesis. Photochem Photobiol 1991; 53:707–716.
82. Rook AH, Jaworsky C, Nguyen T, Grossman RA, Wolfe JT, Witmer WK, Kligman AM. Beneficial effect of low-dose systemic retinoid in combination with topical tretinoin for the treatment and prophylaxis of premalignant and malignant skin lesions in renal transplant recipients. Transplantation 1995; 59:714–719.
83. Vainio H, Bianchini F, eds. IARC Handbook of Cancer Prevention. Vol. 5. Sunscreens. Lyon, France: International Agency for Research on Cancer, 2001.

10

Biotechnology in Hair Care (I): Overview

Daniela Kessler-Becker

Henkel KGaA, Corporate Biological Research, Dusseldorf, Germany

INTRODUCTION: HAIR FUNCTION

The hair appendage is an important part of human skin. Nearly the whole surface (approximately 90%) of the human body is covered with hair, and the total number of hairs on the body surface of an adult is impressive: Approximately 5,000,000 hairs can be found there of which 100,000 to 110,000 cover the scalp at a density of 175–300 hairs/cm^2 (1). During mammalian evolution, hair had an outstanding biological importance in regulating various physiological processes (Table 1). As stratified epithelium, hair generally provides protection against heat loss and environmental influences, such as mechanical injuries or ultraviolet (UV) irradiation from sunlight. Other important functions of hair are the indication of sexual development of an individual, enhancement of attractiveness, and social communication. Hair also functions as a sensory organ, which can be deduced from the fact that various hair follicles are connected with a complex nerve network that provides sensory information about the environment.

However, for human beings these primary biological functions nowadays are less important. Due to social aspects and cosmetic considerations, secondary functions of hair are in the focus of interest today: Hair styling, treatment, and modification have a long history in different cultures (2), and hairstyles even mark the identification of an individual with a certain part of society. Furthermore, human hair growth generally is regarded as a sign of vitality, power, and individuality, and such dysfunctions as regression and loss of scalp hair often evoke negative associations, for example, aging aspects and diseases that can

Table 1   Functions of the Human Hair Shaft

Functions of the hair shaft
Decoration; social communication and camouflage
Protection against trauma and insect penetration
Protect against electromagnetic radiation
Provide a sensory "antennae" to feel the environment
Insulation against heat loss and heat gain
Mechanisms of cleansing skin surface
Mechanisms of outward transport of environmental signals: sebum, pheromones

Source: From Ref. 11.

lead to stress conditions with diminished body image satisfaction and altered psychological functioning of an individual (3).

All these examples show that hair and hair care are important parts of many people's lives, and, therefore, hair is an important topic of personal care. But what does that imply? On the one hand, development of hair-care products primarily deals with the visible but biologically "lifeless" part of the hair, namely the hair shaft or hair fiber. From a cosmetic point of view, there is a strong desire to protect the hair shaft from external influences or to modify and enhance hair color, hair volume, and its manageability (4). On the other hand, the "living" part of the hair, the hair root, has come more and more into focus of interest due to enormous progress in biological and medical sciences. Stimulation or modification of this specialized, metabolically active part, may in the future, offer unlimited possibilities to influence hair growth, color, and structure in a biological manner. However, the complex mode of hair formation is still not fully understood. A basic insight into hair in its entirety—that is, the mechanisms that govern growth, structure, and pigmentation of human hair, as well as the morphology and composition of the fibrous structures of the visible part of human hair— facilitates proper development of innovative and effective hair-care products adapted to the biological characteristics of this specialized structure. This chapter shall give a basic overview of human hair physiology, function, and properties of the living as well as the lifeless components of this, fascinating "miniorgan" (5). Furthermore, examples of current hair-care applications will be introduced to elucidate interesting topics and problems in hair care. Last but not least, integration of biotechnological approaches, the challenges, and the future perspectives of novel products developed by biotechnological means will be discussed.

HAIR: MORPHOLOGICAL STRUCTURE, PROPERTIES, AND PHYSIOLOGY

The term "hair" describes a complex biological unit consisting of a visible hair shaft and a hair root that is located under the surface of the skin. Within these different compartments, a variety of highly complex biological and biochemical processes are coordinated. The visible hair shaft, a thin keratinized structure with specialized fiber properties, is very often regarded as the lifeless part of the hair because it lacks cellular activities, whereas the hair root contains the living hair follicle, which is home to numerous cellular and biochemical interactions responsible for proper fiber formation (Fig. 1). The hair follicle consists of different specialized epithelial and connective tissue layers, surrounded by vascular structures, nonstriated muscles (musculus arrector pili), and nerve endings forming a neuronal network (reviewed in 6). In the hair follicle, most biological activities, such as cell growth, differentiation, and proliferation as well as many biochemical processes (e.g., pigment formation), are located. Additionally, on many sites of the body hair follicles are associated with sebaceous glands.

Between different body regions, size and distribution of hair follicles and the type of hair fibers being produced varies, although the basic morphology of hair generally is similar (7). Differences occur in terms of size, length, diameter, formation cycle, structural variations of the fiber, and response to steroidal

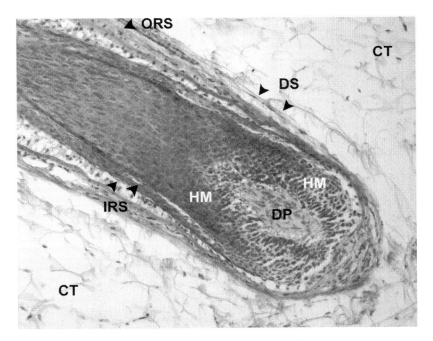

Figure 1 Vertical cross-section of a human scalp hair follicle in anagen stage showing a large vascularized DP located within the lowest part of the follicle, HM, IRS, and parts of the ORS. The whole follicle is enclosed by the DS and embedded into the CT of the surrounding dermis (picture: M. Giesen, Henkel KGaA). *Abbreviations*: DP, dermal papilla; HM, hair matrix; IRS, inner root sheath; ORS, outer root sheath; DS, dermal sheath; CT, connective tissue.

hormones. A classification according to the parameters size and length distinguishes the following types of human hair (8):

> Lanugo hair is the first hair fiber produced by a hair follicle in an embryo. It is soft and thin, without medulla, and of variable length. Later on, it is replaced by vellus hair.
> Vellus hair can be described as short, fine, and rarely pigmented hair that generally covers the body surface. It is usually not longer than 2 cm.
> Terminal hair derives from larger hair follicles. It is coarse, thick (30–120 μm), usually pigmented, and of variable length. During the lifetime of an individual, a hair follicle is capable of producing vellus hair first before switching to the production of terminal hair. Also, the reverse process can be found: The switch from terminal to vellus-like structure is a typical sign of hair regression during male-pattern baldness.

Another interesting fact is that hair follicles from different body sites differ in their response to hormonal factors (9). Many hair follicles show no or only little response to female or male hormones (e.g., eyebrows, lashes, hair of hand or feet, nonbalding scalp hair), but follicles from other regions are extremely sensitive to varying concentrations of male and female hormones (e.g., beard hair, pubic hair).

Hair Follicle: The Living Part of Human Hair and Its Properties

Hair Follicle Morphology

The hair follicle (Fig. 1) develops as a derivative from the embryonic epidermis. During embryogenesis, epithelial–mesenchymal interactions lead to formation of an epithelial peg migrating downward into the dermis. Later on, this peg forms the hair shaft as well as the epithelial structures of the hair follicle. It is important to know that hair follicle formation occurs only once in the lifetime of an individual, that is, a mammal is born with a fixed number of follicles that potentially give rise to visible hair fibers (5).

The specialized morphological structure, the inherent biochemical processes, as well as the particular protein composition of the mature hair follicle have been the subject of many very detailed investigations (reviewed in 10–12). From the morphological point of view, the hair follicle appears as a complex tissue consisting of several different cell layers in a cylindrical, concentric arrangement.

Following a cross-section along the horizontal axis, the outermost component is an epidermal cell layer termed "outer root sheath" (ORS) that encloses the whole follicular structure. Its thickness varies from the top of the follicle to the bottom. It is followed by the "inner root sheath" (IRS). Both living cell layers, ORS and IRS, encase the growing hair fiber that is composed of flattened, overlapping scale cells of the cuticle and the spindle-shaped cells of the cortex. Except for the ORS, hair follicle epithelial cells derive from a germinative hair follicle keratinocyte cell portion residing in the bulblike part of the follicle.

Proliferation and differentiation of these specialized cells during the growth phase of the hair cycle results in a continuous fiber formation.

At the bottom of the hair follicle, the dermal papilla (DP), a fingerlike protrusion adjacent to the connective tissue of the dermis, is located. The dermal papilla contains condensed dermal papilla cells, a specialized fibroblast-like cell type, and extracellular matrix proteins, such as laminin, collagen IV, and versican. It is separated from the epithelial cell portions by a prominent basement membrane that covers the interfaces between epidermal and mesenchymal cells. The dermal papilla possesses unique hair-inductive properties and is a key element in the cyclic regulation of hair growth (13). The whole follicular apparatus is embedded into connective tissue of the surrounding skin: Adjacent to the outermost layers, the so-called glassy layer is formed by orthogonally arranged collagen fibrils, and the connective tissue external to this is termed "dermal sheath."

Along its longitudinal axis, three hair follicle zones with distinct cellular and biochemical activities can be distinguished:

1. The lowest part of the follicle (hair bulb) is the zone with the highest biosynthetic activity. Epithelial cells in this zone are characterized by a high nuclear to cytoplasmic ratio and repeated cell divisions. The high rate of cell proliferation leads to the formation of a constant stream of new hair cells migrating upward to produce hair fiber and IRS. The close vicinity of mesenchymal and epithelial tissue provides cell–cell and cell–matrix interactions playing a major role in hair follicle maintenance, growth, and cycling. It is also the region of hair color formation: Melanocytes produce pheo- or eumelanin pigments that are transferred to hair follicle keratinocytes (14).
2. In the medium regions of the follicle, a zone of keratinization is located. Here, the hardened hair fiber is formed by partial dehydration and formation of disulfide linkages of cystine residues.
3. The most distal part of the hair follicle comprises the zone of permanent hair, comprising the visible fiber, which then emerges from the skin surface.

Hair Follicle Cycling

One of the most fascinating properties of human hair is the fact that it is indeed a self-regenerating system. Hair is continuously subjected to a tightly regulated growth cycle. In contrast to other mammals, in humans it is asynchronous, that is, each hair follicle follows its own, independent cycle. The growth cycle of mature hair follicles can be divided into the following phases (reviewed in 11):

Anagen: During this phase, hair is actively growing, and the hair shaft is elongated. Dependent on the site of the body, this stage lasts approximately from two to six years and extends from the termination of the quiescent phase (telogen) to the beginning of regression. It involves the regrowth of the lower part of the follicle as a whole leading to the production of the (pigmented) hair shaft. The epithelium of the resting follicle grows downward into the dermis and forms the specialized cell types that develop into cylindrical epithelial cell layers. Simultaneously, the dermal papilla changes its morphology, and extracellular matrix proteins, such as laminin, collagen, and versican, are expressed. At the end of anagen, the base of the hair follicle extends deeply into the skin, and hair growth rate is maximal.

Catagen: This term defines a regression or transition stage lasting for a few weeks. Catagen is, again, a highly coordinated process of cellular interactions. It starts with withdrawal of papilla cells from the basement membrane. Due to remodelling of extracellular matrix, the dermal papilla is reduced in its size. Almost simultaneously, pigmentation processes are interrupted, cell division in the epithelial compartment of the hair follicle ceases, and cell number is reduced by apoptotic processes in defined regions of the hair follicle. The lower part of the follicle shrinks and withdraws as epithelial strand, while the surrounding connective tissue thickens and wrinkles. This results in the upward movement of the inferior follicle while the condensed papilla moves distally but remains attached to both the regressing epithelial column as well as to the vascular stalk below. By the end of catagen, the follicle is located in the upper dermis.

Telogen: This term defines the resting or dormant stage of the hair follicle. The hair club and the semi-detached papilla lie close to the so-called bulge region below the sebaceous gland where the arrector pili muscle is attached. This region is thought to contain hair follicle stem cells, which play a central role in the regeneration of a new hair follicle cycle after telogen. The stem cells are dispersed in a basal layer of the outer root sheath, and from this reservoir, cells migrate to the hair matrix and start to divide and differentiate. Their behavior is controlled by a number of inductive signals produced by dermal papilla cells (15). Starting of a new hair cycle after telogen results in epithelial growth, downward movement of follicular structures, and tissue remodeling.

Exogen: Once the growth cycle is completed, the hair shaft is shed. This stage is regarded as a separate stage of hair follicle cycling that occurs independent of the development of a new hair germ (12).

   The hair follicle therefore can indeed be regarded as specialized regenerating biological unit or "miniorgan" that comprises an intense and highly coordinated cross-talk between epithelial components, mesenchyme-derived dermal papilla, and the surrounding connective tissue of the skin. To date, hair biology research has tried to identify the basic mechanistic factors governing cyclic regeneration (e.g., inflammatory and immune stimuli, neural and vascular factors, growth factors, and hormones). Although during the last decade enormous progress in the identification of molecular key players has been made, the complex interactions within the hair follicle are still not fully understood (16).

The duration of different growth phases directly influences the visible part of the hair: It defines the maximal length of the hair shaft that varies between different body sites (Table 2). On a normal, healthy scalp approximately 80% to 85% of the hairs are in anagen phase, 1% to 2% in catagen, and 10% to 20% in telogen stage; the hair shedding is 60 to 80 hairs per day (18). Healthy scalp hair grows 0.35 mm, beard hair 0.38 mm, and eyebrows only 0.16 mm per day (19).

However, malfunctions and disorders of hair follicle cycling can provoke such phenomenons as loss of scalp hair or baldness (alopecia). A common feature of alopecia is a shortening of anagen period, which diminishes the number of hairs in growth stage while the percentage of hairs in catagen and telogen stage increases. As a consequence, in most forms of alopecia, changes in anagen/telogen ratio, miniaturization of hair follicles, and transition from terminal hair to hair with vellus-like appearance indicates regression of hair follicles and balding. Androgenetic alopecia (AGA), a common form of baldness, occurs in both sexes but with distinct hair loss patterns (20,21). The percentages of human beings affected by common baldness varies and depends on sex, age, ethnic background, and individual genetic predisposition. It is known that among different androgens, dihydrotestosterone (DHT), which is produced from testosterone by the enzymatic activity of 5α-reductases, mediates AGA by continuous miniaturization of androgen-sensitive hair follicles. Treatment with antiandrogens or inhibitors of 5α-reductase activity was shown in some cases to prevent hair loss (22–24). Also other forms of hair loss are known. Among them, the term alopecia areata describes a patchy type of baldness that is believed to be a nonscarring inflammatory disease of the hair follicle associated

Table 2 Growth and Resting Phases of Human Hair in Different Regions of the Human Body

Region	Phase	Duration (months)
Scalp	Anagen	24–72
	Catagen	0.5
	Telogen	3–4
Eyebrows	Anagen	1–2
	Telogen	3
Beard	Anagen	10
	Telogen	2
Back of the hand	Anagen	2.5
	Telogen	1.75

Source: From Ref. 17.

with an autoimmune pathogenesis (25). Although some reasons for hair loss have been found so far, many aspects of these phenomenons that affect large percentages of the population are still unclear. Therefore, detailed investigation of the biological processes that regulate hair growth and hair cycling is necessary to develop new, effective treatments for medical as well as cosmetic hair care.

Melanogenesis and Pigmentation

Hair color is determined by pigment content of the hair shaft (reviewed in 26). The color palette of human hair ranges from yellow and red, to black, gray, and white. This is due to a single family of pigments, the melanins, whose structure and composition is under the genetic control of a few genes (27). Melanins provide hair with a broad spectrum of color and determine absorption and reflection, which are cosmetically relevant properties.

The pigment-producing cells form a bicompartment system consisting of follicular melanocytes within the hair follicle and epidermal melanocytes located in the skin. Although melanin synthesis is based on similar biochemical mechanisms in both compartments, there are characteristic differences between skin and hair follicle melanocytes (28). Upon melanin production and pigmentation, hair follicle melanocytes can be divided into two major cell portions. Melanin-producing, so-called melanotic melanocytes are found in the upper part of the follicle close to the epidermis as well as in the part neighboring the upper dermal papilla, whereas amelanotic melanocytes with no or reduced melanin production are located in the middle and lower follicle. Further, melanogenesis and cell proliferation of hair follicle melanocytes is strictly dependent on the hair follicle cycle; that is, hair bulb melanocytes produce and transfer pigments only during anagen stage. As a consequence, synthesis of tyrosinase, a key enzyme in pigment production, occurs only during this phase of the hair cycle (29), and only during this stage is a pigmented hair shaft produced. The fate of melanocytes in the regressing and resting hair follicle during catagen and telogen stages is still unclear. Several investigations suggest that similar to epithelial stem cells a reservoir of "surviving," undifferentiated melanocytes acts as a "perpetuating" system. It is suggested that melanogenic activity is strictly coupled to epithelial–mesenchymal interactions of the hair follicle, and, therefore, melanogenesis is reinitiated at the onset of a new hair follicle cycle (30).

Despite these differences, hair follicle and epidermal melanocytes share some common characteristics. In both, the main processes of melanin synthesis and pigment transfer are similar. Pigment synthesis occurs in highly organized cell organelles, the melanosomes. After synthesis, the ellipsoidal, membrane-bound cell organelles are translocated to epithelial cells in a process of pigment transfer. (31). However, in contrast to the epidermal melanin unit, pigment synthesis in hair follicles is independent of UV exposure, and follicular melanosomes are larger than epidermal ones (28).

The production of various amounts of different melanins is under genetic control. Human hair contains two major types of melanins, eumelanin and pheomelanin, both of which occur in human hair (32). Eumelanins are black to brown and insoluble in all solvents, while the reddish-brown pheomelanins are alkali-soluble.

On a biochemical level, melanogenesis is controlled by several key enzymes exclusively expressed in melanocytes (reviewed in 33). The amino acid tyrosine serves as pigment precursor and is processed via specialized biochemical pathways. One of these enzymes is tyrosinase, a copper-containing enzyme catalyzing the rate-limiting initial steps of melanogenesis. Its activity determines the level of the melanogenic activity of follicular melanocytes (34).

The resulting hair color depends on content and ratio of melanin types. In red hair, melanocytes containing pheomelanin are prominent, while hairs of other colors exhibit an increased content of eumelanin. In human beings, aging often leads to greying and whitening of hair. The term "gray hair" describes a blend of pigmented and nonpigmented hair. The precise mechanisms that lead to changes and finally loss of hair color are still not fully understood, but in greying hair a decreased number of hair follicle melanocytes has been reported. However, even in white hair a portion of functionally active, but amelanotic, melanocytes is detectable (35). It therefore seems that the reason for loss of pigmentation in aging hair follicles may be uncoupling of hair follicle cycling and melanogenesis.

In the last few years, several mechanisms and factors regulating pigmentation and hair follicle melanocyte biology have been identified. For example, it has been shown in a mouse model, that loss of bcl2 protein, a cellular factor normally involved in the regulation of controlled cell death, leads to premature graying (36). Further, the growth factor "stem cell factor" (SCF) and its cellular receptor c-kit, are required for cyclic regeneration of the hair pigmentation unit. Blocking this pathway in mice leads to depigmentation of hairs and decreased melanocyte proliferation (37). This shows that important steps towards the understanding of the molecular pigmentation mechanisms have been made, which may be in future also important for the development of a new generation of hair-care products.

Hair Shaft: The Lifeless, Keratinized Part of Human Hair

Morphology of Cuticle, Cortex, and Medulla

Close examination of a cross-section of the lifeless human hair fiber from outside-in reveals that it consists of three basic layers: cuticle, cortex, and medulla. The outermost layer, the cuticle, is formed by flattened overlapping scale cells with a platelike shape of approximately 45 μm length and a thickness of 0.5–1 μm (18). These scales are remnants of terminally differentiated hair keratinocytes and have lost their ability to divide. Their specific orientation—scales are attached at the root end and orientate toward the tip of the fiber—is responsible for the frictional properties of hair. The cells sometimes show a laminar structure, comprising the so-called exo- and endocuticle (38). Characteristically, the cuticle has a high content of cystine residues and is, at least to some extent, resistant to chemicals and proteolytic digestion (39). Each cuticle cell is surrounded by a thin, hydrophobic outer membrane, the epicuticle. Within this structure, proteins are highly cross-linked by disulfide and isopeptide bonds and further contain a prominent lipid portion (14,40). All cuticular interactions contribute to the stability and resistance of the hair fiber, against chemical influences or mechanical forces, for example. Loss of cuticular integrity results in breaking of fibers and split hair. Therefore, preservation of the cuticular structure is important for the physical properties of the hair fiber and for its cosmetic value.

The cortex, the inner layer adjacent to the cuticle, represents the largest portion of the hair shaft. It contains the structural proteins, which are responsible for the mechanical properties of the hair fiber. It consists of densely packed and interconnected cortical cells as well as intercellular binding material (18). These terminally differentiated cortical cells are spindle shaped and orientate along the longitudinal axis. They are $1-6$ μm thick and up to 100 μm long (41) and contain spindle-shaped keratinous structures called macrofibrils. Within the cortical cells, pigment granula are dispersed as small, spherical particles with a diameter of approximately 0.2 to 0.8 μm. The fibrillar cortex units are embedded in amorphous matrix whose structure still is not completely solved, but it has been shown that it contains a high content of cystine components. Cortical cells are separated from cuticle cells by a membrane complex containing lipidlike chemical components (referred to as cell membrane complex, CMC; 14). The composition of the CMC varies between the different parts of the hair shaft: Close to the skin surface, that is, in an early differentiation stage, cortical cells are connected via numerous desmosomes, gap junctions, and phospholipid-like structures (42). In later stages of differentiation, these components are exchanged for new intercellular material: In distal parts of the hair shaft they show a higher content of free fatty acids, sterols, cholesterol and desmosterol, as well as glycoproteins (43). The intercellular structures represent a kind of intercellular glue surrounding each cuticle and cortex cell to provide cellular adhesion. For the mechanical integrity, especially for the tensile properties of the fiber, the intercellular layers are almost as important as the keratin filaments and keratin-associated proteins.

The innermost layer located in the core of animal hair shafts with a larger diameter is referred to as medulla. It consists of loosely packed medullary cells and has insulating capacities. In human hair, however, insulating functions are nowadays of minor importance, and, therefore, the medulla is often discontinuous or even missing (18).

The Molecular Structure of the Hair Fiber

Hair keratins: The physical properties of the hair shaft are directly determined by the composition and the molecular organisation of its major constituents. This fact should also be kept in mind in the discussion of cosmetic properties of the hair fiber.

Keratins, the major structural proteins of hair and wool, are products of gene families with closely related family members. The term "hair keratin" defines a complex group consisting of approximately 50 to 100 different proteins (reviewed in 14).

This protein class is an excellent example of how protein primary structure, namely the amino acid sequence, provides all information for typical fiberlike building units that define the function and the physical and chemical properties of a macroscopic structure, such as human hair, in a modular manner.

Structural studies of keratins during the early 1950s revealed a periodic polypeptide structure in a right-handed helical conformation, which was designated as α-helix (44). Keratins generally contain about 3.6 amino acid residues per turn, stabilized via hydrogen bonds between NH- and CO-groups of every third amino acid. Two or more α-helices coil around each other in a left-hand manner and form a coiled-coil, rodlike structure. The unusual physical stability partly is increased by covalent cross-links between protein chains by the formation of cystine disulfide bonds resulting from the oxidation of cysteine residues.

Due to their great range of amino acid compositions, different types of hair keratins with different chemical properties can be distinguished (18). Keratins within the hair shaft differ in their content of cystine and cysteine: For example, keratins of the cuticle are rich in cystine and highly cross-linked by disulfide bonds and, therefore, rather tough and resilient, whereas keratin microfibrils with small amounts of cystine but high amounts of leucine and glutamic acid are important structural components of the hair cortex.

Water and lipids, fundamental hair components: Besides its polypeptide composition, the amount of moisture determines physical and cosmetic properties of the hair fiber (reviewed in 18). Within the polymeric fiber, water is bound by hydrogen bonds. Binding occurs most likely to hydrophilic side chains of amino acids and also, but probably to a lesser extent, to the polar peptide bond backbone of the peptide chain. Moisture content depends on the relative humidity of the surroundings and determines several important physical and cosmetic properties of hair. For example, increased relative humidity and higher moisture content lead to enhanced extensibility and increased fiber diameters. It influences torsional and static charge properties. Also, wet friction for human hair is higher than dry friction. The properties of water-soaked hair influence its manageability, and fiber's ability to absorb water and form hydrogen bonds can be used to put hair into a certain shape that will temporarily, but not permanently, retain its setting.

Furthermore, lipids are important components of hair (18). Their composition is rather complex; they contain saturated and unsaturated fatty acids with straight and branched chains of varying length. Surface lipids are mainly derived from sebum produced by sebaceous glands, but internal lipids also exist in the cell membrane complex. The amount of lipid is thought to be regulated by steroid hormones, for example, androgens, but environmental conditions, for example, daily or seasonal variations, also have an influence on the lipid content of human hair. Surface lipids can be easily removed by shampoo treatment, but internal lipids are part of the hair structure and entrapped in the membraneous structures of the cuticle and the cortex.

CURRENT TECHNOLOGIES USED IN HAIR CARE: COSMETIC STRATEGIES IN TREATMENT OF SCALP HAIR

Molecular composition and complex cellular and biochemical interactions determine "macroscopic" properties of human hair and, therefore, play a central role in daily care. Although several aspects of hair care are discussed, for example, treatment or removal of unwanted body hairs, a large part of cosmetic treatment today focuses on the most prominent portion of visible hair, namely on human scalp hair. Here, one takes a close look at hair in its entirety, the living as well as the lifeless part of the hair. Both parts are in the focus of intense product development activities: A metabolically active hair follicle is a prerequisite for perpetuating hair growth and pigmentation activity, while treatment of the lifeless part deals with such aspects as conditioning, hair volume and shine, manageability, and modulation of hair color and style. Therefore, the personal care industry has a growing interest in this fascinating mini organ and is developing large varieties of hair-care products, such as shampoos, conditioners, tonics, hair styling formulations and fixatives, as well as coloring, bleaching, and waving agents.

If we narrow our view on care aspects, we can ask the question why hair care is so important. The idea to develop effective hair-care products does not derive only from a general desire to enhance the cosmetic value of scalp hair (e.g., efficient cleaning, enhanced volume, and manageability) but is also based on the need to protect the hair shaft from actions of endogenous as well as exogenous factors that affect hair structure. During its lifetime, a human hair shaft repeatedly has to withstand different types of damages: Given that the anagen phase of scalp hair lasts approximately for six years, damage effects can accumulate and negatively influence hair function and manageability. Hair damage occurs due to mechanical, thermal, and chemical "injuries" resulting in an altered fiber morphology and changes in the molecular structure and altered physical interactions at molecular level (reviewed in 45). All types of damage attack the molecular constituents of the visible hair fiber. Mechanical damage can be caused by heat drying, combing, brushing, and stretching and also by other forms of hair styling that often result in cuticular abrasions or cuticle loss, scale abrasion, and loss of such important hair components as water and lipids. Chemical damage can occur after exposure to environmental factors (also known as "weathering"), for example UV irradiation (sun light etc.), air pollutants, sea water, and also after extensive chemical bleaching, dyeing, and waving. All these processes influence hair structure, most likely cause degradation of cystine cross-links, and affect amino acids in the protein backbone. Application of hair-care products significantly improves the condition and visible perception of the fiber and partly reverses hair damage (45,46).

Development of hair-care applications tries to meet these cosmetic requirements and, therefore, combines different aspects, such as adaptation to natural fiber conditions and improvement of its cosmetic properties. "Classical" types of treatment, for example, shampoos, tonics, or conditioners, function as cleansers or conditioners in rinse-off or leave-on applications. Their ingredients must be safe in terms of toxicology and ecology. Important functions of shampoos lie in the removal of soil—such as lipids, soils from previous hair-care preparations, protein soils from scalp skin, and environmental soils—and in providing maximal cleansing flexibility. That is, they should be capable of removing a variety of different soils without affecting the hair substance. Further, a combination with active ingredients (e.g., antidandruff agents) or conditioning agents ("2-in-1 shampoo") should be possible. Current shampoo formulations typically contain such ingredients as primary and secondary surfactants, thickening agents and solvents, conditioning agents, pH regulators, and active ingredients (e.g., antidandruff components, vitamins and provitamins, panthenol, or protein hydrolysates) (18, chap. 5).

Conditioning agents are applied to temporarily improve combing conditions and to prevent the so-called "flyaway." They provide hair with shine and volume and are usually liquids, creams, or pastes that mimic sebum in making the hair manageable, glossy, and soft, and are easily removed by cleansing agents (46). Conditioning agents aim at the improvement of fiber properties, such as increased shine, decreased static electricity, enhanced fiber strength, and protection from harmful UV irradiation. Conditioners mainly act on the hair cuticle, because an intact cuticle is responsible for the strength, shine, smoothness, and manageability of healthy hair (45,47). Currently used conditioner formulations therefore typically contain cationic surfactants, often long-chain quaternary ammonium salts, long-chain fatty alcohols, thickening agents, lipids, pH regulators (e.g., citric acids), and polymers or film-forming agents. These components directly influence cosmetic properties of the fiber: Treatment with film-forming polymers leads to fill-in spaces in the surface area of the cuticle and refines adherence of cuticle scales. This results in increased light reflection producing a visible shine that is associated with "healthy" hair. Application of positively charged substances decreases static electricity of negatively charged hair fiber and improves manageability of fine hair. As active ingredients, current conditioner formulations often contain panthenol, vitamins, and native or hydrolysed proteins from different sources with a positive effect on hair strength. They temporarily bind to the hair surface to provide increased volume and better manageability or enter the hair shaft by penetration. Interestingly, the source of the protein seems not to be as important as the protein particle size (46). However, as mentioned before, interactions are only temporal, and protein components can be removed by shampoos. To protect the hair shaft from UV irradiation, which can cause protein degradation, oxidation of stabilizing cystine bonds, and oxidation of color pigments, photoprotective agents are often added.

CHALLENGES FOR BIOTECHNOLOGICAL PRODUCTS AND FUTURE PERSPECTIVES

Although in the past a lot of different hair-care formulations have been developed, there still is a strong requirement for innovative materials and effective compounds improving hair-care formulations. Identification of agents that adapt to specific hair properties, that is, development and choice of appropriate active ingredients inducing particular cosmetic effects, is a key element in product development. In order to meet these challenges, modern technologies, such as biotechnological methods, are often applied. Indeed, some examples show that use of one particular class of biopolymers, namely proteins or their derivatives, as structural or enzymatically active ingredients for treating the lifeless part of the hair has already led to perceptible effects.

Proteins as Hair-Care Ingredients

From a historical point of view, proteins from various natural sources, for example, gelatin, milk or eggs (45) have been used successfully as materials in cosmetics for a long time: This class of biopolymers generated through the formation of peptide bonds between amino acids, fulfils both structural as well as functional roles in vivo. The conformation of the peptide chain determines inherent biochemical properties, for example, maintenance of enzymatic activity, or interstructural binding characteristics. For use in cosmetic products, proteins and their derivatives are generally classified according to terms of origin, amino acid profile, derivatization, and molecular weight. Molecular weight, or rather molecular weight distribution, is especially important: Proteins with high molecular weight ($>$80,000 Da) preferably possess good film-forming properties, while medium-chain (2000–5000 Da) or low-molecular weight proteins ($<$1000 Da) have higher penetration capacity within the hair shaft. Furthermore, the specific molecular amino acid composition influences substantivity or solubility to a large extent (48).

Structural Proteins

Structural proteins from natural sources and their derivatives are common ingredients of current hair-care formulations. In the past, the vast majority of proteins used to be of animal origin, but vegetable proteins today are gaining importance as ingredients of hair-care formulations (49). Within a cosmetic formulation, proteins are often applied as hydrolysates: Hydrolysis is common step within protein purification to separate protein units, to enhance solubility of structural proteins in cosmetic formulations, and to increase their effectiveness. The types of hydrolysate derived from natural origin ranges from relatively crude materials with broad molecular weight distribution to refined preparations with well-defined properties. Additionally, chemical modification of the products obtained, for example, quaternization of protein preparations, is a preferred step to enhance substantivity of compounds to hair fibers by increasing the cationic character of the protein molecules.

The following natural proteins and their derivatives are known as hair-care ingredients to strengthen the fiber, restore damaged spaces or prevent hair damages due to chemical treatments (permanent waving, coloring etc.): For example, collagen hydrolysates of different hydrolysis preparations are widely used today as structural components. At medium molecular weight, hydrolysates (5000–15,000 Da) preferably function as moisturizers and film formers, while at lower molecular weight their partial penetration into the hair shaft and their enhanced binding capacity, especially to damaged regions of the fiber, are predominant characteristics. Other animal-derived structural proteins, such as elastin hydrolysates, keratin hydrolysates, or silk proteins and their derivatives, which are also good film formers but less hygroscopic than collagen derivatives, are also known as hair-conditioning agents (50–54).

As already mentioned, vegetable proteins from renewable resources are valued as beneficial hair-care ingredients and gain importance: For example, proteins and hydrolysates of sweet almond, oat, and wheat have been described as beneficial hair care conditioning components. Due to their amino acid composition, which is different from that of animal-derived materials, they are supposed to interact with the human hair fiber in a slightly different manner. One potential mechanism of interaction between plant biopolymers and keratin structures at molecular level is supposed to be mediated by disulfide interchanges (50). Furthermore, plant protein preparations often contain additional plant components (e.g., oligosaccharides), which are supposed to have additional effects on hair. In particular, native wheat proteins and wheat hydrolysates have been intensively investigated and are valued for their beneficial effects on hair protection. Wheat hydrolysates with high molecular masses have good coating properties, whereas hydrolysed wheat oligopeptides with low molecular weight (<1000 Da) actively penetrate into the cuticle and cortex, where they are temporarily retained (55). Furthermore, additional attractive properties of hydrolysed wheat proteins, such as an anti-inflammatory effect that can relieve skin irritations, have been described (48).

Enzymes

Beside structural polypeptides, proteins with inherent enzymatic activity were intensively investigated for their potential in hair-care preparations, especially for application in hair dyeing and waving procedures. Generally, there is a broad repertoire of enzymatic applications within the industry (56). With respect to hair-care applications, the majority of known protein-based formulations is designed for treatment and modification of the lifeless part of the hair. Numerous patent applications claiming the use of enzymes produced by biotechnological procedures have been issued so far. Examples are the use of oxidative enzymes as substitutes for hydrogen peroxides contributing to a milder hair coloring process, such as oxidases, peroxidases, phenoloxidases, and tyrosinases, or enzyme preparations for bleaching, hair waving, and decoloration (57–63). Despite many research activities within this field, biotechnological products are not frequently used in hair-care formulations, and, therefore, cosmetic products containing enzymes are still relatively rare. Potential reasons lie in the relatively higher price of enzymatic formulations compared to conventional synthetic or naturally derived raw materials, lack of availability in industrial scale, and just a comparable, but not higher, performance as conventional ingredients (50,64).

Future Perspectives of Biotechnological Materials in Hair Care

It is obvious that biotechnological products offer many advantages and completely new perspectives for the use in hair care: The development of fermentation processes during the second half of the last century made it possible to manufacture enzymes and protein compounds as purified, well-characterized preparations even on a larger scale. This development enhanced the introduction of biotechnologically produced proteins into many industrial applications and processes (56). Especially the use of recombinant gene technology has further improved manufacturing processes: This progress has made it possible to provide biotechnological materials with specialized, custom-made functions and tailored properties, enabling new activities and adaptation to the field of use. For the use of such ingredients in hair care, this means, for example, that based on recombinant gene technology and knowledge of corresponding nucleic acid sequences, inherent protein properties can be actively modulated: Among them are such properties as chain length, amino acid composition, molecular weight distribution, polarity and charge of amino acid side chains, penetration properties, maintenance of native conformation and inherent enzymatic activity, as well as substantivity to the hair fiber. Introduction of the latest development within modern biotechnology, for example, protein engineering and directed evolution, further contribute to the development of protein compounds (55). Another advantage is that fermentation procedures are more or less independent of the availability of natural sources for protein extraction. Furthermore, uncountable possibilities of modifications, for example, chemical or enzymatic processing, as well as amino acid exchanges and point mutations within active sites, are conceivable. Production via fermentation further contributes to a high product quality by decreasing the content of impurities and avoidance of remnants (e.g., varying levels of inorganic materials) or artifacts of derivatization. Other examples of biotechnological procedures for refining and modifying raw materials, such as removal of lipids from cosmetic collagen preparations and proteolytical hydrolysis of collagen from tendon, have already been described (65).

Beyond that, there are many perspectives for hair-care ingredients from the field of biotechnology: Combination of novel findings in the rapidly growing fields of human hair research and new delivery systems with the latest progress in biotechnological fermentation procedures and genetic engineering may lead to innovative functional materials contributing to new concepts in terms of resources, custom-made or nature-identical biopolymers, reduction of irritation, and sensitization potential of ingredients for new, as well as improved, current applications (50). Based on this knowledge, biotechnological products could also be successfully used to actively modify hair in its entirety, that is, both the living and the lifeless part of this complex but interesting "miniorgan." Indeed, there is an infinite number of targets and possibilities for influencing hair metabolism, for example, by directly influencing cellular processes, such as signaling, gene expression, and other functions via direct targeting. Intensified research activities on proteins and custom-made peptides and their derivatives may yield a broad product range with high performance and unique properties adapted to the customer's desires and needs, and hair will become just more than a kind of "textile" attached to the human body.

REFERENCES

1. Szabo G. The regional frequency and distribution of hair follicles in human skin. In: Montagna W, Ellis RA, eds. The Biology of Hair Growth. New York: Academic Press, 1958:33–38.
2. Van Neste D. Hair and nits in the museum. In: Van Neste D, ed. Hair science and technology. Proceedings of the 9th Annual Meeting of the European Hair Research Society held in Brussels, Belgium, June 2002. Tournai: Skinterface, 2003: 11–16.
3. Cash TF. The psychosocial consequences of adrogenetic alopecia: a review of the research literature. Br J Dermatol 1999; 141:398–405.
4. Schueller R, Romanowski P. Introduction to conditioning agents for hair and skin. In: Schueller R., Romanowski P, eds. Conditioning Agents for Hair and Skin. New York: Marcel Dekker, 1999:9–11.
5. Philpott M, Paus R. Principles of hair follicle morphogenesis. In: Cheng-Ming Chuong, ed. Molecular Basis of Epithelial Appendage Morphogenesis. Austin: R.G. Landes Company, 1998:75–110.
6. Hashimoto K, Ito M, Suzuki Y. Innervation and vasculature of the hair follicle. In: Orfanos CE, Happle R, eds. Hair and Hair Diseases. Berlin, Heidelberg: Springer-Verlag, 1990:117–147.
7. Otberg N, Richter H, Schaefer H, Blume-Peytavi U, Sterry W, Lademann J. Variations of hair follicle size and distribution in different body sites. J Invest Dermatol 2004; 122:14–19.

8. Serri F, Cerimele D. Embryology of the hair follicle. In: Orfanos CE, Happle R, eds. Hair and Hair Diseases. Berlin: Springer-Verlag, 1990: 1–17.

9. Randall VA, Hibberts NA, Thornton MJ, Hamada K, Merrick AE, Kato S, Jenner TJ, De Oliveira I, Messenger AG. The hair follicle: a paradoxical androgen target organ. Horm Res. 2000; 54:243–250.

10. Messenger AG. The control of hair growth: an overview. J Invest Dermatol. 1993; 101(Suppl):4S–9S.

11. Stenn KS, Paus R. Controls of hair follicle cycling. Physiol Rev 2001; 81:449–494.

12. Stenn KS, Parimoo S, Prouty SM. Growth of the hair follicle: A cycling and regenerating system. In: Cheng-Ming Chuong, ed. Molecular Basis of Epithelial Appendage Morphogenesis. Austin: R.G. Landes Company, 1998:111–130.

13. Jahoda CA, Horne KA, Oliver RF. Induction of hair growth by implantation of cultured dermal papilla cells. Nature 1984; 311:560–562.

14. Powell BC, Rogers GE. The role of keratin proteins and their genes in the growth, structure and properties of hair. EXS 1997; 78:59–148.

15. Alonso L, Fuchs, E. Stem cells of the skin epithelium. Proc Natl Acad Sci 2003; 100(suppl 1):11830–11835.

16. Botchkarev VA, Kishimoto J. Molecular control of epidermal-mesenchymal interactions during hair follicle cycling. J Investig Dermatol Symp Proc 2003; 8:46–55.

17. Umbach W. Kosmetik. Vol 2. Aufl. Stuttgart: Thieme, 1995.

18. Robbins CR. Chemical and Physical Behavior of Human Hair. 3rd ed. New York: Springer Verlag, 1994.

19. Pelfini C, Cerimele D, Pisanu G. Aging of the skin and hair growth in man. In: Montagna W, Dobson RL, eds. Hair Growth. London: Pergamon Press, 1969:153–160.

20. Hamilton JB. Patterned loss of hair in man; types and incidence. Ann NY Acad Sci 1951; 3:708–728.

21. Ludwig E. Classification of the types of androgenetic alopecia (common baldness) occurring in the female sex. Br J Dermatol 1977; 3:247–254.

22. Schweikert HU, Wilson JD. Regulation of human hair growth by steroid hormones. I. Testesterone metabolism in isolated hairs. J Clin Endocrinol Metab 1974; 5: 811–819.

23. Kaufman KD. Androgen metabolism as it affects hair growth in androgenetic alopecia. Dermatol Clin 1996; 4:697–711.

24. Dallob AL, Sadick NS, Unger W, Lipert S, Geissler LA, Gregoire SL, Nguyen HH, Moore EC, Tanaka WK. The effect of finasteride, a 5 alpha-reductase inhibitor, on scalp skin testosterone and dihydrotestosterone concentrations in patients with male pattern baldness. J Clin Endocrinol Metab 1994; 3:703–706.

25. McDonagh AJ, Messenger AJ. The pathogenesis of alopecia areata. Dermatol Clin 1996; 14:661–670.

26. Cesarini JP. Hair melanin and hair color. In: Orfanos CE, Happle R, eds. Hair and Hair Diseases. Berlin: Springer-Verlag, 1990:165–197.

27. Ortonne JP, Prota G. Hair melanins and hair color: ultrastructural and biochemical aspects. J Invest Dermatol 1993; 105:82S–89S.

28. Castanet J, Ortonne JP. Hair melanin and hair color. EXS 1997;78:209–225.

29. Burnett JB, Holstein TJ, Quevedo WC. Electrophoretic variations of tyrosinase in follicular melanocytes and during the hair growth cycle in mice. J Exp Zool 1969; 171:369–376.

30. Tobin DJ, Slominski A, Botchkarev V, Paus R. The fate of hair follicle melanocytes during the hair growth cycle. J Investig Dermatol Symp Proc 1999; 3:323–332.

31. Jimbow K, Quevedo WC, Fitzpatrick TB. Biology of melanocytes. In: Fitzpatrick TB, Eisen AZ, Wolff K, Freedberg IM, Austen KF, eds. Dermatology in General Medicine. 4th ed. New York: Mac Graw-Hill Inc., 1993: 261–271.

32. Prota G. Progress in chemistry of melanins and related metabolites. Med Res Rev 1988; 8:525–526.

33. Hearing VJ. Biochemical control of melanogenesis and melanosomal organisation. J Investig Dermatol Symp Proc 1999; 4:24–28.

34. Hearing VJ, Tsukamoto K. Enzymatic control of pigmentation in mammals. FASEB J 1991; 5:2902–2909.

35. Takada K, Sugiyama K, Yamamoto I, Oba K, Takeuchi T. Presence of amelanotic melanocytes within the outer root sheath of senile white hair. J Invest Dermatol 1992; 99:629–633.

36. Veis DJ, Sorenson CM, Shutter JR, Korsmeyer SJ. Bcl-2-deficient mice demonstrate fulminant lymphoid apoptosis, polycystic kidneys, and hypopigmented hair. Cell 1993; 75:229–240.

37. Botchkareva NV, Khlgatian M, Longley BJ, Botchkarev VA, Gilchrest BA. SCF/c-kit signaling is required for cyclic regeneration of the hair pigmentation unit. FASEB J 2001; 3:645–658.

38. Baden HP. Hair keratin. In: Orfanos CE, Happle R, eds. Hair and Hair Diseases. Berlin: Springer-Verlag, 1990:45–71.

39. Bradbury JH. The structure and chemistry of keratin fibers. Adv Protein Chem 1973; 27:11–211.

40. Zahn H, Messinger H, Hocker H. Covalently-linked fatty acids at the surface of wool: Part of the cuticle cell envelope. Textile Res J 1994; 64:554–555.

41. Randebrock R. Electron-microscopic photographs of human hairs. J Soc Cosmet Chem 1962; 13:404–415.

42. Orwin DFG. An ultrastructural study of the membranes of keratinizing wool follicle cells. J Cell Sci 1972; 11:205–219.

43. Herrling J, Zahn H. Investigations of the cell membrane complex and its modification during industrial processing of wool. Proceedings of the 7th International Wool Textile Research Conference, Tokyo, Japan, 1985; 1:181–193.

44. Pauling LC, Corey RB, Branson, HR, The structure of proteins: Two hydrogen-bonded helical configuration of the polypeptide chain. Proc Natl Acad Sci USA 1951; 37:205–211.

45. Draelos, ZD. Biology of the hair and skin. In: Schueller R, Romanowski P, eds. Conditioning Agents for Hair and Skin. New York: Marcel Dekker Inc, 1999:13–34.

46. Draelos ZD. Conditioning hair: creams, lotions, and potions, part I. Cosmet Dermatol 2003; 16:61–64.

47. Goldemberg RL. Hair conditioners: the rationale for modern formulations. In: Frost P, Horwitz SN, eds. Principles of Cosmetics for the Dermatologist. St. Louis: Mosby, 1982:157–159.

48. Huetter I. Hair care with depth effects by low molecular proteins, SÖFW-Journal 2003; 129:12–16.

49. Burmeister F, Brooks GJ, O'Brien KP. Vegetable/plant proteins in shampoos. Cosmet Toilet 1991; 106:41–46.

50. Neudahl GA. Proteins for conditioning hair and skin. In: Schueller R, Romanowski P, eds. Conditioning Agents for Hair and Skin. New York: Marcel Dekker Inc., 1999:139–166.

51. Yoshioka I, Kamimura Y. Keratin hydrolyzate useful as hair fixatives. US Patent 4,279,996, September 25, 1979, Seiwa Kasei Co. Ltd.

52. Yoshioka I, Kamimura Y. Keratin hydrolyzate useful as hair fixatives. US Patent 4,390,525, January 6, 1981, Seiwa Kasei Co. Ltd.

53. Oshika M, Naito S. Acylated silk proteins for hair care. US Patent 5,747,015, April 24, 1996, Kao Corporation.

54. Schulze zur Wiesche E, Zuedel N, Kleen A, Rohland C. Synergistic combination of silk proteins. WO2004/024176, August 21, 2003, Henkel KGaA.

55. Vollhardt J. Native hydrophobic wheat proteins with intelligent hair care properties. SÖFW Journal 1999; 125:2–9.

56. Kirk O, Borchert TV, Fuglsang CC. Industrial enzyme applications. Curr Opin Biotechnol 2002; 13:345–351.

57. Takada K, Uozumi T, Kimura A, Someya K, Yoshino T. Influence of oxidative and/or reductive treatment on human hair (III): Oxidative reaction of polyphenol oxidase (laccase) to hair dyeing. J Oleo Science 2003; 52:557–563.

58. Kleen A, Meinigke B, Saettler A, Howorka W, Suenger G. Cosmetic agents containing protein disulfide isomerase. WO03/099242, May 20, 2003, Henkel KGaA.

59. Beck H. Mittel und Verfahren zur natuerlichen Entfaerbung von gefaerbtem Haar. DE10108393, February 21, 2001, Wella AG.

60. Lang G, Cotteret J. Keratinous fibre oxidation dyeing composition containing a laccase and dyeing method using the same. WO99/36041, January 13, 1998, L'Oreal.

61. Saettler A, Kleen A, Weiss A, Rose D. Colouring agents with enzymes. WO00/21497, October 14, 1998, Henkel KGaA.

62. Rozzell D, Sauter G, Braun HJ. Agent and method for dyeing keratin fibres. WO02/47633, October 5, 2001, Wella AG.

63. Onuki T, Noguchi M, Mitamura J. Hair dye compositions. WO00/37030, December 22, 1998, Lion Corporation.

64. Aehle W, ed. Enzymes in Industry: Production and Applications. 2nd ed. Weinheim: VCH-Wiley, 2004.

65. Langmaier F, Mladek M, Kolomaznik K, Sukop S. Collagenous hydrolysates from untraditional sources of proteins. Int J Cosmet Sci 2001; 23:193–199.

11

Biotechnology in Hair Care (II): Growth Modulation

Tsutomu Soma, Kiichiro Yano, and Jiro Kishimoto
Shiseido Research Center, Yokohama, Japan

OVERVIEW

The hair growth promotion product market is rapidly growing and a very competitive area in the personal care market. The efficacy of these products dictates their success in the marketplace. Therefore, research on hair growth promotion products is possibly one of the most basic science-based, R&D-mediated areas among personal care product development. However, even with tremendous efforts being made for decades, a very small number of marginally effective compounds have been developed. At present, only two products are categorized as FDA-approved active compounds, one of which was found accidentally from its side effect during a clinical trial for another purpose. This demonstrates how complicated and difficult it is to develop hair growth promoting compounds solely based on strategy and common science knowledge/techniques without any breakthroughs and innovative tools. In this context, biotechnology would provide hair biology researchers the potential technology to develop novel effective products. Within the biotechnology field, rapid progress in molecular biology in the last two decades has given birth to recombinant DNA technologies, or so-called genetic engineering. Recent completion of the worldwide genome project also seems to provide additional potential information for genetic manipulation. In the personal care field, hair growth promotion research may benefit the most from these innovative technologies. Until now, because no active compound for hair promotion has been made by genetic engineering (i.e., biofermentation), this chapter will mainly discuss utilizing this technology to investigate basic biological mechanism of hair growth and establish novel evaluating systems for hair growth modulation. In the future, once an active compound is found, a biofermentation process may be used to produce it. In this chapter, we describe basic terms of hair biology and the potential application of recombinant DNA technology to hair research, especially the use of genetically engineered trans-genic model systems, and provide future direction, including use of state-of-art microarray and proteomics technology for the development of hair growth promotion products.

MECHANISM OF HAIR GROWTH CYCLE

Hair Growth and Cycle

Hair grows from epithelial matrix cells at the bottom of the follicle and these matrix cells differentiate and become specialized within each follicular layer. The uniqueness of the hair follicle as a miniorgan within a mature adult body is that the healthy normal hair growth in each hair follicle occurs in a cyclic manner (Fig. 1). There are three main phases of hair growth cycle: anagen, catagen, and telogen. Anagen is the active growth phase during which hair fiber is produced and hair shaft is elongated (1). Melanogenesis occurs within pigmented hair follicles during this phase. Completion of first anagen phase from hair embryogenesis is followed by the catagen phase, which controls regression of the hair follicle. After a relatively short transient period of catagen phase, the hair

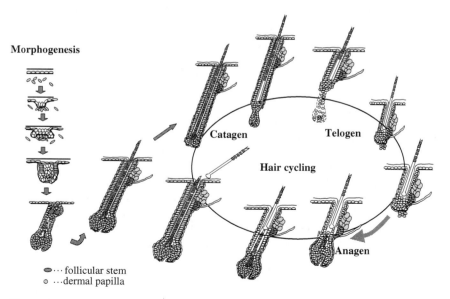

Figure 1   Hair morphogenesis and hair cycling.

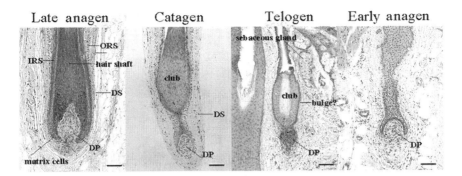

Figure 2 Morphological changes in human hair cycle. Scale bars: 50 μm. *Abbreviations*: DP, dermal papilla; DS, dermal sheath; IRS, inner root sheath; ORS, outer root sheath.

follicle enters telogen, during which the follicles stay in a resting condition for a longer period. Details of each stage will be described later in this chapter.

In the human hair cycle (Fig. 2), anagen lasts about 5 to 10 years and is the longest of the three phases. Therefore, usually more than 90% of the follicles in a normal scalp are in the anagen phase and the remaining 10% in telogen. Catagen is transient, lasting only for two to three weeks, whereas telogenasts for one to three months (2). Hair growth is best studied in mice because their hair cycles are highly synchronized, especially during development and following the first hair cycle, and they have shorter hair cycles than humans. In most mouse strains, the hair bud first appears at embryonic (E) day 13–15 and reaches the hair bulb structure by day E17. Hair elongation, a later part of hair embryogeneis, persists until two weeks after birth. The catagen phase starts about postnatal (P) day 16 and goes into telogen by day P19. The onset of the second anagen phase (as a strict definition this is the time of the first hair cycle) occurs around four weeks after birth and lasts for two weeks (3). After completion of this first hair cycle, mice have a relatively longer resting period of about a month. In young mice particularly, the anagen growth phase occurs in a wave pattern across the skin surface, but in humans the hair cycle patterns for each hair follicle are entirely independent from neighboring follicles.

Follicular Stem Cells

Follicular stem cells have been extensively studied. Initial evidence for these came from carefully designed histochemical techniques, which showed slow cycling stem cells (label retaining cells; LRC) localized to a very restricted area of the follicle called "bulge," located in the upper one-third portion of the hair follicle (4). The bulge area is best recognized by the hair-associated smooth muscle called the arrector pilli muscle (4). Several histochemical and biological studies have proved that follicular epithelial cells in this region show slow cycling in vivo but, once isolated, show high proliferative potential in culture and differentiate into several different cell lineages (5,6). These studies suggest that allowing stem cells to enter a more actively dividing stage (transient amplifying cells; TA cells) could initiate anagen hair cycle from the telogen phase. Hair stem cells are obviously one of the major target cells in which hair growth-modulation compounds act directly to induce hair, but the detailed mechanism for their activation is virtually unknown.

Dermal Papilla Cells

Dermal papilla (DP) cells are thought to be differentiated and specialized from dermal fibroblasts, but their precise origin or characteristic biological markers are yet unknown. DP directs the embryonic generation of a hair follicle and also retains the instructive ability throughout life. Under the influence of the DP, follicular epidermal cells differentiated at anagen produce keratinized hair fibers and associated products, such as keratin-associated protein (KAP). Therefore, in spite of sometimes being thought of as the outside of the hair follicle structural unit, DP cells function as a center for hair growth and cycling. Unlike several follicular epithelial cell-specific gene markers, such as hair keratins and KAP, there is no clear marker for DP. One candidate molecule is nexin, which is a serine protease inhibitor and is localized in anagen DP in mice (7). In the 1950s, accumulation of glycosaminoglycan in DP was reported (8), and later in 1980s, immunohistochemical studies with several proteoglycan-specific antibodies demonstrated their abundance in the DP, especially chondroitin sulfate proteoglycan (CSPG) (9). Molecular cloning of CSPG identified one unique core protein molecule of CSPG, versican (10), and immunostaining with antiversican-specific antibody showed DP-specific staining (11). The use of DP-specific versican expression in transgenic system to study hair cycle mechanism and search for hair growth-modulating compound will be discussed later in this chapter.

Anagen: Initiation of New Follicle Induction by Epithelial–Mesenchymal Interaction

The two distinct cell types, epithelial cells and mesenchymal cells, form many organs, such as lung, kidney, heart, and various types of appendages, such as teeth. Interaction between these two types of cells is termed epithelial–mesenchymal interactions (EMI) EMI plays a central role in the organogenesis in many organs, including hair follicles. EMI has a powerful influence not only during the developmental stage, but also on the hair follicle cycling process, especially during anagen induction. Hair cycle of the follicles is governed by the signaling cascade between follicular keratinocyte stem cells in the bulge (epithelial cells) committed to hair follicle-specific differentiation, and DP (mesenchymal cells) (1,12). At the onset of anagen induction, follicular stem cells and degenerated DP cells come closest (Fig. 1 at telogen phase).

Table 1 List of Growth Modulators' Potential to Affect the Human Hair Cycle

Growth modulators	Mode of action	Selected references
Bone morphogenic protein (BMP)	induction	(27)
Sonic hedgehog (shh)	induction	(110)
Basic fibroblast growth factor (bFGF)	induction	(111)
Fibroblast growth factor 5 (FGF5)	inhibition	(112)
Hepatocyte growth factor (HGF)	induction	(113)
brain-derived neurotrophic factor (BDNF)	induction	(114)
Wnt 3a/7/10a	induction	(70)
Insulin-like growth factor-I (IGF-I)	induction	(115)
Transforming growth factor-β (TGF-β)	inhibition	(21)
Vascular endothelial growth factor (VEGF)	induction	(40)

This closeness is believed to allow the effective interaction between these two cells (bulge theory) (4). Anagen entry is thought to occur by initiating signal secretion either from degenerated papilla or follicular stem at bulge, but the actual molecule has not been identified. However, several morphogenic-patterning genes, which are known to be involved in development for other appendages, are most likely candidates. These morphogens include fibroblast growth factor (FGF), sonic hedgehog (shh), wnt, and transforming growth factor (TGF-β). The signaling cascade in EMI is thought to be highly organized and most likely more than a single master molecule is thought to be involved in this process in addition to these above morphogen molecules (13,14). Major candidate molecules for EMI in hair follicles are listed in Table 1. Many of these signaling pathways interact and modulate activity of each other on different levels. A recent report also suggests that signaling exchange between the epithelium and mesenchyme is modulated by extracellular matrix (ECM) molecules (15), which may significantly enhance or reduce biological activity of the secreted growth stimulators. In any case, clarifying the complicated and sequential EMI process during hair induction period at a molecular level will be the center theme for hair biology research (reviewed in 16).

Catagen: Apoptotic Force to Cessation

Once hair follicles enter into the regressing phase (catagen), follicular epithelial cells stop their proliferation, followed by their apoptosis (17). Several recent studies have revealed that TGF-β is a strong candidate that terminates anagen to initiate catagen in the nonpathological process of mammalian hair cycling. The endogenous TGF-β1 is mainly seen in the outer root sheath (ORS) of the late anagen hair follicles, and is increased during the anagen–catagen transition (18). Active TGF-β responses, which were monitored by phospho-Smad2/3-specific antibodies, were observed throughout anagen and catagen period (19). In contrast to TGF-β, expression of growth factors that stimulate follicular epithelial cells, such as insulin growth factor (IGF)-1 (20), is significantly decreased during anagen–catagen transition. These studies may support that TGF-β works as a negative regulator of follicular epithelial cell, and the balance between stimulation and inhibition signals are critical to maintain the anagen-growing phase. TGF-β also works in the catagen development of human hair follicles as well as mice (21). TGF-β2 accumulation in the boundary area of the bulb matrix and the DP was characteristic of early catagen phase in humans. TGF-β2 treatment causes the inhibition of DNA synthesis and the induction of catagen in vitro (22).

The catagen phase is also characterized by the rapid and highly controlled process of organ involution with massive epithelial cell apoptosis (22–24). In the mouse hair cycle, apoptotic cells in the bulb matrix were detected in catagen I hair follicles but not anagen VI hair follicles (24). An increased number of apoptotic cells were detected in the follicular epithelial cells at late catagen. Apoptosis was not detectable in the DP throughout the hair cycle. DP cells, as well as the stem cells, in the bulge area may be protected from apoptosis by dominant Bcl-2 expression (25). TGF-β strongly inhibits the growth of epithelial cells and can induce their apoptosis, accompanied with activation of caspases 3 and 9 (26). But the exact mechanism of apoptosis induced by TGF-β is complicated and still remains unclear. It is more useful to maintain hair growth by inhibiting the levels of TGF-β elevated in late anagen prior to the apoptosis that occurs in catagen. Other members of the TGF-β superfamily, such as bone morphogenetic proteins (BMP), are well known to be important in morphogenesis of hair follicles (see review article, 27).

Other features of the catagen phase are termination of melanogenesis, proteolysis of ECM, and remodeling of blood vessels (17) (Also see angiogenesis paragraph in this chapter). Some of the endothelial cells are also eliminated by apoptosis from the hair follicles at catagen phase (28).

Telogen: Resting Phase of Hair Cycle

Telogen hair follicles are relatively quiescent when the expression level of various genes is low or diminished. DP in telogen is compactly packed and contains lower amounts of ECM molecules, compared to the anagen stage. In addition, the proteoglycan versican, which plays important roles for inducing and maintaining anagen phase (see next section), is not detectable in the telogen phase (29). The hair shaft is attached to the club hair above the secondary hair germ. Plasminogen activator inhibitor type 2 (PAI-2), which is a serine protease inhibitor, is expressed in the attachment of the club hair to prevent premature hair shedding in telogen phase (30). Desmoglein-3, a molecule involved in cell adhesion, is also localized at the boundary area between the club hair and the ORS in telogen hair (31). In human terminal hairs, re-entry into anagen phase with cellular growth and gene expression probably occurs before shedding of the club hair. For example, activinβA, which belongs to TGF-β super family, is predominantly expressed in the DP of telogen (or initiated anagen) hair follicles but not anagen (Fig. 3) (32).

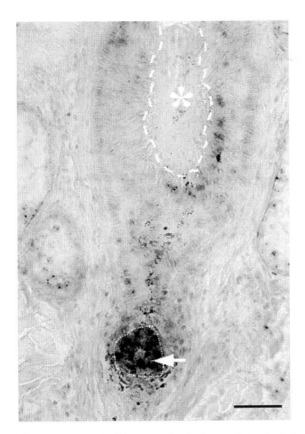

Figure 3 Activin βA expression in human hair. Scale bar: 50 μm. Activin βA gene is predominantly expressed in the dermal papilla of telogen hair follicles. Arrow indicates dermal papilla. Asterisk, club hair.

Angiogenic Factors: Key Modulators for Hair Growth

Cutaneous vascular system plays a critical role in the maintenance of skin homeostasis, and the existence of massive microvascular network surrounding hair follicles suggest its pivotal role for hair growth modulation. Hair cycle-dependent vascular remodeling (angiogenesis) is thought to be controlled by endogenous angiogenesis-related factors, such as vascular endothelial growth factor-A (VEGF-A) and thrombospondin-1 (TSP-1), based on their role in skin angiogenesis.

VEGF-A, released by epidermal keratinocytes, is a major skin angiogenesis factor (33). VEGF-A is a secreted glycoprotein that has four isoforms derived from different splicing variants (34) that interact with the receptors—such as FLK-1/KDR (35), FLT-1 (36), or neuroplin-1 (37)—on endothelial cells, leading to new blood vessel formation from pre-existing vessels.

TSP-1 is a 450-kDa matricellular protein (33) produced by epidermal keratinocytes, endothelial cells, and some dermal fibroblasts. A potent angiogenesis inhibitor, TSP-1 inhibits endothelial cell proliferation and migration—angiogenesis—in vitro and in vivo by the interaction between distinct sequences, the type I repeats in TSP-1, and CD36 receptor on endothelial cells, leading to endothelial cell apoptosis (38). TSP-1-is constitutively expressed in the skin and contributes to the normal quiescence of the cutaneous vasculature (39).

It has been previously reported that dramatic angiogenesis occurs during the murine hair cycle, with a significant increase in perifollicular vessel size and endothelial cell proliferation (Fig. 4) during the anagen growth phase and a

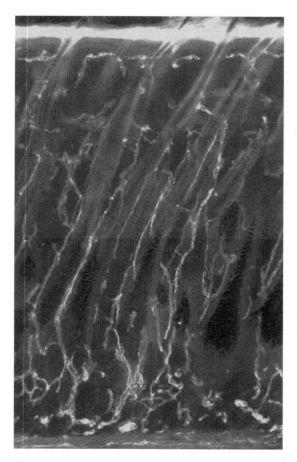

Figure 4   Three-dimensional reconstruction of perifollicular vascularization during mid-anagen phase. Dermal bright signal represents CD31-positive cells.

rapid decrease during the catagen and telogen phases (40). The changes in vessel size coincided temporally with cyclic changes in follicle size, and perifollicular angiogenesis was temporally and spatially correlated with upregulation of VEGF mRNA expression by follicular keratinocytes of the ORS (40) On the other hand, the mRNA and protein expression of the endogenous angiogenesis inhibitor, TSP-1, are highly upregulated in the DP and follicular keratinocytes and during the catagen and telogen phase leading to apoptosis-driven vascular regression (28) and absent from the hair bulb during the anagen growth phase. Taken together, these studies imply that cyclic changes of perifollicular vascularization are precisely regulated by hair follicle–derived angiogenesis factors and inhibitors, such as VEGF and TSP-1, during hair cycling (28,40).

Hormonal Reaction: Cause of Major Hair Loss

Hair loss is caused by various factors, including biological, genetic, environmental, and social. Each cause has a name, such as alopecia areata (immunological and genetic hair loss), androgenic alopecia (male-pattern baldness; MPB), anagen effluvium (chemical and radiation-induced hair loss), telogen effluvium (stress-related hair loss), and self-induced hair loss (tearing out one's own hair). Among these, androgenic alopecia and MPB are priority targets in hair biology research for hair growth products. Androgens have profound effects on scalp and body hair in humans (41), and the major androgenic hormones in humans is testosterone. Many lines of evidence implicate testosterone in the pathogenesis of MPB (42). In androgen-targeted tissues the steroid 5alpha-reductase (5aR) converts testosterone to dihydrotestosterone (DHT), which is the more potent androgen. Two distinct genes, coding type I and type II 5aR have been identified in humans (43,44). Type I 5aR has a pH optimum at neutral pH, whereas type II 5aR shows a maximum activity at acidic pH. While type I 5aR is predominantly detected in liver, skin, and sebaceous gland, type II 5aR is relatively abundant in prostate, foreskin, and beard (45). Expression of type II 5aR is also found in the DP cells of frontal scalp hair but not occipital scalp hair (46). Some observations, including the genetic type II 5aR deficiency, (44) indicate that type II 5aR is closely related to MPB rather than the type I isozyme.

CURRENT SCREENING METHODS AND PRODUCTS FOR HAIR GROWTH MODULATION

Traditional Screening Approaches for Hair Growth Modulator

In Vivo Animal/Human Test

Several in vivo and in vitro evaluation methods have been developed for the traditional screening of hair growth promoting compounds. Mice, rabbits, monkeys, and humans have been generally used for in vivo experiments.

Among these, other than humans, mice have been mainly utilized for years (47). For evaluation, after shaving the center of the back skin, compounds to be tested, which are often dissolved in either alcohol or dimethyl sulfoxide (DMSO) solution, are topically applied. Specific pigmented strains, such as C3H/He or C57BL/6, are commonly used as their melanocytes are recruited when new hair follicles are generated at the onset of anagen from telogen, and they exhibit clear dark skin color, which is easily visible over the surface without surgical procedure. As a positive hair growth stimulator control, cyclosporin A, which is an immunosuppressive compound, or vasodilator molecule minoxidil (48) are widely used, although only cyclosporin A induces nearly 100% hair growth when applied at appropriate concentrations. Because of the relatively short hair cycle period and its synchronicity, this handy experimental system is still very popular. However, one major risk for in vivo hair growth test on mouse skin is that compounds found by this method do not always show hair promotion activity in humans. One possible explanation is the differential hormonal control mechanisms of hair growth between humans and mice, and the other is that sometimes inflammatory stimuli initiate pathological hair growth, which often differs from normal human hair growth. Therefore, alternative supplementary approaches have been developed in vitro using human-derived cells.

Cell Culture System

Culturing dissociated, hair follicle–related cells on multiwell dishes and measuring such parameters as growth rate, dissolved oxygen amount, or specific biomarkers, such as hair keratins, in response to candidate compounds are some of the in vitro assay systems developed to screen for hair growth-promoting compounds. Types of cells preferentially cultured are the ORS cells (ORS: follicular epithelial cells), DP cells, and dermal sheath cells (DS), which are believed to be DP-derived mesenchymal cells. Primary or two- to three-times passaged DP cells are rarely used because the number of cells are very limited; usually cultured cells passaged 6 to 10 times are used because or sometimes established stable cell lines.

In Vitro Organ Culture Method

Dissected human anagen follicles from intact skin specimens can be successfully grown for a certain period in cultured medium. Thus, follicles truncated below dermis and subcutaneous tissue are placed in appropriate medium, usually serum-free, in order to test selected compounds (24). These isolated human follicles often grow for a week, and compounds can be tested during this period by measuring the expanded length of the follicles, but because they do not enter the next hair cycle, the induction of anagen hair is difficult to assess with them. Such organ culture systems are ranked between whole animal/human systems and cell culture systems and are the only assay systems that use cells from human origin.

Hair Growth Modulation Products

5aR Inhibitor

Finasteride, an orally active type II-selective 5aR inhibitor, is being used for the treatment of benign prostate hyperplasia (49–51). Clinical trials with oral administration of this compound showed a significant improvement in hair growth in men with MPB (52–54). In addition to finestride, both 6-azasteroid and 10-azasteroid have the activity of type II 5aR inhibition (55,56). Episteroid and 17ß-N,N-diethylcarbamoyl-4-methyl-4-aza-5-androstan-3-one (4MA) can inhibit not only type II 5aR but also type I 5aR (57). Topical application of 4MA stimulated hair growth in the bald scalps of stumptailed macaques (58). In contrast, a topical treatment using type I selective 5aR, LY191704 had no effect on hair growth in bald macaques (59). MK-386 (4,7 β-dimethyl-4-aza-5 α-cholestan-3-one) showed the selective inhibition of type I 5aR, which is useful for treatments of acne but not MPB (60). These clinical and experimental attempts also suggest that type II 5aR plays an important role in the development and progression of MPB, and the selective inhibition of this isozyme is more effective for treatments of MPB.

Although many steroids and their analogues can work as competitive inhibitors of 5aR, (61), it is difficult to apply them as inhibitors of transformation from testosterone to DHT because of their other bioactivities. Another approach for inhibiting 5aR is noncompetitive inhibition of nicotinamide adenine dinucleotide phosphate (NADPH) binding to 5aR (or dissociation from 5aR) because 5aR requires NADPH as a coenzyme (62). Several unsaturated fatty acids inhibited 5aR of hamster flank organs through a noncompetitive action, which emphasized an important role of fatty acids metabolism in androgen target cells (63). Recombinant human type I 5aR has been successfully expressed by baculovirus systems in Sf9 insect cells in an active form and is associated with the nuclear membrane (64).

Vasomodulator

Minoxidil (generic name) is a piperidinopyrimidine derivative compound and now widely used to prevent hair loss or in some cases improve hair growth rate in both men and women. Minoxidil is the first FDA drug approved for the treatment of male-type baldness. Minoxidil itself is a stable compound, but when it is applied to the scalp tissue it is converted to an active product minoxidil sulfate by the enzyme called sulfonyl transferase. Mode of action of minoxidil sulfate is virtually unknown, but it may activate potassium channels in target follicular cells leading to hair growth (65,66). It has also been suggested that minoxidil dilates blood vessels surrounding hair follicles, increasing oxygen and nutrient supply, which produces increased hair growth. However, this hypothesis is somewhat controversial, as other vasodilator drugs do not promote hair growth.

APPLICATION OF BIOTECHNOLOGY FOR HAIR GROWTH MODULATING COMPOUNDS

In Vitro Assay System Using Genetically Engineered Cell Lines

A reporter assay system is based on measuring the transcriptional activity of promoters by linking an easily detectable reporter gene to the regulatory sequence of interest. Reporter genes encoding chloramphenicol acetyltransferase, bacterial β-galactosidase (lacZ), or firefly luciferase are conventional and easy to handle. Fluorescent proteins, such as green fluorescent protein (GFP), have become more popular reporter markers for detection within living cells. (See the transgenic section in detail for each reporter gene.) These conventional systems are designed for transient expression. The advanced vectors contain both the selective marker gene and the episomal replication signal in mammals in addition to reporter genes (67,68).

After preparation of plasmid combined with the regulatory sequence of interest, the constructed reporter plasmids are transfected into cells by chemical or physical treatments. After addition or withdrawal of bioactive reagents to the reporter assay system, effects are evaluated by changes of the reporter gene expression. Both colorimetric and chemiluminescent substrates are available for measuring lacZ and luciferase activity. Quantitative fluorometric assay of GFP is performed using known amounts of purified GFP protein with fluorometric illuminate. GFP systems have some advantages over the other two reporter systems. In some expression systems, GFP can be detected directly without cell disruption. The cells, which express GFP, can be monitored with fluorescence microscopy. In addition, GFP-expressing cells can be successfully sorted by flow cytometry (69). Various transgenic mice have been already generated using LacZ or GFP reporter gene (see the next section), and DP cells and follicular epithelial cells from transgenic mice may be available for reporter assay systems (70). Introduction of the gene of interest into hair follicle cells has been reported; for example, an androgen receptor gene was transiently transfected and successfully overexpressed in DP cells (71). In contrast, low rates of the gene transfer using an adenovirus were found in DP and follicle epithelial cells (72). Compared to the transient expression system, established cell lines are helpful to run a bioassay system without preparation of primary cells for every experiment. Rat vibrissa DP cell lines, which retain hair-inductive ability, have been generated with a polyomavirus large T gene inserted into a retrovirus vector (73). If the DP cell lines maintain hair-inductive ability, they would also be useful for screening molecules that affect the hair-inductive ability of DP combined with in vitro grafting, although the biological character of immortalized cells is unknown. The immortalized DP cell lines are expected as better host cells for overexpression study because they can uptake exogenous DNA more efficiently than primary or cultured DP cells isolated from human or mouse tissues. Also keratinocyte cell lines transfected with a reporter plasmid have been constructed and used for screening of bioactive compounds (73).

Use of Transgenic Models and Gene Targeting for Studying Hair Growth Mechanism

Transgenic Techniques

Since the 1980s, hair biology is being studied using recombinant DNA techniques through skin-related research for several reasons. First, the hair provides the most obvious phenotype, which is easily detectable without surgical dissection or specific equipment, and so hair abnormalities were reported in many gene-manipulated mouse models (mostly gene knockout model). Secondly, several skin-specific gene regulatory elements (promoter) have been developed especially for the keratin gene family. These keratin promoters provide very useful tools to overexpress the genes of interest, specifically in the skin epidermis and follicular epithelium. Using this technique many genes have been proved to be essentially involved in hair follicle development, growth, and cycling. Table 1 lists such genes revealed by these techniques. A transgenic approach artificially introduces genetic information, mostly DNA, into the germ cell line of mammals and plants to study the effect of the foreign protein expression. Among several species, mice are most widely used for such studies (74–76). There are three routes for transgene expression in mammals: retroviral vectors, pronuclear injection, and, the most recently developed, manipulation of embryonic stem cells. Among these, until recently, injection of foreign DNA into the pronucleus of a fertilized egg has been the most popular approach. The DNA that is integrated into the genome structure can be passed through the germ line as stable genomic information. The kind of integrated DNA varies dependent on the purpose of the transgenic line generation. Oocyte injections can deliver as much as several hundred kilobase of DNA into germ line but normally 1–10 kbp fragments are used. This injection technique allows genes with associated regulatory (promoter) sequences to integrate into the genome (Fig. 5).

Overexpression of Proteins in Hair Follicle Through Transgenic Delivery

If one wants to pursue the effect of gene dosage on the expression of product in a particular cell type or tissue, that gene sequence is put under a certain cell/tissue-specific regulatory promoter, so that the expression rate of the target gene of interest is controlled by that promoter. Fortunately, because several skin epidermis and hair follicles specific keratin genes are known, we can use the regulatory regions of these genes to construct transgene fragment (Table 2).

Transgenes are often found in multicopies in the genomic structure and are often in a head-to-tail tandem repeat order. The number of the insertions varies from a single copy to 50 copies. Often these tandem-repeat multiple insertions contribute to the amplification of total gene expression. Therefore, one reason to generate this type of transgenic expression is to study gene dosage effect so that amplification of gene expression makes it easy to detect phenotypic alteration when compared with endogenous single-copy gene expression. However,

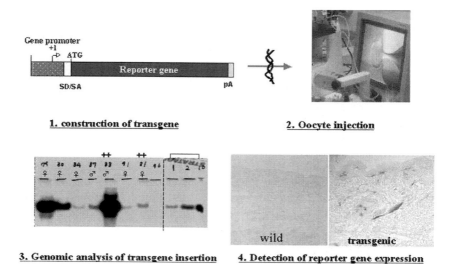

Figure 5 Summarized scheme of transgenic generation and detection of transgenic gene expression. *Abbreviations*: SD/SA, splicing signal sequence; PA, polyadenylation signal sequence.

many reports indicate that the site of integration of the transgene in the genome can greatly affect the expression efficiency so that sometimes hundred copies of transgene insertion may result in no signal, while, at times, only a single copy insertion is enough to exhibit detectable signals (77). Thus, postanalyses of generated transgenic lines are essential.

Usage of VEGF/TSP-1 Transgenic Mice

To investigate the biological function of VEGF (40) or TSP-1(28)-mediated angiogenesis, mice with skin specific overexpression of VEGF or TSP-1 in the basal layer of keratinocytes and ORS keratinocytes of hair follicles using Keratin 14 promoter cassettes (K14/VEGF, K14/TSP-1) were enrolled for hair studies.

Table 2 Promoter Used for Hair Follicle Specific Expression

Keratin used for promoter	Site of expression	Gene expressed
Ultrahigh sulfur keratin	cortex/cuticle	CAT (reporter) (93)
Keratin 5	basal/ORS	CD44 (116), PKC-α (117), integrin β4 (118)
Keratin 6	epidermis/ORS	ODC (119)
Keratin 14	basal/ORS	Agouti (120), thrombomodulin (121), Desmocollin-1 (122), Smad2 (123), COX (124)

K14/VEGF transgenic mice induced pronounced perifollicular vascularization resulting in accelerated hair regrowth after depilation and an increased size of hair follicles and hair shafts, as compared to wildtype littermates (40). Conversely, blockade of VEGF by systemic treatment with a neutralizing anti-VEGF antibody led to hair growth retardation and size reduction of hair follicles. No effects of VEGF treatment or VEGF blockade were observed in mouse vibrissa organ cultures, in the absence of a functional vascular system. These results identify VEGF as a major mediator of hair follicle growth and cycling and provide the first direct evidence that improved follicle vascularization promotes hair growth and increases hair follicle and hair size (40).

In TSP-1-deficient mice, the follicle growth phase was significantly prolonged, associated with increased perifollicular vascularization and vascular proliferation (28). Conversely, hair follicle growth was delayed in K14/TSP-1 transgenic mice that expressed high levels of TSP-1 in ORS keratinocytes, associated with reduced perifollicular vascularization (28). These effects were most likely mediated via its antiangiogenic effects because TSP-1 did not affect the growth of cultured murine vibrissae in the absence of a functional vascular system. These results identify a critical role for TSP-1 in the induction of anagen follicle involution, with potential implications for the therapeutic modulation of hair follicle growth (28).

Targeting Gene Ablation (Gene Knockout) Mouse Model

Disruption of the gene of interest by homologous recombination in embryonic stem cell (ES cells) and subsequent germ line transmitting produce a transgenic mouse in which the gene of interest has completely lost its function in vivo, so that the significance and role of the gene are undoubtedly clear. This approach is often referred to as gene knockout or gene targeting and is one of the most popular and advanced research tools in molecular biology. In hair biology research, many gene knockout mice are available. For example, in TGF-β1 knockout mice, catagen development was notably delayed. In contrast, TGF-β1 overexpressing mice exhibited a reduction in the number of hair follicles, (18) and subcutaneous injection of TGF-β1 in mice induced catagen phase (18,78). These results clearly indicate a stimulating role of TGF-β1 in hair regression. Because the appearance or existence of the hair follicle is the most obvious phenotype for knockout analysis, some studies reported the unexpected involvement of the targeted gene for hair follicle development. In most extreme cases, disruption of the signaling molecule, wnt inhibitor completely shut down the inductive ability of the hair follicle germ in embryonic skin during development (79). More recently, inducible turn-on or turn-off gene knockout systems have been developed, which make it possible to produce normal hair follicle formation until the developmental stage is finished but inactivate each hair cycle stage, so that involvement of the gene of interest in hair cycling is distinguishable from hair embryogenesis (80–83).

Power of Transgenic Approach for Monitoring Gene
Expression and Novel Evaluation Methods for Hair
Growth Compounds

Advantages of reporter type transgenic expression: The transgenic
approach in basic hair biology is mainly used in two ways as discussed in previous section: overexpression with hair-specific promoter or inactivation of
endogenous gene by gene targeting of ES cells. Both experimental designs
affect gene manipulation, resulting in phenotypic alteration, such as abnormal
hair growth, prolonged anagen period, and cessation of hair cycle re-entry.
These are very striking and clear results and bring impressive pictures to the
reader's mind, but these mouse strains themselves are often categorized as unu-
sable strains for further bioactive compound search. Completely different from
gene targeting approach, the reporter type transgenic approach, which designs
the transgene with reporter gene whose expression is controlled by the regulatory
element of the gene of interest, should not be expected to provide dramatic phenotypic changes at all; instead, changes in the reporter gene expression are very
close to the endogenous gene expression pattern. This type of transgenic model is
particularly useful when the level of endogenous product is difficult to detect by
immunohistochemistry (for protein) and in situ hybridization (mRNA, gene transcription level) because of low levels of the gene expression. Following are the
common reporter genes widely used to generate this type of transgenic animals.

Type of reporter gene: *CAT.* CAT gene encodes a converting enzyme
chloramphenicol acetyltransferase (CAT), which transfers an acetyl group (a
CH3CO-group) to chloramphenicol. CAT is a classical reporter and was extensively used in the early era of transgenic research (84). CAT shows a higher
sensitivity, but its measurement requires either a liquid scintillation method or
thin layer chromatography, which employ a radioisotope, or specific equipment
such as high performance liquid chromatography (HPLC); therefore, it is rarely
used to generate new transgenic lines in recent studies (85).

lacZ. β-galactosidase, a product of the lacZ gene, is the most popular reporter gene and particularly useful for studying precise localization of the desired
protein by tissue histochemistry. Detection of lacZ is usually achieved by the
enzymatic histochemical staining procedure using exogenous substrate, X-gal
(5-bromo-4-chloro-3-indolyl-β-D-galactopyranoside). Insoluble, precipitated
X-gal product retains very precisely within the original β-galactosidase-produ-
cing cells, so that lacZ-positive cells are easily distinguishable from other negative cells. To measure the β-galactosidase activity quantitatively, colorimetric
assay method is available using homogenated tissue supernatant. Although this
colorimetric measurement would not be very sensitive, some researchers still
prefer to generate their transgenics with lacZ reporter because of its superior
resolution on tissue sample compared to other reporters.

Luciferase. Firefly luciferase is similar to CAT, but no radioactive compounds are necessary for its detection, as the signal is usually detectable by

chemiluminescence. Usages of luciferase reporter in transgenic model are also documented in recent publications (86,87). The disadvantage of using CAT or luciferase as reporters is that these do not allow visualization of the signal in tissue in situ.

   Fluorescent protein. Perhaps in the last few years, fluorescent proteins as reporters have overtaken lacZ as a useful marker for monitoring gene expression. Green fluorescent protein (GFP) or enhanced GFP (EGFP) is most widely used for transgene construct and stable expression (88). GFP is a spontaneously fluorescent protein isolated from marine-living jellyfish (*Aquaria Victoria*). GFP has chromophore at its center and emits fluorescence by transducing the blue chemiluminescence into green fluorescent light by energy transfer. Now there are several fluorescent protein derivatives available from different marine creatures, (89,90). A characteristic feature of these fluorescent proteins is that they do not require cofactors to emit fluorescence. The ability to simply clone the cDNA of GFP protein, and successfully express it in transfected mammalian cells by vector DNA as a reporter gene, greatly enhances the application of this protein in biological research. Advantages of using fluorescent proteins as reporters for hair follicle research are: (*i*) cells derived from fluorescent protein transgenics can be easily isolated for example, by fluorescent-activated cell sorting (FACS), and (*ii*) expression of fluorescent protein can be visualized under living conditions without dissecting or homogenizing tissues, therefore, without an enzymatic reaction or radioactive detection.

Versican reporter transgenic model for the study of active status of DP: Versican is a member of a large chondroitin sulfate proteoglycan family and is specifically expressed in DP, especially during anagen onset period (11,29). The expression of versican in active DP was further confirmed by gene expression using in situ hybridization (29,91). Transgenics with lacZ and GFP reporter genes under human versican regulatory element (promoter) have been generated, and their expression pattern has been confirmed to be nearly identical with endogenous versican messenger ribonucleic acid (mRNA) by in situ hybridization (29). Because the degree of reporter gene expression (either lacZ or GFP) correlates with versican gene expression, and versican expression correlates with anagen hair induction in hair cycle, the reporter gene activity should represent active (inductive) status of DP cells. To test this hypothesis, DP cells from this versican-GFP transgenic mouse were isolated by FACS and grafted with undifferentiated neonatal epidermal cells by cellular grafting procedure in an immunodeficient mouse strain. The results consistently showed that reporter-positive (GFP-positive) cells have hair inductive ability, whereas negative cells do not (29). These results proved that the degree of reporter gene expression, which is easily visible or quantitative, could be used for measuring hair inductive ability of potential hair growth-modulating compounds (data not shown). We have tested several bioactive compounds, including those listed in Table 1, and most of them showed no effect alone, suggesting that possibly single isolated molecules are not enough to promote hair growth modulation. However, one of patterning morphogen molecules, wnt, could maintain hair inductive ability of isolated DP cells (70), and this induction occurred only with certain subtype of wnt family, such as wnt-3 and wnt-7 (70). These results indicate the usefulness of the versican transgenic system to assess hair follicle modulating compounds as well as for basic hair research. We examined the effect of a known hair follicle inducing compound, cyclosporin A, using the versican transgenic system. Firstly, topical application of cyclosporin A in vivo on the back skin of transgenic animals showed upregulation of GFP fluorescence in newly generated DP cell region (91) (Fig. 6). Induction of versican gene expression by cyclosporin A was also monitored utilizing versican-reporter transgenic mouse skin-derived cells. When cyclosporin A was added in unsorted dermal cells (i.e., containing follicular and other dermal cells) derived from versican–GFP reporter transgenic mouse skin, a significant response of increased versican expression was observed as assessed by GFP reporter gene expression. However, when sorted GFP-positive cells were used alone (i.e., purified DP fraction without follicular epithelium), they

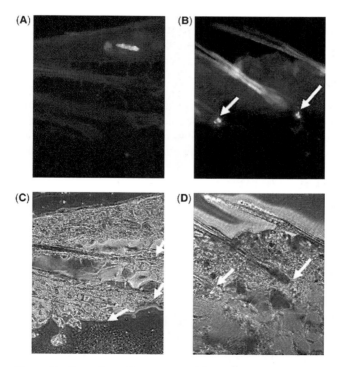

Figure 6 Detection of anagen-specific marker (versican) induction in vivo. Control mouse skin of the versican transgenic mouse (**A** & **C**), and 10 days after topical application of 10 μmoles cyclosporin A (**B** & **D**). Fluorescent microscopy images (**A** & **B**) and bright field (Nomarski) of unfixed, nonstained tissue. Arrows indicate specific fluorescent signals in newly generated hair dermal papilla for versican gene induction.

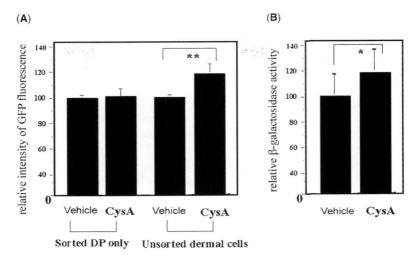

Figure 7 A known hair growth promotion compound-upregulated versican expression. Cyclosporin A (CysA; 5 μM)–induced versican expression assessed by GFP (**A**) or lacZ reporter (**B**) in isolated (sorted) and nonisolated (unsorted) dermal papilla cells.

failed to respond, indicating that cyclosporin A may act on versican gene induction via non-GFP-positive cells, perhaps follicular epithelium cells (Fig. 7) (91). This response was also observed when versican–lacZ reporter transgenic-derived dermal cells were used (Fig. 7) (91). These results imply the potential application of a novel screening approach for hair growth promoting compounds by monitoring versican expression as a positive indicator. A schematic representation for the screening system is illustrated in Figure 8.

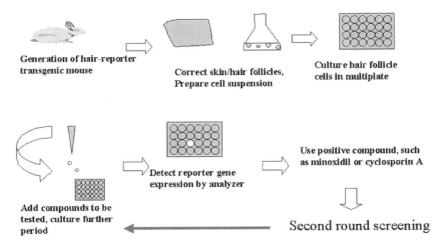

Figure 8 Schematic diagram of drug screening procedure using reporter transgenic mice.

VEGF-Reporter Transgenic Mouse

VEGF is only expressed at low levels in vivo in skin compared with abundant expression in cultured keratinocytes in vivo. (See previous section of angiogenetic factor in this chapter.) In order to monitor VEGF in vivo, VEGF-reporter transgenic mice were generated, and these showed bright GFP signal both in the epidermis and ORS of the hair follicles (92). In order to monitor GFP reporter in vivo, transgenic mice were anathesitized and placed on confocal microscopy (92). Although this experiment model needs substantial improvement for actual use in monitoring the effect of compounds in vivo, the specific signal generated was enough for detection on the confocal monitor. So far, using this model, we have monitored the effect of hair modulating compounds for a few hours, but the results demonstrate the possibility of monitoring in vivo for longer periods of time in order to confirm its effects on morphogenetic changes.

Other Transgenic Lines Useful for Hair Growth Research

Transgenic mice with CAT gene expression under the control of hair-specific ultrahigh sulfur keratin protein (UHSK) promoter have been generated (93). This transgenic system showed specific CAT activity in hair follicle by in situ hybridization with cortex and cuticle-specific endogenous UHSK gene expression demonstrating correct expression site of the reporter gene. Moreover, this transgenic model showed hair cycle–specific CAT activity. Regeneration of transgenic lines with fluorescent protein under the control of the same promoter could be useful, both, to isolate specific hair follicle epithelial cell types and monitor hair epithelial cell proliferation.

FUTURE DIRECTION: HOW DOES BIOTECHNOLOGY CONTRIBUTE TO UNDERSTANDING THE MECHANISM, IDENTIFYING TARGETS, AND DEVELOPING NEW PRODUCTS FOR HAIR GROWTH PROMOTION?

Bioproduction of Hair Growth Modulators by Biotechnology

Both minoxidil and finasteride, two FDA-approved hair growth modulation compounds are relatively small molecules and do not need to be produced by bioproduction. However, other potential compounds, for example, cyclosporin-related compounds, are good target molecules for a biofermentation process for mass production as hair growth modulators. Cyclosporin A is an immunosuppresant and is a well-known strong hair growth promotion compound (94). In fact, cyclosporin A itself has been already produced by biofermentation using *Tolypocladium inflatum* as a production strain (95). Also other growth modulation molecules such as small molecular size peptides FGF, shh, and wnt are potential candidates for future recombinant bioproduction using animal cell culture systems. However, in some of these, the presence of peptide signaling molecules are known to make these inactive when produced as recombinant proteins in culture system, or perhaps the three-dimensional structure or cross-linking at cytokine residues are inappropriate compared with naturally synthesized ones (96). Also some of the vitamins may work for androgenic alopecia, such as B12 and vitamin H (biotin) (97). For biotin production, biofermentation with genetically manipulated bacterial strains in which biotin-synthesized gene cluster is harbored as a vector plasmid in order to achieve higher bioconversion yield of vitamin from the substrate has been demonstrated (98).

Systematic Approach: Microarray Analysis, Proteomics, and SNP Genetic Approach

Recent completion of the human genome project has led to a new era of comprehensive genome-wide research. This research field includes microarray technology, in which either oligonucleotide or cDNA of more than 10,000 genes complementary to individual genes in the genome are attached within a tiny (mostly less than 10 mm) printed area, called DNA chip or DNA microarray. DNA microarray is one DNA hybridization technique to detect the degree of temporal mRNA gene expression at once, using normally two fluorescent dyes, Cy3 and Cy5. The most commonly used microarrays are affymetryx oligo array and agilent array. DNA microarray has now been used in the dermatological research field, and a few studies have been reported in the hair biology research field (99–101). So far, these reports focus on comprehensive gene profiling in pathological conditions of hair follicles, such as alopecia areata. However, accumulated evidence for normal hair, MPB, and each hair cycle–specific gene profiling by microarray analysis, will lead us to elucidate the complicated, comprehensive set of gene expression changes for key molecules and could reveal the fundamental mechanism of hair growth and hair cycling. For example, one research group that has shown comprehensive gene expression profiling data specific in mouse bulge area, could impact our understanding on how communication between hair epithelium stem cell and hair DP cells occurs in EMI (102). Compared with DNA microarray, comprehensive protein profiling combined with the analytical technology, called proteomics, could take time to use routinely, and it may be difficult to judge, at present, whether this technology could become the default standard for searching key molecules that modulate hair growth (103–106). In the postgenome phase of research, the most attractive theme and perhaps longest awaited area is whether genetic factors affect MPB. Analysis of single nucleotide polymorphisms (SNP) between normal and MPB patients could lead to deciding whether genetic factors are directly involved in MPB. When this evidence becomes clear, tailor-made hair growth modulation compounds, dependent on individual set of SNP, which improve individual hair growth more effectively, could be developed.

Regeneration of Hair Follicle: Transplantation of Genetically Engineered Hair Follicle Cells and Gene Therapy

Different from topical application of hair growth modulation compounds, the latest hope to cure baldness is to develop transplantation technology, so that self-follicle (or other part) tissue could be transplanted back to the scalp skin, with the expectation that hair follicle would regenerate without immuno-rejection. Hair follicle organ transplantation has been already developed in the United States, but disadvantages of this approach are the limited number of follicles available as well as the pain associated with the procedure, making the use of this technology limited. Alternatively, cellular grafting of hair follicles, preferentially hair mesenchymal DP or DS cells, and hair follicular epithelial cells (stem cells) are expected to overcome the disadvantages of the current transplantation procedure. So far, successful hair generation by cellular grafting is limited to rodent species (29), mainly because of the limited source of human cells that possess the hair inductive ability or the hair follicle differentiation property. This could be due to the loss of the essential signaling cascade of EMI during cell culture period that is necessary to obtain enough number of cells for grafting. Delivering appropriate genes for hair induction either in cultured human cells or at the grafting site may solve this dilemma. One such delivering method is the delivery of the gene or protein of interest by a liposomal vector. Hair follicles are thought to be the first candidate place where such delivered liposomal vector is able to integrate into the skin (107–109).

CONCLUSION

During the last 20 years or so, hair biology research in basic science and developmental biology field has progressed significantly on molecular levels. We now definitely know that hair growth requires not only molecular signals between follicular epithelial stem and follicular papilla, but also angiogenic factors, appropriate cycling control including the manipulation of apoptotic force in catagen to telogen phase. Furthermore, melanogenesis, neurotropic factors, and the endocrine system should also considerably contribute to hair growth modulation. Also several in vivo transgenic and in vitro cellular-based approaches have been developed to test for screening hair growth modulating compounds, as described in this chapter. This combination, elucidation of the basic mechanism of hair growth and the hair cycle, and renovation of more effective and reliable screening methods based on knowledge of basic science, should facilitate to develop real effective hair growth modulating compounds, or alternatively more clinical-oriented procedures, such as cellular transplantation. Biotechnology and recombinant DNA technology would become a vital tool for putting this research forward and hopefully this would lead to enjoying our health with a higher level of quality of life (QOL) condition in the near future.

REFERENCES

1. Stenn KS, Paus R. Controls of hair follicle cycling. Physiol Rev 2001; 81:449–494.
2. Saitoh M, Uzuka M, Sakamoto M. Human hair cycle. J Invest Dermatol 1970; 54:65–81.
3. Muller-Rover S, Handjiski B, van der Veen C, Eichmuller S, Foitzik K, McKay IA, Stenn KS, Paus R. A comprehensive guide for the accurate classification of murine hair follicles in distinct hair cycle stages. J Invest Dermatol 2001; 117:3–15.
4. Cotsarelis G, Sun TT, Lavker RM. Label-retaining cells reside in the bulge area of pilosebaceous unit: implications for follicular stem cells, hair cycle, and skin carcinogenesis. Cell 1990; 61:1329–1337.
5. Taylor G, Lehrer MS, Jensen PJ, Sun TT, Lavker RM. Involvement of follicular stem cells in forming not only the follicle but also the epidermis. Cell 2000; 102:451–461.
6. Oshima H, Rochat A, Kedzia C, Kobayashi K, Barrandon Y. Morphogenesis and renewal of hair follicles from adult multipotent stem cells. Cell 2001; 104:233–245.
7. Yu DW, Yang T, Sonoda T, Gaffney K, Jensen PJ, Dooley T, Ledbetter S, Freedberg IM, Lavker R, Sun TT. Message of nexin 1, a serine protease inhibitor, is accumulated in the follicular papilla during anagen of the hair cycle. J Cell Sci 1995; 108(Pt 12):3867–3874.
8. Montagna W, Chase HB, Malone HJD, Melarango HP. Cyclic changes in polysaccharides of the papilla of the hair growth. J Micros Sci 1952; 93:241–245.
9. Westgate GE, Messenger AG, Watson LP, Gibson WT. Distribution of proteoglycans during the hair growth cycle in human skin. J Invest Dermatol 1991; 96:191–195.
10. Shinomura T, Nishida Y, Ito K, Kimata K. cDNA cloning of PG-M, a large chondroitin sulfate proteoglycan expressed during chondrogenesis in chick limb buds. Alternative spliced multiforms of PG-M and their relationships to versican. J Biol Chem 1993; 268:14461–14469.
11. du Cros DL, LeBaron RG, Couchman JR. Association of versican with dermal matrices and its potential role in hair follicle development and cycling. J Invest Dermatol 1995; 105:426–431.
12. Hardy MH. The secret life of the hair follicle. Trends Genet 1992; 8:55–61.
13. Botchkarev VA, Kishimoto J. Molecular control of epithelial-mesenchymal interactions during hair follicle cycling. J Investig Dermatol Symp Proc 2003; 8:46–55.
14. Millar SE. Molecular mechanisms regulating hair follicle development. J Invest Dermatol 2002; 118:216–225.
15. Wallner EI, Yang Q, Peterson DR, Wada J, Kanwar YS. Relevance of extracellular matrix, its receptors, and cell adhesion molecules in mammalian nephrogenesis. Am J Physiol 1998; 275:F467–F477.
16. Fuchs E, Merrill BJ, Jamora C, DasGupta R. At the roots of a never-ending cycle. Dev Cell 2001; 1:13–25.
17. Ebling FJ. The biology of hair. Dermatol Clin 1987; 5:467–481.
18. Foitzik K, Lindner G, Mueller-Roever S, Maurer M, Botchkareva N, Botchkarev V, Handjiski B, Metz M, Hibino T, Soma T, Dotto GP, Paus R. Control of murine hair follicle regression (catagen) by TGF-beta1 in vivo. FASEB J 2000; 14:752–760.
19. Soma T, Dohrmann CE, Hibino T, Raftery LA. Profile of transforming growth factor-beta responses during the murine hair cycle. J Invest Dermatol 2003; 121:969–975.

20. Rudman SM, Philpott MP, Thomas GA, Kealey T. The role of IGF-I in human skin and its appendages: morphogen as well as mitogen? J Invest Dermatol 1997; 109:770–777.

21. Soma T, Tsuji Y, Hibino T. Involvement of transforming growth factor-beta2 in catagen induction during the human hair cycle. J Invest Dermatol 2002; 118:993–997.

22. Weedon D, Strutton G. Apoptosis as the mechanism of the involution of hair follicles in catagen transformation. Acta Derm Venereol 1981; 61:335–339.

23. Lindner G, Botchkarev VA, Botchkareva NV, Ling G, van der Veen C, Paus R. Analysis of apoptosis during hair follicle regression (catagen). Am J Pathol 1997; 151:1601–1617.

24. Soma T, Ogo M, Suzuki J, Takahashi T, Hibino T. Analysis of apoptotic cell death in human hair follicles in vivo and in vitro. J Invest Dermatol 1998; 111:948–954.

25. Stenn KS, Lawrence L, Veis D, Korsmeyer S, Seiberg M. Expression of the bcl-2 protooncogene in the cycling adult mouse hair follicle. J Invest Dermatol 1994; 103:107–111.

26. Tsuji Y, Denda S, Soma T, Raftery L, Momoi T, Hibino T. A potential suppressor of TGF-beta delays catagen progression in hair follicles. J Investig Dermatol Symp Proc 2003; 8:65–68.

27. Botchkarev VA. Bone morphogenetic proteins and their antagonists in skin and hair follicle biology. J Invest Dermatol 2003; 120:36–47.

28. Yano K, Brown LF, Lawler J, Miyakawa T, Detmar M. Thrombospondin-1 plays a critical role in the induction of hair follicle involution and vascular regression during the catagen phase. J Invest Dermatol 2003; 120:14–19.

29. Kishimoto J, Ehama R, Wu L, Jiang S, Jiang N, Burgeson RE. Selective activation of the versican promoter by epithelial-mesenchymal interactions during hair follicle development. Proc Natl Acad Sci USA 1999; 96:7336–7341.

30. Lavker RM, Risse B, Brown H, Ginsburg D, Pearson J, Baker MS, Jensen PJ. Localization of plasminogen activator inhibitor type 2 (PAI-2) in hair and nail: implications for terminal differentiation. J Invest Dermatol 1998; 110:917–922.

31. Hanakawa Y, Matsuyoshi N, Stanley JR. Expression of desmoglein 1 compensates for genetic loss of desmoglein 3 in keratinocyte adhesion. J Invest Dermatol 2002; 119:27–31.

32. Nakamura M, Matzuk MM, Gerstmayer B, Bosio A, Lauster R, Miyachi Y, Werner S, Paus R. Control of pelage hair follicle development and cycling by complex interactions between follistatin and activin. FASEB J 2003; 17:497–499.

33. Detmar M. The role of VEGF and thrombospondins in skin angiogenesis. J Dermatol Sci 2000; 24(suppl 1):S78–S84.

34. Tischer E, Mitchell R, Hartman T, Silva M, Gospodarowicz D, Fiddes JC, Abraham JA. The human gene for vascular endothelial growth factor. Multiple protein forms are encoded through alternative exon splicing. J Biol Chem 1991; 266:11947–11954.

35. Quinn TP, Peters KG, De Vries C, Ferrara N, Williams LT. Fetal liver kinase 1 is a receptor for vascular endothelial growth factor and is selectively expressed in vascular endothelium. Proc Natl Acad Sci USA 1993; 90:7533–7537.

36. de Vries C, Escobedo JA, Ueno H, Houck K, Ferrara N, Williams LT. The fms-like tyrosine kinase, a receptor for vascular endothelial growth factor. Science 1992; 255:989–991.

37. Soker S, Takashima S, Miao HQ, Neufeld G, Klagsbrun M. Neuropilin-1 is expressed by endothelial and tumor cells as an isoform-specific receptor for vascular endothelial growth factor 1998; Cell 92:735–745.

38. Jimenez B, Volpert OV, Crawford SE, Febbraio M, Silverstein RL, Bouck N. Signals leading to apoptosis-dependent inhibition of neovascularization by thrombospondin-1. Nat Med 2000; 6:41–48.

39. Yano K, Kajiya K, Ishiwata M, Hong YK, Miyakawa T, Detmar M. Ultraviolet B-induced skin angiogenesis is associated with a switch in the balance of vascular endothelial growth factor and thrombospondin-1 expression. J Invest Dermatol 2004; 122:201–208.

40. Yano K, Brown LF, Detmar M. Control of hair growth and follicle size by VEGF-mediated angiogenesis. J Clin Invest 2001; 107:409–417.

41. Randall VA. Androgens and human hair growth. Clin Endocrinol (Oxf) 1994; 40:439–457.

42. Hamilton JB. Effect of castration in adolescent and young adult males upon further changes in the proportions of bare and hairy scalp. J Clin Endocrinol Metab 1960; 20:1309–1318.

43. Andersson S, Russell DW. Structural and biochemical properties of cloned and expressed human and rat steroid 5 alpha-reductases. Proc Natl Acad Sci USA 1990; 87:3640–3644.

44. Andersson S, Berman DM, Jenkins EP, Russell DW. Deletion of steroid 5 alpha-reductase 2 gene in male pseudohermaphroditism. Nature 1991; 354: 159–161.

45. Thigpen AE, Silver RI, Guileyardo JM, Casey ML, McConnell JD, Russell DW. Tissue distribution and ontogeny of steroid 5 alpha-reductase isozyme expression J Clin Invest 1993; 92:903–910.

46. Sawaya ME, Price VH. Different levels of 5alpha-reductase type I and II, aromatase, and androgen receptor in hair follicles of women and men with androgenetic alopecia. J Invest Dermatol 1997; 109:296–300.

47. Ogawa H, Hattori M. In: Seiji M, Bernstein IA, eds. Normal and Abnormal Epidermal Differentiation. Tokyo: Tokyo Univ. Press, 1983:159–170.

48. Buhl AE, Waldon DJ, Miller BF, Brunden MN. Differences in activity of minoxidil and cyclosporin A on hair growth in nude and normal mice. Comparisons of in vivo and in vitro studies. Lab Invest 1990; 62:104–107.

49. Stoner E. The clinical development of a 5 alpha-reductase inhibitor, finasteride. J Steroid Biochem Mol Biol 1990; 37:375–378.

50. Tempany CM, Partin AW, Zerhouni EA, Zinreich SJ. Walsh PC. The influence of finasteride on the volume of the peripheral and periurethral zones of the prostate in men with benign prostatic hyperplasia. Prostate 1993; 22:39–42.

51. Peters DH, Sorkin EM. Finasteride. A review of its potential in the treatment of benign prostatic hyperplasia. Drugs 1993; 46:177–208.

52. Kaufman KD, Olsen EA, Whiting D, Savin R, DeVillez R, Bergfeld W, Price VH, Van Neste D, Roberts JL, Hordinsky M, Shapiro J, Binkowitz B, Gormley GJ. Finasteride in the treatment of men with androgenetic alopecia. Finasteride Male Pattern Hair Loss Study Group. J Am Acad Dermatol 1998; 39:578–589.

53. McClellan KJ, Markham A. Finasteride: a review of its use in male pattern hair loss. Drugs 1999; 57:111–126.

54. Leyden J, Dunlap F, Miller B, Winters P, Lebwohl M, Hecker D, Kraus S, Baldwin H, Shalita A, Draelos Z, et al. Finasteride in the treatment of men with front male pattern hair loss. J Am Acad Dermatol 1999; 40:930–937.

55. Russell DW, Wilson JD. Steroid 5 alpha-reductase: two genes/two enzymes. Annu Rev Biochem 1994; 63:25–61.

56. Mellin TN, Busch RD, Rasmusson GH. Azasteroids as inhibitors of testosterone 5 alpha-reductase in mammalian skin. J Steroid Biochem Mol Biol 1993; 44:121–131.

57. Andriole GL, Rittmaster RS, Loriaux DL, Kish ML, Linehan WM. The effect of 4MA, a potent inhibitor of 5 alpha-reductase, on the growth of androgen-responsive human genitourinary tumors grown in athymic nude mice. Prostate 1987; 10:189–197.

58. Uno H, Kurata S. Chemical agents and peptides affect hair growth. J Invest Dermatol 1993; 101:143S–147S.

59. Neubauer BL, Gray HM, Hanke CW, Hirsch KS, Hsiao KC, Jones CD, Kumar MV, Lawhorn DE, Lindzey J, McQuaid L, et al. LY191704 inhibits type I steroid 5 alpha-reductase in human scalp. J Clin Endocrinol Metab 1996; 81:2055–2060.

60. Schwartz JI, Tanaka WK, Wang DZ, Ebel DL, Geissler LA, Dallob A, Hafkin B, Gertz BJ. MK-386, an inhibitor of 5alpha-reductase type 1, reduces dihydrotestosterone concentrations in serum and sebum without affecting dihydrotestosterone concentrations in semen. J Clin Endocrinol Metab 1997; 82:1373–1377.

61. Voigt W, Fernandez EP, Hsia SL. Transformation of testosterone into 17 beta-hydroxy-5 alpha-androstan-3-one by microsomal preparations of human skin. J Biol Chem 1970; 245:5594–5599.

62. Liang T, Liao S. Inhibition of steroid 5 alpha-reductase by specific aliphatic unsaturated fatty acids. Biochem J 1992; 285(Pt 2):557–562.

63. Liang T, Liao S. Growth suppression of hamster flank organs by topical application of gamma-linolenic and other fatty acid inhibitors of 5alpha-reductase. J Invest Dermatol 1997; 109:152–157.

64. Iehle C, Delos S, Filhol O, Martin PM. Baculovirus-directed expression of human prostatic steroid 5 alpha-reductase 1 in an active form. J Steroid Biochem Mol Biol 1993; 46:177–182.

65. Buhl AE, Waldon DJ, Baker CA, Johnson GA. Minoxidil sulfate is the active metabolite that stimulates hair follicles. J Invest Dermatol 1990; 95:553–557.

66. Buhl AE, Waldon DJ, Conrad SJ, Mulholland MJ, Shull KL, Kubicek MF, Johnson GA, Brunden MN, Stefanski KJ, Stehle RG, et al. Potassium channel conductance: a mechanism affecting hair growth both in vitro and in vivo. J Invest Dermatol 1992; 98:315–319.

67. Margolskee RF, Kavathas P, Berg P. Epstein-Barr virus shuttle vector for stable episomal replication of cDNA expression libraries in human cells. Mol Cell Biol 1988; 8:2837–2847.

68. Belt PB, Groeneveld H, Teubel WJ, van de Putte P, Backendorf C. Construction and properties of an Epstein-Barr-virus-derived cDNA expression vector for human cells. Gene 1989; 84:407–417.

69. Galbraith DW, Anderson MT, Herzenberg LA. Flow cytometric analysis and FACS sorting of cells based on GFP accumulation. Methods Cell Biol 1999; 58:315–341.

70. Kishimoto J, Burgeson RE, Morgan BA. Wnt signaling maintains the hair-inducing activity of the dermal papilla. Genes Dev 2000; 14:1181–1185.

71. Inui S, Fukuzato Y, Nakajima T, Yoshikawa K, Itami S. Androgen-inducible TGF-beta1 from balding dermal papilla cells inhibits epithelial cell growth: a clue to understand paradoxical effects of androgen on human hair growth. FASEB J 2002; 16:1967–1969.

72. Rohr UP, Kronenwett R, Grimm D, Kleinschmidt J, Haas R. Primary human cells differ in their susceptibility to rAAV-2-mediated gene transfer and duration of reporter gene expression. J Virol Methods 2002; 105:265–275.

73. Filsell W, Little JC, Stones AJ, Granger SP, Bayley SA. Transfection of rat dermal papilla cells with a gene encoding a temperature-sensitive polyomavirus large T antigen generates cell lines retaining a differentiated phenotype. J Cell Sci 1994; 107(Pt 7):1761–1772.

74. Bernstein A, Breitman M. Genetic ablation in transgenic mice. Mol Biol Med 1989; 6:523–530.

75. Katsuki M. Transgenic mice as systems for analyses of biological functions. J Toxicol Sci 1988; 13:287–289.

76. Roemer K, Johnson PA, Friedmann T. Knock-in and knock-out. Transgenes, development and disease. A Keystone Symposium sponsored by Genentech and Immunex, Tamarron, CO, January 12–18, 1991. New Biol 1991; 3:331–335.

77. Ramirez A, Milot E, Ponsa I, Marcos-Gutierrez C, Page A, Santos M, Jorcano J, Vidal M. Sequence and chromosomal context effects on variegated expression of keratin 5/lacZ constructs in stratified epithelia of transgenic mice. Genetics 2001; 158:341–350.

78. Mori O, Hachisuka H, Sasai Y. Effects of transforming growth factor beta 1 in the hair cycle. J Dermatol 1996; 23:89–94.

79. Andl T, Reddy ST, Gaddapara T, Millar SE. WNT signals are required for the initiation of hair follicle development. Dev Cell 2002; 2:643–653.

80. Xie W, Chow LT, Paterson AJ, Chin E, Kudlow JE. Conditional expression of the ErbB2 oncogene elicits reversible hyperplasia in stratified epithelia and up-regulation of TGFalpha expression in transgenic mice. Oncogene 1999; 18:3593–3607.

81. Diamond I, Owolabi T, Marco M, Lam C, Glick A. Conditional gene expression in the epidermis of transgenic mice using the tetracycline-regulated transactivators tTA and rTA linked to the keratin 5 promoter. J Invest Dermatol 2000; 115:788–794.

82. Liu X, Alexander V, Vijayachandra K, Bhogte E, Diamond I, Glick A. Conditional epidermal expression of TGFbeta 1 blocks neonatal lethality but causes a reversible hyperplasia and alopecia. Proc Natl Acad Sci USA 2001; 98:9139–9144.

83. Li M, Chiba H, Warot X, Messaddeq N, Gerard C, Chambon P, Metzger D. RXR-alpha ablation in skin keratinocytes results in alopecia and epidermal alterations. Development 2001; 128:675–688.

84. Katchman SD, Del Monaco M, Wu M, Brown D, Hsu-Wong S, Uitto J. A transgenic mouse model provides a novel biological assay of topical glucocorticosteroid potency. Arch Dermatol 1995; 131:1274–1278.

85. Waldon DJ, Kubicek MF, Johnson GA, Buhl AE. A HPLC-based chloramphenicol acetyltransferase assay for assessing hair growth: comparison of the sensitivity of UV and fluorescence detection. Eur J Clin Chem Clin Biochem 1993; 31:41–45.

86. Zhang J, Tan X, Contag CH, Lu Y, Guo D, Harris SE, Feng JQ. Dissection of promoter control modules that direct Bmp4 expression in the epithelium-derived components of hair follicles. Biochem Biophys Res Commun 2002; 293:1412–1419.

87. Chen J, Kelz MB, Zeng G, Steffen C, Shockett PE, Terwilliger G, Schatz DG, Nestler EJ. Inducible, reversible hair loss in transgenic mice. Transgenic Res 2002; 11:241–247.

88. Kawakami N, Sakane N, Nishizawa F, Iwao M, Fukada SI, Tsujikawa K, Kohama Y, Ikawa M, Okabe M, Yamamoto H. Green fluorescent protein-transgenic mice: immune functions and their application to studies of lymphocyte development Immunol Lett 1999; 70:165–171.

89. Karasawa S, Araki T, Yamamoto-Hino M, Miyawaki A. A green-emitting fluorescent protein from Galaxeidae coral and its monomeric version for use in fluorescent labeling. J Biol Chem 2003; 278:34167–34171.

90. Tu H, Xiong Q, Zhen S, Zhong X, Peng L, Chen H, Jiang X, Liu W, Yang W, Wei J, et al. A naturally enhanced green fluorescent protein from magnificent sea anemone (Heteractis magnifica) and its functional analysis. Biochem Biophys Res Commun 2003; 301:879–885.

91. Kishimoto J, Souma T, Burgeson RE, Hibino T. Versican-expression by dermal papilla regerated hair follicles–A promising tool for hair regrowth products. IFSCC Magazine 2004; 7:21–28.

92. Kishimoto J, Ehama R, Ge Y, Kobayashi T, Nishiyama T, Detmar M, Burgeson RE. In vivo detection of human vascular endothelial growth factor promoter activity in transgenic mouse skin. Am J Pathol 2000; 157:103–110.

93. McNab AR, Andrus P, Wagner TE, Buhl AE, Waldon DJ, Kawabe TT, Rea TJ, Groppi V, Vogeli G. Hair-specific expression of chloramphenicol acetyltransferase in transgenic mice under the control of an ultra-high-sulfur keratin promoter. Proc Natl Acad Sci USA 1990; 87:6848–6852.

94. Paus R, Handjiski B, Czarnetzki BM, Eichmuller S. A murine model for inducing and manipulating hair follicle regression (catagen): effects of dexamethasone and cyclosporin. A J Invest Dermatol 1994; 103:143–147.

95. Agathos SN, Parekh R. Enhancement of cyclosporin production in a tolypocladium inflatum strain after epichlorohydrin treatment. J Biotechnol 1990; 13:73–81.

96. Hsieh JC, Rattner A, Smallwood PM, Nathans J. Biochemical characterization of wnt-frizzled interactions using a soluble, biologically active vertebrate wnt protein. Proc Natl Acad Sci USA 1999; 96:3546–3551.

97. Shelley WB, Shelley ED. Uncombable hair syndrome: observations on response to biotin and occurrence in siblings with ectodermal dysplasia. J Am Acad Dermatol 1985; 13:97–102.

98. Ifuku O, Haze S, Kishimoto J, Yanagi M. Biotin production by using recombinant DNA technology. J Nutr Sci Vitaminol (Tokyo) 1992; 263–266.

99. Xu X, Lyle S, Liu Y, Solky B, Cotsarelis G. Differential expression of cyclin D1 in the human hair follicle. Am J Pathol 2003; 163:969–978.

100. McElwee KJ, Hoffmann R. Alopecia areata – animal models. Clin Exp Dermatol 27:410–417.

101. Carroll JM, McElwee KJLEK, Byrne MC, Sundberg JP. Gene array profiling and immunomodulation studies define a cell-mediated immune response underlying

the pathogenesis of alopecia areata in a mouse model and humans. J Invest Dermatol 2002; 119:392–402.

102. Tumbar T, Guasch G, Greco V, Blanpain C, Lowry WE, Rendl M, Fuchs E. Defining the epithelial stem cell niche in skin. Science 2003; 303:359–363.

103. Goldstein AM. Changing paradigms in dermatology: proteomics: a new approach to skin disease. Clin Dermatol 2003; 21:370–374.

104. Gromov P, Skovgaard GL, Palsdottir H, Gromova I, Ostergaard M, Celis JE. Protein profiling of the human epidermis from the elderly reveals upregulation of a signature of interferon-{gamma}-induced polypeptides that includes manganese-superoxide dismutase and the p85{beta} subunit of phosphatidylinositol 3-kinase. Mol Cell Proteomics 2003; 2:70–84.

105. Moshell AN. The changing face of cutaneous biology as seen from the National Institutes of Health. J Investig Dermatol Symp Proc 2002; 7:4,5.

106. Boxman IL, Hensbergen PJ, Van Der Schors RC, Bruynzeel DP, Tensen CP, Ponec M. Proteomic analysis of skin irritation reveals the induction of HSP27 by sodium lauryl sulphate in human skin. Br J Dermatol 2002; 146:777–785.

107. Raghavachari N, Fahl WE. Targeted gene delivery to skin cells in vivo: a comparative study of liposomes and polymers as delivery vehicles. J Pharm Sci 2002; 91:615–622.

108. Li L, Hoffman RM. Model of selective gene therapy of hair growth: liposome targeting of the active Lac-Z gene to hair follicles of histocultured skin in vitro. Cell Dev Biol Anim 1995; 31:11–13.

109. Gupta S, Domashenko A, Cotsarelis G. The hair follicle as a target for gene therapy. Eur J Dermatol 2001; 11:353–356.

110. Sato N, Leopold PL, Crystal RG. Induction of the hair growth phase in postnatal mice by localized transient expression of sonic hedgehog. J Clin Invest 1999; 104:855–864.

111. Ozeki M, Tabata Y. Promoted growth of murine hair follicles through controlled release of basic fibroblast growth factor. Tissue Eng 2002; 8:359–366.

112. Ota Y, Saitoh Y, Suzuki S, Ozawa K, Kawano M, Imamura T. Fibroblast growth factor 5 inhibits hair growth by blocking dermal papilla cell activation. Biochem Biophys Res Commun 2002; 290:169–176.

113. Jindo T, Tsuboi R, Imai R, Takamori K, Rubin JS, Ogawa H. Hepatocyte growth factor/scatter factor stimulates hair growth of mouse vibrissae in organ culture. J Invest Dermatol 1994; 103:306–309.

114. Botchkarev VA, Botchkareva NV, Peters EM, Paus R. Epithelial growth control by neurotrophins: leads and lessons from the hair follicle. Prog Brain Res 2004; 146:493–513.

115. Su HY, Hickford JG, Bickerstaffe R, Palmer BR. Insulin-like growth factor 1 and hair growth. Dermatol Online J 1999; 5:1.

116. Kaya G, Rodriguez I, Jorcano JL, Vassalli P, Stamenkovic I. Selective suppression of CD44 in keratinocytes of mice bearing an antisense CD44 transgene driven by a tissue-specific promoter disrupts hyaluronate metabolism in the skin and impairs keratinocyte proliferation. Genes Dev 1997; 11:996–1007.

117. Wang HQ, Smart RC. Overexpression of protein kinase C-alpha in the epidermis of transgenic mice results in striking alterations in phorbol ester-induced inflammation

and COX-2, MIP-2 and TNF-alpha expression but not tumor promotion. J Cell Sci 1999; 112(Pt 20):3497–3506.

118. van der Neut R, Cachaco AS, Thorsteinsdottir S, Janssen H, Prins D, Bulthuis J, van der Valk M, Calafat J. Sonnenberg A. Partial rescue of epithelial phenotype in integrin beta4 null mice by a keratin-5 promoter driven human integrin beta4 transgene. J Cell Sci 1999; 112(Pt 22):3911–3922.

119. Soler AP, Gilliard G, Megosh LC, O'Brien TG. Modulation of murine hair follicle function by alterations in ornithine decarboxylase activity. J Invest Dermatol 1996; 106:1108–1113.

120. Kucera GT, Bortner DM, Rosenberg MP. Overexpression of an agouti cDNA in the skin of transgenic mice recapitulates dominant coat color phenotypes of spontaneous mutants. Dev Biol 1996; 173:162–173.

121. Raife TJ, Lager DJ, Peterson JJ, Erger RA, Lentz SR. Keratinocyte-specific expression of human thrombomodulin in transgenic mice: effects on epidermal differentiation and cutaneous wound healing. J Investig Med 1998; 46:127–133.

122. Henkler F, Strom M, Mathers K, Cordingley H, Sullivan K, King I. Trangenic misexpression of the differentiation-specific desmocollin isoform 1 in basal keratinocytes. J Invest Dermatol 2001; 116:144–149.

123. Ito Y, Sarkar P, Mi Q, Wu N, Bringas P Jr, Liu Y, Reddy S, Maxson R, Deng C, Chai Y. Overexpression of Smad2 reveals its concerted action with Smad4 in regulating TGF-beta-mediated epidermal homeostasis. Dev Biol 2001; 236:181–194.

124. Bol DK, Rowley RB, Ho CP, Pilz B, Dell J, Swerdel M, Kiguchi K, Muga S, Klein R, Fischer SM. Cyclooxygenase-2 overexpression in the skin of transgenic mice results in suppression of tumor development. Cancer Res 2002; 62:2516–2521.

12

Biotechnology in Hair Care (III): Hair Coloring and Gray Hair

Desmond J. Tobin

Department of Biomedical Sciences, University of Bradford, Bradford, U.K.

BIOLOGY OF HAIR PIGMENTATION

The Significance of Hair Color in Society

As social beings we communicate significantly via our physical appearance. Of all our visible features, skin and hair color contribute disproportionately to our overall visual appearance and highlight striking variations between different human subgroups. The main contributor to this phenotypic palette is a complex class of mixed indole-rich compounds called melanins. Unlike skin color, where hemoglobins and carotenoids contribute also to color perceived at the skin surface, pigmentation of hair relies on the presence or absence of different types of melanins alone. These melanins, whether deposited in skin or hair fiber, are formed within cytoplasmic organelles called melanosomes that are produced within neural crest–derived pigment cells called melanocytes via a complex, phylogenetically ancient, biochemical pathway called melanogenesis.

Evolution of Skin and Hair Color

Evolutionary selective pressures are thought responsible for the bewildering array of natural hair shades ranging from yellows, reds, and browns to black in humans. Though not formally testable, evolutionary selective pressures may also account for the hair color "biologic clock," as gray/white hair is almost universally a harbinger of lost youth! Recent advances in molecular genetics have started to yield clues to explain the dramatic diversity of human scalp hair color, especially among northern Europeans. Both skin and hair pigmentation phenotypes appear to be linked to degree of variability (polymorphism) in the melanocortin-1 receptor (MC1-R) gene and perhaps others. This receptor is activated through binding of the peptide α-melanocyte-stimulating hormone (α-MSH), an interaction competitively inhibited by agouti signaling protein (ASP). Most northern European individuals with red hair are homozygotes or compound heterozygotes for a few MC1-R mutations (1). Natural selection pressures may have restrained mutation of this gene in the hot, humid, and sunny tropics, ensuring dark hair and skin. These pressures may have been less critical as humans migrated to less sunny, less humid, colder northern climes. There, this break on gene mutation may have lifted, resulting in the emergence of functionally relevant mutations in the MC1-R gene.

So what of today? Is there any biologic value in human hair pigmentation and, indeed, its subsequent loss with aging in humans? Although hair growth and pigmentation facilitated evolutionary success in nonhuman mammals, via thermal insulation, camouflage, social and sexual communication, and sensory perception, these do not appear to have been critical for human survival. Having said that, we still should not diminish the role hair (and hair color) plays in social and sexual communications among modern humans, where our relative nakedness draws attention to scalp hair that, uniquely among primates, can be very thick, very long, and very pigmented. The hair follicle pigmentary unit appears to lie too deep in the skin to be influenced, at least directly, by ultraviolet radiation (UVR) (2). One attractive possibility may derive from *Homo sapiens*'s littoral evolution by seacoasts and riverbanks where early humans consumed considerable amounts of fish, many of which concentrated heavy metals (3). Thus, the ability to rapidly rid the body of these toxic metals, by selectively binding to melanin (4), would have a selective advantage. Furthermore, long-melanized scalp hair could trap/bind chemicals toxins, and heavy metals, and so prevent access to the living tissue of the highly vascularized scalp. It may be worth a mention here that this avidity of melanin may be very relevant when engineering biotechnologies to affect hair pigmentation (see following text).

Impressive evidence suggests that primary function(s) of melanin may be via the antimicrobial properties of melanocytes, melanosomes, and melanin (5). The reactive quinone intermediates generated during melanin biosynthesis have potent antibiotic properties, and this may be important as hair follicles provide numerous ports of entry into the body for micro-organisms (6). However, we need to avoid linking too tightly our current understanding of human physiology and the concept of natural selection as a perfecting force. This may be particularly important regarding pigmentation, as melanins can be produced by many species of bacteria, fungi, and helminthes that are actually pathogenic to humans. Here, melanin is associated with virulence via hindering host defense mechanisms (7). Melanization of fungi, for example, is particularly associated with subcutaneous infected chromoblastomycosis, for example, and in the yeast infection *Cryptococcus neoformans* (8). Thus, more melanin distributed inappropriately by imperfect biotechnologies may not be compatible with healthy skin and hair. These observations further demand that the development and exploitation of biotechnologies that alter the physical characteristics of hair be based on a sound understanding of the basic biology of the human hair follicle. Biotechnological intervention in hair pigmentation will need to pay due attention to the fact that humans have all but lost our ability to grow hair synchronously (i.e., as a wave). The characteristic mosaic pattern of human scalp hair growth and pigmentation, where autonomy resides mostly within individual hair follicles, makes the human scalp hair follicle somewhat resistant to the influences of solely systemic modifiers, including potential therapeutic modalities.

Origin and Development of the Hair Pigmentary Unit in Humans

Despite their common origin as melanoblasts migrating from the neural crest, epidermal and follicular melanocyte subpopulations are, for the most part, broadly distinct. This can be appreciated instantly by the objective beholder when observing gray or white-haired Black individuals and conversely, raven-haired white-skinned Eurasians. This is further supported clinically, by the selective/preferential targeting of epidermal, but not follicular, melanocytes in many cases of vitiligo, while only follicular melanocytes are damaged in the presumptive autoimmune hair disease acute alopecia areata. The importance of melanogenesis to humans is inferred by the phylogenetically ancient nature of this biochemical pathway and its expression very early on during embryologic development. Melanocytes are first detected in human skin around seven weeks (9) and synthesize actual pigment at least five months before birth.

Differences Between Epidermal and Hair Follicle Melanocytes

Epidermal and hair follicular melanocytes are derived from pluripotent neural crest cells that commit to the melanocyte lineage (so-called melanoblasts). They migrate out of the neural crest along stereotypic routes to enter the skin. This involves a long and eventful journey from the dorsal closing neural tube (10) until they enter the dermis. Melanocytes are present in the epidermis about two weeks before hair follicle development (9). After melanocytes reach the human epidermis, some of them leave the epidermis and enter the forming pilosebaceous units, where they distribute randomly as dopa-positive and dopa-negative cells (11). Once hair fiber formation commences, melanocytes concentrate near the basal lamina around the apex of the follicular/dermal papilla and, as amelanotic cells, mainly in the outer root sheath (ORS).

Analysis of mutations that effect differentiation, proliferation, and migration of melanocyte precursors in mice has helped clarify the events involved in the development of melanocyte compartments within the skin and hair follicle (12). Of the more than 90 loci shown to affect hair color in mouse (13), mutations in the receptor tyrosine kinase c-kit and its cognate ligand, stem cell factor (SCF) (14), and the endothelin 3 and its receptor (Ednrb), have been most informative. Mutant homozygotes exhibit an almost complete lack of hair pigmentation. In this way, melanocyte precursors interact with dramatically varying microenvironments (e.g., via integrins, extracellular matrix, cadherins etc.) during their regulated migration to the epidermis and hair follicle (15–17). Similar events are likely to be recapitulated during the reconstruction of the hair follicle pigmentary unit during normal cycling and may become impaired during graying/canities (see following text).

Despite their common origin, follicular melanocytes and epidermal melanocytes differ when in their respective distinct compartments in many important ways. For example, hair bulb melanogenic melanocytes are larger, have longer and more extensive dendrites, contain more developed Golgi and rough endoplasmic reticulum, and produce melanosomes two to four times larger than those in epidermal melanocytes (18). While melanin degrades almost completely in the differentiating layers of the epidermis, eumelanin granules transferred into hair cortical keratinocytes remain minimally digested (18). In this way, a eumelanic Caucasian individual may have raven black hair but very fair skin and blue eyes (e.g., as seen in the so-called "black" Irish). By far the most striking difference between these two melanocyte subpopulations, and one with significant implications for the regulation of hair pigmentation, is the observation that the activity of the hair bulb melanocyte is under cyclical control and that melanogenesis is tightly coupled to the hair growth cycle (19). Epidermal melanogenesis, by contrast, appears to be continuous (20).

Distribution of Melanocytes in the Human Scalp Hair Follicle

The growing anagen VI hair follicle is a useful starting position for a description of the cell biology of the hair pigmentary unit. Dopa-positive melanotic melanocytes occur in only two locations: the ORS of the infundibulum and in the hair bulb around the upper follicular papilla. Dopa-negative amelanotic melanocytes are distributed in the mid-to-lower ORS and also in the peripheral and most proximal hair bulb (Fig. 1A–C). The hair bulb is the only site of pigment production for the hair shaft and contains both highly melanogenic melanocytes and a minor subpopulation of poorly differentiated melanocytes (Fig. 2) (21,22). The role of amelanotic melanocytes in hair pigmentation is unclear (see below), although it has been speculated that these cells represent a pool of "transient" melanocytes that migrate from precursor melanocyte stores in the upper ORS (22–27). This pool may be an important one for targeting in any attempt to intervene biotechnologically in impaired hair pigmentation. Melanogenically active melanocytes are restricted to the upper hair matrix of the anagen hair follicle, just below the precortical keratinocyte population. This location correlates with the fact that melanin is transferred during anagen to the hair shaft cortex, less so to the medulla, and, very rarely, to the hair cuticle.

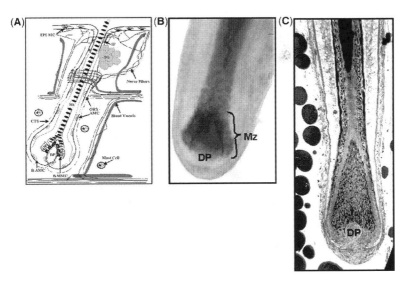

Figure 1 The hair follicle pigmentary unit in human scalp. (**A**) Schematic of a normal intact pigmentary unit in a human scalp hair follicle. (**B**) Isolated whole intact, pigmented anagen hair follicles. Note the location of the intensely pigmented melanogenic zone [MZ] around the DP. (**C**) Longitudinal resin section of human anagen scalp hair follicle from a young adult. Note that melanocytes remain intensely pigmented and transfer melanin only to the precortical keratinocytes. *Abbreviations*: Epi-Mc, epidermal melanocyte; IF, infundibulum; SG, sebaceous gland; ORS-Amc, outer root sheath amelanogenic melanocyte; DP, dermal papilla; B-MMc, bulbar melanogenic melanocyte; B-Amc, bulbar amelanotic melanocyte; HS, hair shaft, MZ, melanogenic zone.

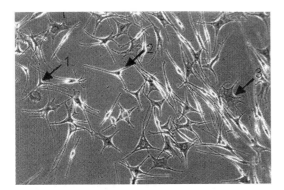

Figure 2 Culture of hair follicle–derived melanocytes. Melanocytes can be isolated and cultured from human hair follicles (21,23). These cells are commonly of three main phenotypic types: poorly pigmented immature (*arrow 1*), moderately differentiated and pigmented (*arrow 2*), and differentiated and intensely pigmented (*arrow 3*) melanocytes.

Regulation of Pigmentation in the Hair Follicle

The process of melanogenesis can be divided into (*i*) the formation of the melanosome: the morphologically and functionally unique organelle in which melanogenesis occurs and (*ii*) the biochemical pathway that converts phenyl-alanine/L-tyrosine into melanin. Both processes are under complex genetic control that encodes a range of enzymes, structural proteins, transcription factors, receptors, and growth factors. Although there is no evidence that melanosome biogenesis in follicular and epidermal melanocytes differs significantly, we must keep an open mind. Melanosome structure correlates with the type of melanin they produce. Melanocytes in black hair follicles contain the largest number and most electron-dense melanosomes (eumelanosomes), each with a fibrillar matrix (27). Brown hair bulb melanocytes contain eumelanosomes that are somewhat smaller but phenotypically similar, whereas blonde hair bulbs produce poorly melanized melanosomes with often only the melanosomal matrix visible. Red hair pheomelanosomes contain a vesicular matrix but with melanin deposited irregularly as blotches. Both eumelanogenic and pheomelanogenic melanosomes can exist in the same normal human melanocytes (28). The formation and maturation of eumelanosomes is currently a subject of intense research and is beyond the scope of this chapter. Less is known about the events involved in the formation of the pheomelanosome that produces the red/yellow melanin. Tyrosinase activity, however, may appear earlier in these melanosomes (29).

The constitutive color of an individual's hair (and for skin) is due to absolute tyrosinase activities, rather than levels of protein expression. Thus, tyrosinase regulation is critical, being controlled not only by the supply of L-tyrosine but also by the stability/activity of tyrosinase and tyrosinase-related proteins. Both L-phenylalanine and L-tyrosine access the melanocyte, the former via the neutral amino acid Na^+/Ca^{++} ATP-ase antiporter system and the latter by facilitated diffusion. L-phenylalanine is converted to L-tyrosine via phenylalanine dehydroxylase (PAH) activity, and PAH activities correlate positively with skin phototypes.

Factors Affecting Hair Pigmentation

The pigmentation of hair fibers is affected by numerous intrinsic factors, including hair cycle–dependent changes, body distribution, racial and gender differences, variable hormone responsiveness, genetic defects, and age-associated change. Study of hair pigmentation is further complicated by the effects of extrinsic variables, including climate and season, infestations, pollutants, toxins, and chemical exposure. The multistep nature of melanosome biogenesis and melanogenesis involves multiple positive and negative regulators/factors of hair follicle melanogenesis, including growth factors, cytokines, hormones, neuropeptides and neurotransmitters, eicosanoids, cyclic nucleotides, nutrients, microelements, and cations/anions (20). These may act via autocrine, paracrine, and endocrine mechanisms, and although much of the available literature pertains to epidermal melanocytes, similar regulators (with the notable possible exception of UVR-induced changes) may also operate in follicular melanogenesis. Examples of positive regulators of melanogenesis include the pro-opiomelanocortin (POMC) peptides α-MSH, ACTH and β-endorphin, endothelin 1 and endothelin 3, and prostaglandin E, while negative regulators include melanin itself, IL-1 and IL-6, TNF-α, and TGF-β (30).

Given the deep location of melanotic follicular melanocytes in the skin, UVB is unlikely to influence the follicular melanin unit directly. To date, the POMC-derived peptides have proven to be the most potent melanogens. α-MSH increases the proportion of black to gray hairs when administered intramuscularly in the guinea pig (31). However, while injection of α-MSH into human skin increased epidermal melanogenesis, particularly of sun-exposed skin, no effect was seen in hair follicles (32). In recent work conducted in my laboratory, we were unable to detect significant expression of α-MSH in pigmented hair bulb melanocytes, in contrast to their epidermal counterparts (33,34). The cognate receptor of α-MSH is the MC1-R, an important positive regulator of hair pigmentation (35). This G protein-coupled membrane receptor is activated upon binding of POMC-derived ACTH, α-MSH, and β-MSH peptides. The resultant signal transduction cascade activates adenylate cyclase, leading to subsequent cAMP production, which results in increased melanocyte proliferation, melanogenesis, and dendrite formation. An important negative regulator of hair pigmentation is ASP, which competitively inhibits the binding of α-MSH to MC1-R. In this way, ASP not only switches melanin synthesis from eumelanogenesis to pheomelanogenesis but also inhibits melanogenesis overall.

Fate of Hair Follicle Melanocytes During the Hair Growth Cycle

Epidermal melanocytes are relatively long-living cells. This may be due to the expression of the antiapoptotic cell survival factor, BCL-2. BCL-2 inhibits cell death particularly in areas where reactive oxygen species (ROS) are generated, as occurs during melanogenesis, by regulating antioxidant pathways (35).

Active pigmentation occurs only during the hair growth phase (anagen), which in human scalp hair can be very long (up to 10 years). The extended anagen of human scalp hair, together with its mosaic pattern of hair growth, hinders systematic analysis of melanocyte dynamics during the human hair cycle. However, the C57BL/6 mouse has proven to be a very useful model for human hair pigmentation, given its short anagen (15–17 days), synchronous hair growth pattern, restriction of melanogenically active truncal melanocytes to the hair follicles (36), and similar linkage of murine melanogenesis with anagen (19).

The relatively quiescent telogen hair germ contains all cell precursors needed to reconstitute a fully developed anagen VI hair follicle (37). Telogen C57BL/6 murine skin does not contain tyrosinase (mRNA or protein), TRP-1 protein and melanin and only very low-level tyrosine hydroxylase activity (38).

During the first one or two days of anagen induction, tyrosinase message and protein becomes barely detectable. At this stage, the follicular papilla pools high concentrations of L-phenylalanine, a potential requirement for the supply of L-tyrosine for melanogenesis (39). Conditions that support the production of high amounts of L-tyrosine from L-phenylalanine, a prerequisite for melanogenesis, include high levels of $6BH_4$, GTP-cyclohydrolase 1, and PAH, all of which are high from earliest anagen through the period of maximum hair follicle activity. Activities of all three drop significantly by anagen III and remain low until the next telogen. Low $6BH_4$ levels may be necessary during pigment production to prevent its allosteric inhibition of tyrosinase. Just prior to this early anagen-associated drop (i.e., anagen II), tyrosinase message, protein, and activity all begin to increase rapidly to peak at early anagen VI (full anagen).

The anagen-associated stimulation of undifferentiated telogen melanocytes/ melanoblasts predates the melanogenic stimulus delivered during anagen III, which is turn is followed by active melanogenesis and subsequent transfer of mature melanosomes into keratinocytes of the pre-cortical matrix. Melanocytes in the S-phase of the cell cycle have been reported as early as anagen II and significant proliferation is clearly apparent in anagen III (40). Bulbar melanocytes during the anagen III to anagen VI transition increase in dendricity, develop more Golgi and rough endoplasmic reticulum, increase the size/number of their melanosomes (41), and begin to transfer mature melanosomes to precortical keratinocytes.

Even before catagen-associated structural changes are apparent in the hair bulb, the earliest signs of imminent hair follicle regression include the retraction of melanocyte dendrites and the attenuation of melanogenesis during late anagen VI (26). Limited keratinocyte proliferation continues for a while, so the most proximal telogen hair shaft remains unpigmented, the functional relevance of which remains enigmatic. One can already detect a dramatic and rapid drop in levels of active tyrosinase beginning during late anagen VI itself, while TRP-2 (dopachrome tautomerase/DCT) activity exhibits moderate reductions from mid to late anagen VI and are lowest during catagen. The termination of melanogenesis may reflect a swamping of a melanogenesis-dependent signaling system or the induction of melanogenesis inhibitory factors, for example, IL-1, IL-6, INF-γ, TGF-β, TNF-α, or corticosteroids (20,30).

A long-enduring enigma of both hair follicle and pigment biology concerns the fate of the hair bulb melanocytes that become undetectable in the proximal catagen hair follicle. Where do these melanocytes go during catagen and telogen, and where do they originate from, when follicular melanogenesis is resumed during the next anagen phase (26)? The long-held view in hair biology is that the hair bulb melanocyte system is a self-perpetuating arrangement, whereby melanocytes involved in the pigmentation of one hair generation are also involved in the pigmentation of the next (42) via multiple cycles of dedifferentiation followed by redifferentiation. Although there is evidence of some plasticity in the hair follicle pigmentary unit, the level invoked by the self-perpetuating theory would imply a degree of plasticity not seen in most nonmalignant cell systems. Moreover, fully differentiated bulbar melanocytes would also need to survive/avoid the extensive apoptosis-driven regression of the hair bulb (43,44) by actively suppressing apoptosis.

Our current view suggests that many of the so-called "redifferentiating" melanocytes in early anagen correspond to newly recruited immature melanocytes derived from a melanocyte reservoir (26,45) and are not reactivated from pre-existing hair bulb melanocytes that were melanogenically active during the previous anagen phase. This is supported by the observation of a population of immature TRP-2$^+$ melanocytes, not affected by blocking anti-c-kit antibody, in the murine bulge (46). It is possible, however, that some new generation melanogenically active melanocytes derive from a population of catagen-surviving melanocytes. Indeed, low numbers of apparently dendritic melanocytes can be detectable in the retreating epithelial strand of catagen hair follicles undergoing active resorption via apoptosis (47). However, these weak or nonmelanogenic cells lack tyrosinase and TRP-1 expression and may in fact represent the poorly differentiated melanocytes that codistribute with pigmented bulbar melanocytes in anagen hair matrix (21).

We recently reported that some highly melanotic (possibly terminally differentiated) hair bulb melanocytes do not survive catagen (48). Deletion of individual melanotic melanocytes by apoptosis was confirmed using well-described ultrastructural features and TUNEL/TRP-1 co-localization. That some, if not most, highly pigmented hair bulb melanocytes may be lost during catagen is further supported by the observation that the vast majority of cells attached to the basal lamina of catagen follicular papilla are of epithelial origin.

Not all the pigment formed during anagen-associated melanogenesis is incorporated into the hair shaft, and this pigment "incontinence" may reflect melanocyte-derived apoptotic bodies that enter the follicular papilla, epithelial strand, or connective tissue sheath of catagen hair follicles. This follicular pigment redistribution is likely to involve phagocytosis, by macrophages (which increase in numbers during hair follicle regression), Langerhans cells, and even by follicular papilla fibroblasts (6). Langerhans cells are also more commonly detected in the graying bulb in canities (27,49), where they contain phagocytosed melanin.

BIOLOGY OF HAIR GRAYING (CANITIES)

Age Effects on Hair Growth and Pigmentation

Our ancient preoccupation with hair and its color is further heightened today as we continue to extend our longevity. Thus, if we are to spend a progressively greater fraction of our lives as adults, we should aim to do this enjoying the greatest possible level of functionality. With this has come the aim to banish "middle age" until our 50s and beyond, while managers of our pension funds would aspire to acknowledge "old age" only when in our 80s and 90s. If this trend continues, we will spend an increasing proportion of our lives sporting signs of our increasingly remote youth. Graying of our scalp hair will play a large part of this loss of a youthful appearance. The hair color market worldwide is already massive, worth seven billion dollars per year (Source: Euromonitor), with some estimates of up to 60% of the adult Western population (men and women) using hair colorants, many to cover gray.

We are born with what appears to be a full complement of approximately five million hair follicles. Only about 2% (i.e., 100,000) of these reside on the scalp. Though the "holy grail" of hair folliculo-neogenesis has some tantalizing secrets to tell in other mammals (e.g., antler velvet in deer), this phenomenon is thought not to occur in humans. The rate of hair growth varies during human aging and when averaged for various sites in post-40-year-old nonbalding individuals, grows most rapidly, and with greater individual fiber thickness, in individuals during the 50s–70s (50). Surface morphology of hair also alters with age, most particularly with reduction in size of cuticular scales in scalp hairs.

Similarly, hair color also shows striking age-related changes in many individuals, particularly in those of Eurasian origin. Hair color in children tends to darken as they grow up, and it is not unusual for a blonde child to be dark-haired after puberty (51). This change is often accompanied by a switch from fairer "intermediate" hair to more deeply pigmented, coarser "terminal" hairs. Hair fiber heterochromia also becomes more apparent with age, most strikingly for scalp and beard (52). However, clearly the most dramatic age-related change in hair pigment is the onset of hair blanching during canities. However, as canities/graying first appears in the 30s, for most of human history this represents already "old" age for average life spans and importantly occurs after reproductive peak age. Graying is only regarded today as "premature" if it appears before the 20s. Thus, the subject of melanocyte aging and functionality is dependent on our concepts of normal functional longevity, and so it is only very recently that the examination of melanocyte aging has been pursued with any particular vigor.

Molecular Aspects of Melanocyte Aging

For every decade after 30 years of age the number of pigment-producing melanocytes in exposed/unexposed epidermis decreases by 10–20% (53,54). This age-associated loss of dopa-positive epidermal melanocytes occurs bodywide and is associated with a very gradual reduction in skin color. By contrast, age-linked loss of color from hair is dramatic, suggesting that the hair pigmentary unit has a different "melanogenetic clock." It has been observed that loss of melanocyte replicative potential in vitro is associated not only with increasing age of the donor but also with the melanin content of the cell. This becomes very apparent after long-term continuous exposure to cAMP inducers (e.g., cholera toxin), which induce pigment without directly engaging the MC1-R (55). Similarly, millimolar L-tyrosine (melanin precursor) abrogates proliferation in cultured "presenescent" pigmented melanocytes, with proliferation continuing only in resistant amelanotic cells (55). On reaching senescence, melanocytes express increased levels of cyclin-dependent kinase (CDK) inhibitors, for example, p21 and p16 that inhibit cell cycling.

Accumulation of oxidative damage is an important determinant in the rate of cell aging, although it is unclear whether it is the primary cause of aging. ROS damage DNA (both nuclear and mitochondrial) that leads to the accumulation of mutations, induce oxidative stress, and also induce antioxidant mechanisms. It is possible that this antioxidant system becomes impaired with age, leading to uncontrolled damage to the melanocyte itself from its own melanogenesis-related oxidative stress. In addition, melanin synthesis, by its very nature, produces mutagenic intermediates (56). Thus, the induction of replicative senescence in melanocytes may be an important protective mechanism against cell transformation (57). The extraordinary melanogenic activity of pigmented bulbar melanocytes, which may continue for many years in some scalp hair follicles, is likely to generate large amounts of reactive oxygen species (ROS) via the oxidation of tyrosine and 3,4-dihydroxyphenylalanine (DOPA) to melanin (58). If not adequately removed, an accumulation of these ROS will generate significant oxidative stress in both the melanocyte itself and also in the highly proliferative anagen hair bulb epithelium. Thus, in these circumstances, melanogenic bulbar melanocytes are perhaps best suited to assume a postmitotic, terminally differentiated "(pre)senescence" status to prevent cell transformation.

Pathogenesis of Hair Graying (Canities)

A characteristic feature of bulbar melanocytes is their extremely high melanin load, maintained throughout the entire time that the pigmented hair fiber is growing, up to 10 years in the human scalp anagen hair follicle. This represents a phenomenal synthetic capacity for melanin production (Fig. 1A–C), whereby a relatively small number of melanocytes can, in a single hair growth cycle, produce sufficient melanin to intensely pigment up to 1.5 m of hair shaft. Moreover, they do this within the context of a melanin-laden cytoplasm. In this way, hair bulb melanocytes are very different from melanogenically active epidermal melanocytes, which retain few fully mature melanosomes in their cytoplasm at any one time. This intrinsic ability of bulbar melanocytes to "pool" melanin may make them more vulnerable than epidermal melanocytes to the toxic elements of melanogenesis.

The synthetic capacity of bulbar melanocytes is greatest during youth when the scalp follicular melanin unit is only a few cycles old and are able to avail of the full postpuberty hormonal stimulus. On average, an individual scalp hair follicle will experience less than 15 melanocyte seedings from the presumptive reservoir in the ORS to the hair bulb in the average fully "gray-free" life span of 35 years for Caucasians (59). Interestingly, repeated plucking of hair from vibrissae follicles leads to the eventual regrowth of gray hair (60), again suggesting limited capacity of the pigmentary reservoir. However, the associated tissue injury during plucking complicates the interpretation of this finding. In any event, the onset and progression of hair graying correlates closely with chronological aging and occurs to varying degrees in all individuals, regardless of gender or race. Age of onset also appears to be genetically controlled and inheritable (61). Thus, the average age for Caucasians is mid-30s, for Asians late-30s, and for Africans mid-40s. Similarly, hair is said to gray *prematurely* if it occurs before the age of 20 in whites, before 25 in Asians, and before 30 in Africans. The progress of canities is entirely individual: A good rule of thumb is that by 50 years of age, 50% of people have 50% gray hair (61). Clearly, the darker the hair the more noticeable early graying will be. However, graying can be more extensive in dark hair before total whitening is apparent; the reverse is true for blond hair. Graying first appears usually at the temples, and spreads to the vertex and then the remainder of the scalp, affecting the occiput last. Beard and body hair is usually affected later. Graying often follows a wave that spreads slowly from the crown to the occiput.

Histopathology of Canities

While "gray" hair may be illusory—a mere impression of gray provided by an admixture of fully white and fully pigmented hair—canities indeed can affect individual hair follicles (Fig. 3). This hair follicle–specific change may result in either a gradual loss of pigment over time and over several cycles, a gradual loss of pigment along the same hair shaft (i.e., within the anagen phase of a *single* hair cycle), or the hair fiber may appear to grow in fully depigmented. While few pigment granules are present in truly white hair shafts, melanin granules can be readily detected within the precortex of gray hair follicles.

Pigment loss in graying hair follicles is due to a marked reduction in melanogenically active melanocytes in the hair bulb of gray anagen hair follicles (62). True gray hairs show a much reduced, but detectable, dopa reaction as an indicator of tyrosinase activity, whereas white hair bulbs are broadly negative. However, there appears also to be a specific defect of melanosome transfer in graying hair follicles, as keratinocytes may fail to contain any melanin granules despite being in close proximity to melanocytes with a moderate number of melanosomes (Tobin et al., unpublished observations). Further evidence of some defect in melanocyte–keratinocyte interaction is provided by the observation of significant melanin debris both in the graying hair bulb and sometimes also in the surrounding dermis. This abnormality is due to either defective melanosomal transfer to the cortical keratinocytes and/or melanin incontinence due to melanocyte degeneration. The remaining hair bulb melanocytes in canities-affected anagen hair follicles often appear hypertrophic, although this may reflect a reduction in dendricity rather than an overall increase in cell volume (62).

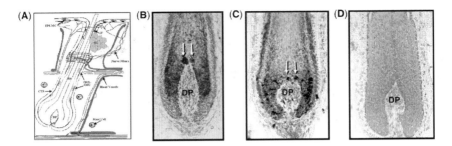

Figure 3 Progress of canities. (**A**) Schematic of an end-stage canities-affected pigmentary unit in a human scalp hair follicle. Note that melanocytes appear to be retained in all hair follicle locations except the most proximal bulb. (**B–D**) Longitudinal cryosection of canities-affected human scalp anagen hair follicle immunostained for tyrosinase protein (not activity). Note the retention of amelanotic melanocytes in the outer longitudinal cryosections of canities-affected human scalp anagen hair follicles immunostained for the (pre)melanosomal marker gp100. This figure shows early (**B**), intermediate (**C**), and late (**D**) stages of canities in three adjacent anagen scalp hair follicles in a 56-year-old individual. (**B**) Early stage: Melanocytes located above the dermal papilla appear exhibit abnormality first and become hypertrophic, lose their dendrites and fill with pigment. Melanosome transfer to precortical keratinocytes is interrupted in this location but continues in the more lateral aspects of the hair bulb. (**C**) Intermediate stage: Most melanogenically active melanocytes have reduced pigment production and more pronounced interruption of melanosome transfer. (**D**) Late stage: No melanogenically active melanocytes remain in this hair bulb. Note that a prominent medulla is now visible in this fully white follicle, but this keratinocyte differentiation product is not apparent in the adjacent follicles. *Abbreviations*: Epi-Mc, epidermal melanocyte; IF, infundibulum; SG, sebaceous gland; ORS-AMc, outer root sheath amelanogenic melanocyte; DP, dermal papilla; HS, hair shaft.

Ultrastructural analysis of the human gray hair matrix reveals melanocytes with highly variable levels of melanogenesis (62). In gray/white hair bulbs, remaining melanocytes contain fewer and smaller melanosomes and less supporting organelles, for example, Golgi apparatus. Interestingly, the remaining melanosomes may be packaged within autophagolysosomes, suggesting that these melanosomes are defective, perhaps even leaking reactive melanin metabolites. Autophagolysosomal degradation of melanosomes is usually followed by the degeneration of the melanocyte itself (63,64). The involvement of ROS in the histopathology of canities is supported by the observation that melanocytes in graying and white hair bulbs may be vacuolated, a common cellular response to increased oxidative stress (65). Degenerative change in canities-affected hair bulbs may resemble apoptosis and is reminiscent of melanocyte degeneration in acute alopecia areata where pigmented hair follicles are preferentially targets by an aberrant immune response (Fig. 3) (66).

Loss of melanocytes from canities-affected hair bulbs can apparently occur very rapidly. Evidence for this can be found in the pigment incontinence located in the follicular papilla and/or connective tissue sheath of hair follicles that lack any morphologic evidence of melanogenesis or melanocytes in their hair bulb. The presence of pigment debris in an amelanotic hair follicle would appear to indicate the recent nature of events responsible for loss of previously melano-genic melanocytes. The loss of active melanocytes from the hair bulb of graying and white hair follicles may be associated with a parallel increase there in dendritic cells (including Langerhans cells) (62). The relocation of these antigen-presenting phagocytic cells from the upper hair follicle to the lower follicle may be in response to degenerative change within the melanocyte population.

Impact of Melanocyte Loss on Hair Growth

Given their close interaction, it is likely that bulbar melanocytes influence precor-tical keratinocyte behavior in several ways. Melanin transfer to keratinocytes appears to reduce their proliferative potential and increase their terminal differ-entiation. Indeed, white beard hair has been shown to grow faster than adjacent pigmented hair (67,68). In this way melanosomes donated to keratinocytes may act as "regulatory packages" (69). Melanocyte may also influence neighboring keratinocytes via the production of various cytokines, growth factors, eicosa-noids, adhesion molecules, and extracellular matrix (70). Similarly, the ability of melanins to provide a buffer for calcium is likely to have implications for cell function, given the critical second messenger/cell signaling role for calcium in melanogenesis, melanosome transfer, and keratinocyte differentiation. The saturation binding of transition metals (e.g., iron, copper, etc.) to melanin provides yet another effective antioxidant defense mechanism for the melano-some-receiving keratinocyte.

Further clinical evidence of melanocyte–keratinocyte interactivity can be seen in the anecdotal impressions that gray hair is coarser, wirier, and more unmanageable than pigmented hair. This may reflect different chemical and phys-ical properties of pigmented and nonpigmented (i.e., gray) hair (71). Indeed, gray hair is often unable to hold a permanent or temporary set and is more resistant to incorporating artificial color. These observations suggest significant change to the underlying substructure of the hair shaft, whereby aging hair follicles may reprogram their matrix keratinocytes to increase production of medullary, rather than cortical, keratinocytes.

In the absence of natural regimens to recover lost hair color, many individ-uals turn to hair colorants (18) (see section "Current Status of Hair Color Tech-nologies"). Such products are used very successfully and safely by millions of individuals worldwide. Some studies however, have raised the possibility that long-term usage of permanent hair dyes (particularly black dyes) may be associ-ated with a very small increased risk of developing certain pathologies (see section "Current Status of Hair Color Technologies"). It would appear prudent, therefore, to evaluate ways of improving strategies to restore hair color, not only by further improving hair dye safety but also by considering ways to block/reverse the process of hair graying itself.

CURRENT STATUS OF HAIR-COLOR TECHNOLOGIES

Of all the products used for hair care, the aging population has ensured that growth in sales has been greatest for hair colorants, with the principal application being to cover gray hair. Additionally, the increasing "cosmetication" of young adult males in western societies has been another significant factor in this growth. Both target groups seek to either add color to their hair (original or different) or to lighten/bleach their hair to generate a preferred, lighter color or to permit subsequent addition of color(s) shades lighter than their natural color. Despite this increasing use of hair colorant products, technological developments in this area have been sluggish, with most focus centering on improvements in the safety profiles of the formulations. Consumer preference for all things "natural," however, have begun to stimulate interest in pursuing the development of more natural hair coloring agents. In the subsequent paragraphs, I restrict my discussions to the categories of colorants/hair dyes, including bleaching agents, permanent dyes, semipermanent dyes, temporary dyes, metallic dyes, vegetable dyes, and the potential for more natural dyes.

Bleaching

Hair can be bleached by both chemical and photochemical (i.e., sunlight) oxidative mechanisms.

Chemical Bleaching

Hair is bleached by hydrogen peroxide-containing systems that also include an alkaline hair lightener base, with additional persulfate salts to accelerate or boost the reaction. To adequately destroy the melanin, the hydrogen peroxide bleach may also degrade hair proteins due to the numerous oxidizable cysteine groups in the hair cortex and cuticle (72). Indeed, normal bleaching may break up to 25% of the fibers' disulfide bonds, while bleaching from black to blond may break as many as 50% of these bonds (73). The high pH values of currently used hair aqueous alkaline bleaches (pH 9–11) are also likely to increase the rates of hydrolysis of resultant oxides to compete with that of oxidation, such that cleavage of cysteine occurs via an S–S fission route to yield principally sulfonic acid. Moreover, hydrolysis of peptide bonds within hair protein (cystine, methionine, tyrosine, histidine, and lysine) may also occur during severe bleaching episodes using higher concentrations of bleach and for longer exposure times (74).

Photo/Sunlight Bleaching of Hair

Hair pigments, hair proteins, and hair lipids are also susceptible to degradation by visible light and UVR. Indeed, lipids making up the membrane complexes holding the hair cortex together may be even more sensitive to light radiation than UVR (75) and may degrade to cause stepped fractures in the fiber. This may be particularly severe if the hair has already been pre-exposed to chemical bleaching. As expected, sunlight affects the amino acids of the hair fiber's cuticular covering more so than its bulk cortex. Hair proteins appear to absorb light principally between 254 and 350 nm, and so most light degradation may occur between those wavelengths (76) affecting cystine, methionine, phenylalanine, tryptophan, histidine, proline, and leucine. Interestingly, amino acids in darker hair may be more resistant to photodamage than paler shades. Chronic exposure to sunlight is likely to cause fiber brittleness which, if further subjected to even relatively mild chemical bleach conditions, that is, aqueous alkalinity and peroxides, may result in marked loss of structural integrity.

Although the substructure of melanin remains in large part enigmatic and unyielding to study, melanins appear to be a tyrosine-based polymer of repeating unit of indole quinones. Oxidation of hair that lacks melanin (senile white hair) occurs much more slowly than that of melanized hair fibers (77,78), suggesting that peroxide reacts preferentially with melanin pigment compared to hair proteins, but only after peroxide gains access to the core of the fiber, that is, after the pigment-free cuticle is bleached. While isolated pigment granules are resistant to a large range of reagents, they are readily dissolved by alkaline hydrogen peroxide at pH 11.75 (77,78).

Permanent Hair Colorants

Despite its very ancient origin, hair coloring technology has struggled to keep up with demand and changes in consumer lifestyles and expectations. The permanent hair colorants or oxidation dyes represent approximately 80% of the hair color market (79) and consist principally of uncolored precursors of *p*-amines and *p*-aminophenols that diffuse into the hair fiber, where they condense with dye couplers (e.g., resorcinol) and are then oxidized into active intermediates (e.g., diiminium or quinonimunium species) by (most commonly) hydrogen peroxide. Other secondary compounds are involved including surfactants, preservatives, pH-adjusting additives (to pH 8–10), and so on. These reactions provide shampoo-fast hair color and a depth of color that can be controlled by adjusting relative amounts of the three principal agents. Most dyes are diffusion-controlled so that ring dyeing is achieved, whereby the dye is restricted to the surface of the hair fiber. However, this is variably achieved, as dye will penetrate more deeply into some hair fibers than others. Somewhat surprisingly, this variability does not always correlate with fiber caliber.

The chemistry involved in these permanent dyes is complex but can be summarized briefly as follows. The dye precursor (e.g., *p*-phenylenediamine) is oxidized to its diiminium ion, and this active intermediate condenses with an electron donating coupler (e.g., resorcinol) to form a dinuclear product. This is then oxidized to an indo dye. More detailed discussion of associated chemistry is beyond the scope of this chapter, but the reader is directed to an excellent and comprehensive treatment of this subject by Robbins (76). Permanent dyes are formulated for the client in two parts, consisting of the precursor-coupler base (with secondary agents for texture etc. as described in preceding text) and the oxidizing agent (with associated secondary products for stabilization etc.). Strand testing allow for interindividual variability to be minimized. However, avoidance of allergy is also of concern, and so testing is recommended prior to full application of these products. Brown to black shaded compounds are formed when dye precursors are oxidized in the absence of couplers, while couplers can modify the color formed by the precursor. Highly colored indo dyes can fade, possibly due to the addition of aromatic moieties to the dinuclear indo dyes.

Semipermanent Hair Colorants

People may choose to change their hair color in a nonpermanent way, and hair colorants are available that can be removed after about four to six shampoos (80). These dyes do not involve the use of hydrogen peroxide and usually contain multiple dyes in combination (81). As with permanent dye, several secondary compounds are also included in these dyes, for example, surfactants, pH adjusters, and so on. These hair dyes consist of highly polar agents, including neutral aromatic amines, nitro aromatic amines, or antraquinone derivatives (74). Rinse-out rates of these dyes correlate with size of the dye molecules used but also depend on the region of the hair fiber. For example, dye is removed most readily from weathered hair fiber tips than the scalp end, and so accommodation needs to be built into the formulations to ensure evenness of tones. Furthermore, some dyes, especially small mononuclear dye molecules, may be washed out more readily from previously bleached hair. As with permanent dyes, ring-dyeing is also observed with this group of hair colorants, consistent with diffusion-controlled reactions.

Temporary Hair Colorants/Rinses

These hair colorants can be washed out of the hair with a single shampoo and contain several (as many as five) color ingredients (e.g., D&C brown No. 1, Acid violet 43 etc.) in order to achieve the desired shade. These reagents can be applied directly to the hair or sprayed onto the hair. More dye can be applied if a more intense color is required, and less dye if only tint addition to gray is desired. The dye molecules used here tend to be larger than those used for semipermanent colorants and are chosen for their maximum water solubility and minimum penetration, thereby facilitating easy rinse-out (82).

Metallic Hair Dyes

Historically, salts of such metals as silver, bismuth, cobalt, copper, iron, mercury, and lead have been used to dye hair. However, only lead salts (e.g., lead acetate with sulfur) are still in use. These are often chosen by men with graying hair as the darkening of the hair shaft occurs very gradually, mostly likely via the formation of lead–sulfur complexes in the periphery of the hair shaft. Users should be aware that these complexes may be unstable, especially when exposed to other chemicals and dyes. Another, less common, group of metal-based hair dyes (or so-called acid dyes) includes the premetalized dyes, where the anionic dyes are complexed with a metal, such as chromium and cobalt.

Vegetable Hair Dyes

While history contains several "colorful" references to the use of vegetable hair colorants, only henna and chamomile are still used to any significant commercial extent, although several patents based on this technology have been filed by major hair colorant companies, for example, Wella Cosmital. Henna (Lawsone) is found in the leaves of the Egyptian privet plant and contains 2-hydroxy-1,4-naphthoquinone. This compound can add red (ionized form) and yellow (nonionized form) shades to protein in hair and nail when applied in acidic media. Deeper henna shades are possible at high concentrations in alkaline media, while acidic pHs are more suitable for hair dyeing. The pH of these may control the chemical bonding of the lawsone to the hair fiber, but levels of color fastness are generally relatively low. Fastness can be improved if lawsone is mixed with the permanent dye precursor, *p*-phenylenediamine, though not without some adverse reactions (83). Chamomile flowers contain an active coloring polyhydroxy flavone called 4′,5,7-trihydroxy flavone that has been used for dyeing of cloth as well as hair.

"Natural" Hair Colorants

The hair colorant industry is actively seeking the development of economical natural hair dyes. Although not yet commercialized, there may be some scope for using DOPA, which, after oxidation, provides a natural brown dye. In the presence of cysteine, natural red pigments (pheomelanins) can be formed from DOPA, while the presence of sulfur-containing nucelophile (rather than cysteine) can increase still further the range of hair color shades possible. Here, hydrogen peroxide is a superior oxidizer, though the reaction can proceed even with basic atmospheric oxygen. Brown colors can be deepened to intense blacks if potassium ferricyanide is added.

SAFETY CONSIDERATIONS IN HAIR-DYE TECHNOLOGY

There is some concern regarding the toxicity of some of the components used in permanent dyes. This concern is particularly focused on the aromatic amines (e.g., *p*-phenylenediamine), involved not only as precursors but also in many dye couplers. There may soon be regulatory attempts to limit or restrict the use of these compounds. For example, the European Union [via *Comité de Liaison*

Européen de Industrie de la Parfumarie de Produits (*COLIPA*)] has taken the lead in regulating oxidizing dye agents. About 25 are listed for use today, down from approximately 150 listed 25 years ago. It is also likely that further testing will eliminate some of those remaining on this list. It is important to note however, that both *p*-phenylenediamine and resorcinol have had significant testing and remain on the proposed list of 25 acceptable ingredients, and such products are used very successfully and safely by millions of individuals world-wide. Despite this, there have been some studies that raised the possibility that long-term usage of permanent hair dyes (particularly black dyes) may be associated with a very small increased risk of developing certain cancers. However, the findings of these small, poorly controlled studies remain highly controversial and, importantly, have not been confirmed in much larger, adequately controlled, recent studies (84,85). In addition, a small number of users may develop chemical and allergic reactions (commonly due to *p*-phenylenediamine), and these may result in dermatitis and even hair loss (86). Thus, it would appear prudent to evaluate ways of improving strategies to restore hair color, for example, by improving further hair dye safety and by reconsidering ways to block/reverse the process of hair graying itself. Although pursuit of more "natural" products for hair colorant biotechnology is a legitimate goal, one should not assume that such "natural" products are, by definition, nontoxic just because they are found in nature.

CELL BIOLOGICAL AND BIOTECHNOLOGICAL MECHANISMS TO IDENTIFY CANITIES TARGETS

Polyphenol Dyes

The desirability to replace the precursors and couplers used in permanent dyes with more "natural" reagents has focused attention on plant-derived compounds, including polyphenols. Polyphenols can be found in many fruits, for example, grapes, in chocolate, and so on. Mostly water-soluble, these molecules bind protein (e.g., hair protein) to form insoluble complexes and so provide fastness and substantivity. Examples of plant polyphenols that may have application in hair colorant technology include hydrolysable tannins (browns to black) and condensed tannins. The former have been used since time immemorial for tanning leather. It is likely that similar effects may be achievable with human hair, given the similarity of proteins found in leather and hair. The condensed tannins are polymers of flavanoid and include the proanthrocyanidins. The proanthrocyanidins are responsible for the wide variety of colors in flowers, for example, reds, purples, and so on. In the case of both hydrolysable and condensed tannins, useful effects may only be obtained if these dyes can be readily extracted from plant sources, if sufficient dye can be added to the hair and if the dyeing process itself can be achieved at temperatures that will not damage human hair or skin. It is not fully clear just how light-fast these dyes will be.

Melanin Delivery to Growing Hair Follicles

The selective delivery of melanin to hair follicles with the view to add color to hair shafts has long been an enticing prospect. Hoffman et al. (87) have reported a method to deliver topically applied liposome-encapsulated melanin to hair follicles in mice and also in 3-D histocultures. These authors reported entry of melanin deep into the hair follicle and also onto/into the hair shaft, albeit nonuniformly. The precise route/mechanism of melanin uptake in this system is unclear but may involve fusion of melanin-containing liposomes with keratinocytes after entry through the lipid-rich coating of the follicular space. For the hair shaft itself to take up pigment, it is likely that differentiating matrix keratinocytes have to take up the liposome cargo and that targeted cells ultimately need to be ones that can differentiate into pigment-bearing cortical keratinocytes. However, there may also be some passive "coating" of the hair shaft with melanin, again via interactions with lipids on the hair fiber surface. This technology can be adapted to deliver not only melanin, but also other molecules relevant to modulating pigmentation of the hair follicle. These may include synthetics, biologics, or even genes to correct deficits or overexpress relevant genes.

Gene Therapy for Hair Pigmentation

There is some evidence that gene therapy through the hair follicle may one day be exploitable for the modification of pigmentation in the hair and also to correct deficits of melanogenesis in graying hair follicles. Recently, Alexeev et al. (88) advanced this prospect significantly when they demonstrated the correction of a genetic defect in the tyrosinase gene via delivery of the correct tyrosinase gene, configured as an RNA–DNA oligonucleotide, using topically applied liposomes and intradermal injection technology. Localized gene correction was still present at least three months after final application. The implications of this work are many and important. However, if the corrected gene is delivered only to progenitor (or transient amplifying cells) and not also to stem cells (here melanoblast/melanocyte stem cells), the correction will only last for the duration of one hair cycle and so will not be propagated. Moreover, the efficiency rates of the current systems are not optimal, especially for liposome delivery system. Delivery via intradermal injection, although providing superior efficiency rates, exhibits much lower hair follicle specificity. Thus, application of the current technologies for cosmetic purposes, where partial success can be less cosmetically acceptable than complete failure, is still some way off.

Cell Biological Approaches

Other opportunities for biotechnological intervention in canities-associated pigment loss may need a greater understanding of melanocyte aging and also the role of melanocytes that are retained in white and gray hair follicles, for example, the limited number of amelanotic melanocytes located in the anagen phase ORS. These cells are, for the most part, not only dopa-negative and but also negative for most melanocyte-specific markers (24). Although the precise role of ORS amelanotic melanocytes in hair and skin biology is unknown, these cells can be recruited for repigmentation/repopulation of the epidermis (e.g., in vitiligo, dermabrasion etc.) (89). Their failure to contribute to the pigmentation of senile white hair follicles may reflect the lack of a permissive environment for their migration to the melanogenic zone during early anagen. Only melanocytes that have successfully migrated to the hair bulb appear to be susceptible to local pigmentation-inducing influences, for example, anagen-induced secretion of follicular papilla-derived factors. The provision of some of these stimuli in vitro may result in the induction of melanogenesis in the amelanotic cells of senile white hair follicles. This finding suggests that these cells retain intact, though inactivated, melanogenic machinery and so could be induced to become active again in more permissive in vivo microenvironments.

The cellular deficit in canities-affected hair follicles is likely to be multifactorial. Primary amongst these may be defective migratory stimuli, particularly during the critical stages of the hair cycle when cell–cell and cell–matrix interactions are highly active. Several factors could theoretically be administered to canities-affected scalp. Basic fibroblast growth factor, leukotriene C4, and endothelin-1 are potent chemotactic factors, at least in Boyden chamber–type in vitro studies (90,91). Along with other potent melanocyte migration factors, for example, stem cell factor, these molecules regulate the expression of integrins on the surface of several cell types, including melanocytes themselves. These growth factors are produced in the skin by keratinocytes (bFGF, endothelin-1) and by fibroblasts, including the follicular papilla fibroblasts (SCF, leukotriene-4) (92). SCF and its receptor c-kit have been directly implicated not only in the migration (via chemokinesis) of melanoblasts into the hair follicle but also their survival and proliferation (93).

Spontaneous Repigmentation in Canities

Spontaneous scalp hair repigmentation has been reported after radiation therapy for cancer (94) or after inflammatory events, for example, erythrodermic eczema and erosive candidiasis of the scalp (95). Here, it is most probable that reversal of canities resulted from radiation/cytokine-induced activation of outer root sheath melanocytes and so raises the attractive possibility that these melanocytes may be induced to migrate and differentiate to naturally repigment graying hair follicles. Another clinical scenario that provides an insight into both the pathomechanism of canities and possibilities for pigment recovery is the not too uncommon partial spontaneous reversal of canities that occur during the early stages of canities. Here, melanogenesis in deactivated bulbar melanocytes may restart during anagen VI of the same hair growth cycle (96). Study of hair follicles at this point in canities may provide several clues to help us identify the subtle changes in the hair follicle's two melanocyte subpopulations.

ACKNOWLEDGMENTS

This manuscript is dedicated to the memory of Prof. Aodán S. Breathnach, mentor and friend. I would like to acknowledge Dr. Eva Peters for the hair follicle schematic.

REFERENCES

1. Rees JL. The melanocortin 1 receptor (MCR1): more than just red hair. Pigment Cell Res 2000; 13:135–140.
2. Slominski A, Pawelek J. Animals under the sun: effects of ultraviolet radiation on mammalian skin. Clin Dermatol 1998; 16(4):503–515.
3. Morgan E. The Ascent of Woman. London: Souvenir Press, 1985.
4. Bertazzo A, Costa C, Biasiolo M, Allegri G, Cirrincione G, Presti G. Determination of copper and zinc levels in human hair: influence of sex, age, and hair pigmentation. Biol Trace Elem Res 1996; 52:37–53.
5. Mackintosh JA. The antimicrobial properties of melanocytes, melanosomes and melanin and the evolution of black skin. J Theor Biol 2001; 211(2):101–113.
6. Paus R. Immunology of the hair follicle. In: Bos JD, ed. The Skin Immune System. Boca Raton, FL: CRC Press, 1997: 377–395.
7. Nosanchuk JD, Casadevall A. The contribution of melanin to microbial pathogenesis. Cell Microbiol 2003; 5(4):203–223.
8. Gomez BL, Nosanchuk JD. Melanin and fungi. Curr Opin Infect Dis 2003; 16(2):91–96.
9. Holbrook KA, Vogel AM, Underwood RA, Foster CA. Melanocytes in human embryonic and fetal skin: a review and new findings. Pigment Cell Res (Suppl) 1988; 1:6–17.
10. Rawles ME. Origin of pigment cells from the neural crest in the mouse embryo. Physiol Zool 1947; 20:248–266.
11. Chase HB, Rauch H, Smith VW. Critical stages of hair follicle development and pigmentation in the mouse. Physiol Zool 1951; 25:1–19.
12. Jackson IJ. Molecular and developmental genetics of mouse coat color. Annu Rev Genet 1994; 28:189–217.
13. Nakamura M, Tobin DJ, Richards-Smith B, Sundberg JP, Paus R. Mutant laboratory mice with abnormalities in pigmentation: annotated tables. J Dermatol Sci 2002; 28:1–33.
14. Fleischman RA, Gallardo T, Mi X. Mutations in the ligand-binding domain of the kit receptor: an uncommon site in human piebaldism. J Invest Dermatol 1996; 107:703–706.
15. Perris R. The extracellular matrix in neural crest cell migration. Trends Neurosci 1997; 20:23–31.
16. Henderson DH, Copp AJ. Role of the extracellular matrix in neural crest cell migration. J Anat 1997; 191:507–515.
17. Hirai Y, Nose A, Kobayashi S, Takeichi M. Expression and role of E- and P-cadherin adhesion molecules in embryonic histiogenesis. II. Skin morphogenesis. Development 1989; 105:271–277.
18. Tobin DJ, Paus R. Graying: gerontobiology of the hair follicle pigmentary unit. Exp Gerontol 2001; 36:29–54.

19. Slominski A, Paus R. Melanogenesis is coupled to murine anagen: Towards new concepts for the role of melanocytes and the regulation of melanogenesis in hair growth. J Invest Dermatol 1993; 101:90S–97S.
20. Nordlund JJ, Ortonne J-P. The normal color of human skin. In: Nordlund JJ, Boissy RE, Hearing VJ, King RA, Ortonne J-P, eds. The Pigmentary System: Physiology and Pathophysiology. New York, NY: Oxford University Press, 1998: 475–487.
21. Tobin DJ, Colen SR, Bystryn J-C. Isolation and long-term culture of human hair-follicle melanocytes. J Invest Dermatol 1995; 104:86–89.
22. Tobin DJ, Bystryn J-C. Different populations of melanocytes are present in hair follicles and epidermis. Pigment Cell Res 1996; 9:304–310.
23. Staricco RG. Amelanotic melanocytes in the outer sheath of the human hair follicle and their role in the repigmentation of regenerated epidermis. Ann NY Acad Sci 1963; 100:239–255.
24. Horikawa T, Norris DA, Johnson TW, Zekman T, Dunscomb N, Bennion SD, Jackson RL, Morelli JG. DOPA-negative melanocytes in the outer root sheath of human hair follicles express premelanosomal antigens but not a melanosomal antigen or the melanosome-associated glycoproteins tyrosinase, TRP-1, and TRP-2. J Invest Dermatol 1996; 106:28–35.
25. Slominski A, Paus R, Plonka P, Chakraborty A, Maurer M, Pruski D, Lukiewicz S. Melanogenesis during the anagen-catagen-telogen transformation of the murine hair cycle. J Invest Dermatol 1994; 102:862–869.
26. Tobin DJ, Slominski A, Botchkarev V, Paus R. The fate of hair follicle melanocytes during the hair growth cycle. J Investig Dermatol Symp Proc 1999; 4:323–332.
27. Tobin DJ. Biology of hair pigmentation. In: Forslind B, Lindberg M, eds. Skin, Hair and Nails. Structure and Function. New York, NY: Marcel Dekker, 2003: 319–364.
28. Inazu M, Mishima Y. Detection of eumelanogenic and pheomelanogenic melanosomes in the same normal human melanocyte. J Invest Dermatol 1993; 100:172S–175S.
29. Jimbow K, Park JS, Kato F, Hirosaki K, Toyofuku K, Hua C, Yamashita T. Assembly, target-signaling and intracellular transport of tyrosinase gene family proteins in the initial stage of melanosome biogenesis. Pigment Cell Res 2000; 13(4):222–229.
30. Slominski A, Tobin DJ, Shibahara S, Wortsman J. Melanin pigmentation in mammalian skin and its hormonal regulation. Physiol Rev 2004; 84(4):1155–1228.
31. Snell RS. Hormonal control of hair color. In: Riley V, ed. Pigmentation: Its Genesis and Biologic Control. New York, NY: Meredith, 1972:193–205.
32. Lerner AB, McGuire JS. Melanocyte stimulating hormone and adrenocorticotrophic hormone: their relation to pigmentation. N Eng J Med 1964; 270:539–546.
33. Kauser S, Schallreuter KU, Thody AJ, Gummer C, Tobin DJ. Regulation of human epidermal melanocyte biology by beta-endorphin. J Invest Dermatol 2003; 120(6):1073–1080.
34. Kauser S, Schallreuter KU, Thody AJ, Gummer C, Tobin DJ. Beta-endorphin as a regulator of human hair follicle melanocyte biology. J Invest Dermatol 2004; 123(1):184–195.
35. Hockenbery DM, Oltvai ZN, Yin XM, Milliman CL, Korsmeyer SJ. Bcl-2 functions in an antioxidant pathway to prevent apoptosis. Cell 1993; 75:241–251.
36. Reynolds J. The epidermal melanocytes of mice. J Anat 1954; 88:45–58.
37. Silver AF, Chase HB. DNA synthesis in the adult hair germ during dormancy (telogen) and activation (early anagen). Devl Biol 1970; 21:440–451.

38. Slominski A, Paus R, Constantino R. Differential expression and activity of melano-genesis-related proteins during induced hair growth in mice. J Invest Dermatol 1991; 96:172–179.

39. Schallreuter KU, Beazley WD, Hibberts NA, Tobin DJ, Paus R, Wood JM. Pterins in human hair follicle cells and in the synchronized murine hair cycle. J Invest Dermatol 1998; 111(4):545–550.

40. Jimbow K, Roth SI, Fitzpatrick TB, Szabo G. Mitotic activity in non-enoplastic mel-anocytes in vivo as determined by histochemical, autoradiographic, and electron microscopic studies. J Cell Biol 1975; 66:666–670.

41. Sugiyama S, Kukita A. Melanocyte reservoir in the hair follicles during the hair growth cycle: an electron microscopic study. In: Biology and Disease of the Hair. Tokyo: University of Tokyo Press, 1976:81–200.

42. Sugiyama S. Mode of re-differentiation and melanogenesis of melanocytes in murine hair follicle. J Ultrastructural Res 1979; 67:40–54.

43. Weedon D, Strutton G. Apoptosis as the mechanism of the involution of hair follicles in catagen transformation. Acta Derm Venerol 1981; 61:335–359.

44. Lindner L, Botchkarev VA, Botchkareva NV, Ling G, van der Veen C, Paus R. Analy-sis of apoptosis during hair follicle regression (catagen). Am J Pathol 1997; 151:1601–1617.

45. Grichnik JM, Ali WN, Burch JA, Byers JD, Garcia CA, Clark RE, Shea CR. KIT expression reveals a population of precursor melanocytes in human skin. J Invest Dermatol 1996; 106:967–971.

46. Botchkareva NV, Khlgatian M, Longley BJ, Botchkarev VA, Gilchrest BA. SCF/c-kit signaling is required for cyclic regeneration of the hair pigmentation unit. FASEB J 2001; 15:645–658.

47. Commo S, Bernard BA. Melanocyte subpopulation turnover during the human hair cycle: An immunohistochemical study. Pigment Cell Res 2000; 13:253–259.

48. Tobin DJ, Hagen E, Botchkarev VA, Paus R. Do hair bulb melanocytes undergo apoptosis during hair follicle regression (catagen)? J Invest Dermatol 1998; 111:6;941–947.

49. Tobin DJ. A possible role for Langerhans cells in the removal of melanin from early catagen hair follicle. Br J Dermatol 1998; 138:795–798.

50. Pelfini C, Cerimele D, Pisanu G. In: Montagna W, Dobson RL, eds. Aging of the Skin and Hair Growth in Man. Advances in Biology of the Skin–Hair Growth. New York, NY: Pergamon Press, 1969:153–160.

51. Allende MF. The enigmas of pigmentation. J Am Med Assoc 1995; 220:1443–1447.

52. Lee WS, Lee IW, Ahn SK. Diffuse heterochromia of scalp hair. J Am Acad Dermatol 1996; 35(5 Pt 2):823–825.

53. Whiteman DC, Parsons PG, Green AC. Determinants of melanocyte density in adult human skin. Arch Dermatol Res 1999; 291:511–516.

54. Medrano EE, Yang F, Boissy R, Farooqui J, Shah V, Matsumoto K, Nordlund JJ, Park HY. Terminal differentiation and senescence in the human melanocyte: repression of tyrosine-phosphorylation of the extracellular signal-regulated kinase 2 selectively defines the two phenotypes. Mol Biol Cell 1994; 5:497–509.

55. Bennett DC. Differentiation in mouse melanoma cells: initial reversibility and an on-off stochastic model. Cell 1983; 34:445–453.

56. Ames BN, Shigenaga MK, Hagen TM. Oxidants, antioxidants, and the degenerative process of aging. Proc Natl Acad Sci USA 1993; 90:7915–7922.

57. Campisi J. The role of cellular senescence in skin aging. J Investig Dermatol Symp Proc 1998; 3:1–5.
58. Hegedus ZL. The probable involvement of soluble and deposited melanins, their intermediates and the reactive oxygen side-products in human diseases and aging. Toxicology 2000; 14:145(2–3):85–1001.
59. Keogh E, Walsh RJ. Rate of graying of human hair. Nature 1965; 207:877–878.
60. Ibrahim L, Wright EA. The long term effect of repeated pluckings on the function of the mouse vibrissal follicles. Br J Dermatol 1978; 99:371–376.
61. Orfanos CE. Das weisse Haar alterer Menschen. Arch Klin Exp Dermatol 1970; 236:368–384.
62. Sato S, Kukita A, Jimbow K. Electron microscopic studies of dendritic cells in the human gray and white matrix during anagen. Pigment Cell 1973; 1:20–26.
63. Weisse I. Changes in the aging rat retina. Ophthalmic Res 1995; 1(suppl 27):154–163.
64. Bowers R, Chun DQ. Ultrastructural study of senescence of regenerating feather melanocytes in the jungle fowl. In: Bagnara K, Schartl M, eds. Biological, Molecular and Clinical Aspects of Pigmentation—Pigment Cell. Tokyo: University of Tokyo Press, 1985:347–357.
65. Westerhof W, Njoo D, Menke KE. Miscellaneous hypomelanoses: disorders characterized by extra-cutaneous loss of pigmentation. In: Nordlund JJ, Boissy RE, Hearing VJ, King RA, Ortonne J-P, eds. The Pigmentary System: Physiology and Pathophysiology. New York, NY: Oxford University Press, 1998:475–487.
66. Tobin DJ, Fenton DA, Kendall MD. Ultrastructural observations on the hair bulb melanocytes and melanosomes in acute alopecia areata. J Invest Dermatol 1990; 94:803–807.
67. Nagl W. Different growth rates of pigmented and white hair in the beard: differentiation vs. proliferation? Br J Dermatol 1995; 132:94–97.
68. Van Neste D, Tobin DJ. Hair cycle and dynamic interactions and changes associated with aging. Micron 2004; 35(3):193–200.
69. Slominski A, Paus R, Schadendorf D. Melanocytes as "sensory" and regulatory cells in the epidermis. J Theor Biol 1993; 164:103–120.
70. Tang A, Eller MS, Hara M, Yaar M, Hirohashi S, Gilchrest BA. E-cadherin is the major mediator of human melanocyte adhesion to keratinocytes in vitro. J Cell Sci 1994; 107:983–992.
71. Hollfelder B, Blankenburg G, Wolfram LJ, Hoecken H. Chemical and physical properties of pigmented and non-pigmented (gray) hair. Int J CoSmet Sci 1995; 17(2):87–89.
72. Wolfram LJJ, Hall K, Hui I. The mechanism of hair bleaching. J Soc Cosmet Chem 1970; 21:875–900.
73. C Robbins, C Kelly. Amino acid analysis of cosmetically altered hair. J Soc Cosmet Chem 1969; 20:555–564.
74. Robbins CR. In: Chemical and Physical Behavior of Human Hair. New York, NY: Springer-Verlag, 2002:153–192.
75. Hoting E, Zimmermann M. Sunlight-induced modifications in bleached, permed, or dyed human hair. J Soc Cosmet Chem 1997; 48(2):79–91.
76. Arnaud J. ESR study of hair and melanin-keratin mixture — the effects of temperature and light. Int J Cosmet Sci 1984; 6:71–83.
77. Hall K, Wolfram LJ. Isolation and identification of the protein component of hair melanin. J Soc Cosmet Chem 1975; 26:247–254.
78. Wolfram LJ, Albrecht L. Chemical-bleaching and photobleaching of brown and red hair. J Soc Cosmet Chem 1987; 38:179–191.

79. Anderson JS. The chemistry of hair colorants. J Soc Dyers Col 2000; 116(7–8): 193–196.
80. Corbett J. The role of meta difunctional benzene derivatives in oxidative hair dyeing. I. Reaction with p-Diamines. Cosmet Toiletries 1973; 24:103–134.
81. Brown K. Hair colorants. J Soc Cosmet Chem 1982; 33:375–383.
82. Wall FE. In: Sagarin E, ed. Cosmetics Science and Technology. New York, NY: Interscience, 1957:486–488.
83. Le Coz CJ, Lefebvre C, Keller F, Grosshans E. Allergic contact dermatitis caused by skin painting (pseudotattooing) with black henna, a mixture of henna and p-phenylenediamine and its derivatives. Arch Dermatol 2000; 136(12):1515–1517.
84. Correa A, Mohan A, Jackson L, Perry H, Helzlsouer K. Use of hair dyes, hematopoietic neoplasms, and lymphomas: a literature review. I. Leukemias and myelodysplastic syndromes. Cancer Invest 2000; 18(4):366–380.
85. Correa A, Jackson L, Mohan A, Perry H, Helzlsouer K. Use of hair dyes, hematopoietic neoplasms, and lymphomas: a literature review. II. Lymphomas and multiple myeloma. Cancer Invest 2000; 18(5):467–479.
86. Xie Z, Hayakawa R, Sugiura M, Kojima H, Konishi H, Ichihara G, Takeuchi Y. Experimental study on skin sensitization potencies and cross-reactivities of hair-dye-related chemicals in guinea pigs. Contact Dermatitis 2000; 42(5):270–275
87. Hoffman RM. Topical liposome targeting of dyes, melanins, genes, and proteins selectively to hair follicles. J Drug Target 1998; 5(2):67–74.
88. Alexeev V, Igoucheva O, Domashenko A, Cotsarelis G, Yoon K. Localized in vivo genotypic and phenotypic correction of the albino mutation in skin by RNA–DNA oligonucleotide. Nat Biotechnol 2000; 18(1):43–47.
89. Cui J, Shen LY, Wang GC. Role of hair follicles in the repigmentation of vitiligo. J Invest Dermatol 1991; 97(3):410–416.
90. Horikawa T, Norris DA, Yohn JJ, Zekman T, Travers JB, Morelli JG. Melanocyte mitogens induce both melanocyte chemokinesis and chemotaxis. J Invest Dermatol 1995; 104(2):256–259.
91. Halaban R, Langdon R, Birchall N, Cuono C, Baird A, Scott G, Moellmann G, McGuire J. Basic fibroblast growth factor from human keratinocytes is a natural mitogen for melanocytes. J Cell Biol 1988; 107(4):1611–1619.
92. Imokawa G, Yada Y, Miyagishi M. Endothelins secreted from human keratinocytes are intrinsic mitogens for human melanocytes. J Biol Chem 1992; 267(34): 24675–24680.
93. Jordan SA, Jackson IJ. MGF (KIT ligand) is a chemokinetic factor for melanoblast migration into hair follicles. Dev Biol 2000; 225(2):424–436.
94. Shetty M. Radiation therapy activates melanocytes in hair. Br Med J 1995; 311:1582.
95. Verbov J. Erosive candidiasis of the scalp, followed by the reappearance of black hair after 40 years. Br J Dermatol 1981; 105:595–598.
96. Tobin DJ, Cargnello JA. Partial reversal of canities in a twenty-two year old Chinese male. Arch Dermatol 1992; 129:789–791.

13

Biotechnology in Oral Care

Diane Cummins
Colgate-Palmolive Company, Piscataway, New Jersey, U.S.A.

William H. Bowen
University of Rochester, Rochester, New York, U.S.A.

INTRODUCTION

Dental caries and the periodontal diseases remain prevalent oral diseases in society today. Each may affect certain individuals at an early age; each will likely impact most individuals during adulthood; together they represent a significant oral health concern. While there are numerous unique aspects to each of these diseases, they share that each is a multifactorial condition with complex and interconnecting elements to its etiology. Dental plaque, as an infection, the interplay between plaque bacteria and the host tissues, and genetic and environmental factors, have each increasingly been recognized for their importance in the pathogenesis of both dental caries and the periodontal diseases.

Dental calculus, tooth staining and oral malodor are also prevalent conditions. Although each of these conditions is cosmetic in nature, each has assumed increasing relevance to the individual over the past decade or so. This is primarily because the impact of each of these conditions is more immediate than that of caries or the periodontal diseases and it is recognized by third parties, thereby affecting the social confidence of the individual.

Together, these oral problems have stimulated extensive research and development over the past four to five decades. Academic research has, primarily, focused on understanding the epidemiology, etiology and pathogenesis of these conditions, as well as on seeking potential routes to their intervention, whereas industrial research has focused on development and validation of professional and consumer products for their treatment and prevention.

New scientific insights have stimulated new research and development. Among these have been breakthroughs in genomics and proteomics. As these, and other, biotechnologies find increasing use, in particular, in disease diagnosis and in determining an individual's disease predisposition, in understanding the complex phenomena associated with the etiology and pathogenesis of disease, and in the evaluation of the delivery and efficacy of therapeutics, it is anticipated that new scientific paradigms will emerge and that these will, ultimately, result in new therapeutic treatments and preventive measures.

This chapter will focus on the disease states, caries and the periodontal diseases, as there is little evidence from the literature to suggest that biotechnological approaches are being investigated, or will be exploited, in the area of oral care cosmetics in the foreseeable future. Comprehensive, though not exhaustive, scientific and patent searches have been conducted pertaining to the potential use of biotechnology in oral care. From these, it is clear that the literature is dominated by approaches to the control of dental plaque formation. Of these, potential routes that may impact the prevention and control of dental caries as their primary outcome are the significant majority. For this reason, this chapter will primarily focus on dental plaque and caries to illustrate key concepts and approaches. Comparison and cross-reference to the periodontal diseases will be made where information is available and appropriate.

PREVALENCE OF DENTAL CARIES AND THE PERIODONTAL DISEASES

Despite a significant decline in the prevalence of dental caries in many segments of society, it remains a major public health problem (1). Dental caries affects more than 95% of the adult population and the public in the United State spends more than $30 billion per year to repair the consequences of this disease. More children develop dental caries than suffer from asthma; dental pain is one of the most common reasons for absence from work and for visits to the emergency room. Dental caries continues to be the major reason for tooth loss.

The periodontal diseases, in one form or another, affect the major proportion of the population. As much as 90% of Americans have been reported to have experienced gingivitis, the early stage of periodontal disease (2). Gingivitis may be prevented or treated by meticulous oral hygiene procedures (3). However, if neglected, it may progress to periodontitis, which requires protracted professional treatment to correct successfully. Periodontitis has been reported to affect 35% of the adult population over the age of 30 (4).

ETIOLOGY AND PATHOGENESIS OF DENTAL CARIES AND THE PERIODONTAL DISEASES

The major oral diseases, dental caries and periodontal disease, have dental plaque in common. They are induced by protracted, essentially undisrupted contact of dental plaque with vulnerable tissues. In dental caries, these tissues are the tooth surfaces, especially the pits and fissures, whereas in gingivitis and periodontitis, these are the gingival margin, and the subgingival soft tissues and periodontal ligament, respectively.

Historically, caries has been assessed by probing the teeth for cavities with a dental probe (5) and X rays have been used in some cases to provide additional information (6). New physical techniques, such as Quantitative Laser Fluorescence (QLF), are now being validated for the detection of precavitated lesions (7), as well as specific probes for *Streptococcus mutans*, using biotechnology tools, such as monoclonal antibodies (Mab), deoxyribonucleic acid (DNA) probes, and polymerase chain reaction (PCR) to assess caries risk (8). In the future, it is anticipated that genetic and proteomic markers of caries risk will likely become available.

Likewise, historically, gingivitis has been assessed by visual inspection of the gingival tissue and probing for bleeding (9), whereas periodontal disease has been assessed by probing subgingivally for periodontal pocket depth and loss of attachment (10). More recently, specific probes have been used to assess multiple marker organisms (11) and host inflammatory markers, such as the interleukins (ILs), tumor necrosis factor (TNF), and prostaglandins (PGs), in gingival crevicular fluid (12). In the future, it is anticipated that genetic and proteomic markers of periodontal disease risk will also become available.

Dental Plaque

Dental plaque is a biofilm. Unlike many natural biofilms, which are largely comprised of a single bacterial species or a relatively small number of different species (13), dental plaque is highly diverse and complex (14). More than 500 bacterial species have been characterized in mature plaque samples from different locations in the mouth (16). Approximately half of these have been identified using classical microbial methods of plating and counting, whereas, more recently, techniques used routinely in biotechnology, such as fluorescent-labeled antibodies, quantum dots, DNA probes, and PCR, have revealed a further 200 to 300 oral species that are noncultivable (15).

Like all biofilms, dental plaque has a highly hydrated exopolysaccharide matrix. Bacteria are enmeshed in the matrix and, indeed, are responsible for its formation and accumulation (16–18).

Supragingival plaque formation commences when a pellicle forms on a clean tooth surface. This pellicle is composed of salivary and bacterial constituents and occurs with extraordinary rapidity. Thus, a completely uncovered tooth surface rarely exists in nature (19). The salivary or mammalian constituents in the pellicle include, for example, amylase, lysozyme, mucin and histatin. Bacterial-derived constituents include glucosyltransferases (Gtf), fructosyltransferase (Ftf), and lipoteichoic acids (20). The orientation and molecular relationship among the various pellicle components are poorly understood. The pellicle undergoes changes in composition over several hours. Bacteria adhere to cleaned tooth surfaces and to pellicle-covered surfaces within hours, but in the earliest stages they do so comparatively poorly (21,22). The earliest colonizers are *Streptococci* and *Actinomyces* species. These may adhere initially through nonspecific physico-chemical forces (23) and subsequently through the specific physical interactions of coaggregation and coadhesion (24,25). The interaction between these early colonizers and the substrata, between bacterial adhesins and their receptors, helps to establish the early biofilm community. *Fusobacteria* species play an important role in plaque maturation and increasing diversity by mediating the transition of anaerobic species (25). New technologies have provided novel insights into dental plaque and its function as a biofilm. Specifically, cell–cell signaling has been widely recognized as an important phenomenon that is likely responsible for key mechanisms of bacterial adhesion, as well as biofilm growth rates and antimicrobial resistance (14).

Following ingestion of food containing even a small amount of sucrose, the Gtfs and Ftfs on the pellicle surface synthesize glucan and fructan, thereby, providing additional binding sites to which bacteria may adhere (26). Many bacteria adhere avidly to the glucan/fructan surface. Bacteria that adhere to the surface are Gtf producers or become coated with Gtf and, thereby, are de facto Gtf producers (27). Glucan comprises about 20% dry weight of dental plaque. Deletion of the Gtf from the genes of *S. mutans* results in marked diminution of the virulence of the prime microbial culprit of dental caries (28). Clearly, as indicated previously, *S. mutans* is not the only micro-organism present in dental plaque, even though it influences the properties of other micro-organisms through apparently coating them with Gtf.

The earliest direct observations of the structure of dental plaque using electron microscopy readily revealed micro-organisms embedded in an abundant matrix of polysaccharide that mediated the coaggregation and coadhesion of the bacteria (29). However, because of the excessive dehydration required for all electron microscopy methods, other than environmental scanning electron microscopy, these early three-dimensional structures were highly compressed (13). The resulting images were erroneously interpreted to be compact matrix structures with limited diffusion of endogenous and exogenous substances into and out of this biofilm matrix. The application of confocal scanning laser microscopy in the early '90s dispelled this illusion and demonstrated that the bacteria grow in microcolonies within the polysaccharide matrix and that this is interspersed with highly permeable water channels that allow access of nutrients from the bulk to the colonized surfaces (13,14,30). Nutrient, and oxygen, gradients can develop in areas of dense biomass and such local environmental heterogeneity may trigger altered patterns of gene expression that significantly influence microbial growth and diversity. Thus, the early observations that dental plaque varies significantly in composition on different anatomical surfaces in the mouth may be rationalized.

Dental Caries

In addition to dental plaque and the tooth surface, the presence of fermentable dietary sugars is a critical etiologic factor in dental caries (31). Following the ingestion of sugars, acid is rapidly produced within plaque; pH values of 4.0 are not uncommonly observed at the tooth surface 10 to 15 minutes following exposure to sugar. Lactic, acetic and formic are the most commonly detected acids (32).

In the absence of adaptive mechanisms, micro-organisms would be unable to survive in such an acid milieu. Several types of organisms, including the two species that are directly implicated in the pathogenesis of caries, *S. mutans* and *Lactobacillus casei*, have evolved sophisticated mechanisms that enable them to be acid-tolerant and, thus, survive and sometimes even dominate the ecology of the plaque (33). Foremost among these mechanisms includes the adenosyltriphosphate (ATP)-ase system which enables acid-tolerant organisms to pump protons from the cytoplasm to maintain a physiological pH within the bacterial cytoplasm (34,35). A second mechanism based is on cell–cell signaling and the involvement in competence-stimulating peptide (CSP) in inducing acid tolerance (14).

The arginine deiminase system is well developed in *Streptococcus sanguis*. In this system, arginine is broken down to ammonia and carbondioxide, which essentially serves in some measure to neutralize the acid found in plaque. The expression of genes that control the arginine deiminase system is suppressed at pH values above 5.5 and is upregulated when most required (36). Ammonia is also generated by urease-producing micro-organisms. This phenomenon is well recognized in patients who have end-stage renal disease. These patients undergo renal dialysis to eliminate elevated levels of urea in their blood and other fluids. The pH value of their plaque is often close to 7.5 or higher and in addition, following the application of sugar solution, the pH value remains elevated. These patients have significantly reduced levels of caries compared with most normal subjects (37).

The pH and amount of acid in dental plaque can also be influenced by the Stickland reaction. In this reaction, the proline ring structure is opened and two protons from lactate are added which results in the formation of δ amino valeric acid. This is found in comparatively high levels in dental plaque (38,39).

The Periodontal Diseases

As undisturbed dental plaque matures at the gingival margin, the first colonizers, mainly *Streptococci*, *Actinomyces*, and *Viellonella* species, are gradually replaced by filamentous bacteria, such as *Fusobacterium*, *Eubacterium*, and *Caphnocytophaga* species, which serve to increase bacterial diversity and to initiate a transition to a predominantly anaerobic flora (14,25,40). The protracted presence of supragingival plaque adjacent to the gingival soft tissues elicits an inflammatory response and the classic symptoms of gingivitis, that is redness, swelling and a propensity to bleed upon probing. When gingivitis persists, the resulting deepened gingival sulcus provides an environment in which anaerobic species, such as spirochetes and motile rods, begin to dominate (41). As plaque begins to extend below the gingival margin, the main nutritional component is GCF and this accounts for the predominance of asaccharolytic species (42).

While it has long been recognized that bacteria are the etiologic agents of periodontal disease, it has only recently been established that a limited number of species are responsible for most periodontal disease destruction (40). Specifically, *Porphyromonas gingivalis*, *Bacteriodes forsythus*, and *Treponema denticola* are strongly associated with chronic periodontitis, whereas *Actinobacillus actinomycetemcomitans* is strongly associated with rapidly progressing periodontitis (43). In contrast to dental caries, a wide range of virulence factors has been proposed as important in the pathogenesis of periodontal disease. Specifically, these periodontopathic organisms have the ability to express antigens, lipopolysaccharide, proteases and other enzymes. While it has been suggested that different clonal types may have different degrees of pathogenicity (43), much remains to be understood in this regard.

Host defense mechanisms are the second critical etiologic factor in periodontal disease pathogenesis (44). Bacterial virulence factors induce an inflammatory response and an elevation of cytokines and other mediators, such as the ILs, TNF, PGs and matrix metalloproteinases (43,44). The complexity of the pathogenic mechanisms is apparent from the simultaneous involvement of multiple host cell types, as well as multiple pathways in a cascade of inflammatory events that ultimately lead to destruction of the periodontal ligament and bone loss (43,44).

Individual host risk factors are the third etiologic factor in periodontal disease and these include environmental factors, such as smoking, as well as genetic factors (43). The latter may be critical to the apparent association between periodontal disease and specific systemic conditions, such as diabetes (45).

It is readily apparent that a plethora of biochemical and physiological interactions occur within dental plaque, both in dental caries and in periodontal disease, which theoretically, at least, could lead themselves to disruption through biotechnology approaches. Likewise, an increased understanding of the complex biological mechanisms that occur within the host in periodontal disease, as well as new insights into genetic risk factors could, in principle, lead through biotechnology approaches to new strategies for prevention and treatment.

CURRENT ROUTES TO PREVENT AND CONTROL DENTAL PLAQUE FORMATION, CARIES, AND EARLY PERIODONTAL DISEASE

As indicated earlier, the primary route to prevent and control all plaque-related oral health problems is meticulous oral hygiene and the mechanical removal of dental plaque from all tooth surfaces (3). However, this is neither practical nor possible for many individuals, as they may lack the motivation and/or dexterity to do so. The use of chemotherapeutic agents to supplement normal mechanical oral hygiene procedures is, therefore, widely accepted (46,47). Many years of research and development have provided a sound understanding of the key biological properties that any chemotherapeutic agent must possess to be clinically effective. The agent must possess inherent biological activity pertinent to the specific mechanism of intervention, it must be delivered to the oral cavity during the application time of the product and it must be retained on the oral tissues after application for a sufficient time period to exert sustained biological activity (48).

Fluoride and the Prevention of Dental Caries

Fluoride is by far the most effective agent in reducing the incidence of dental caries, with benefits proven in all segments of the population. Indeed, fluoride is the only clinically proven anticaries agent that is approved for routine use in oral hygiene (49).

Fluoride extends its protective effect, primarily through its effects on the tooth structure, by promoting the remineralization of very early carious lesions and by reducing the demineralization of sound enamel (50). Fluoride may also exert secondary effects on various bacterial processes. It may modulate the acid tolerance of plaque through inhibition of ATPase (51), it may reduce acid production by inhibiting enolase (52), it may affect membrane transport of glucose (52) and it may reduce the synthesis of Gtf but not necessarily the activity of the enzyme (53).

Clinical and mode-of-action studies have shown that fluoride is clinically effective when a constant low concentration of fluoride is maintained in dental plaque over an extended (12 hour) time period (50). Such elevated levels of fluoride can be maintained in dental plaque and, thus, caries can be prevented by regular intake of fluoridated drinking water (0.1–1 ppm fluoride) (54). The same endpoints have been accomplished by twice daily use of fluoride toothpaste (typically 1000–1500 ppm F). Indeed, the widespread use of fluoride toothpaste has been the most important factor contributing to the decline of caries over the past several decades (55).

As saliva is an effective cleansing agent, normal oral hygiene practices present a paradox; on one hand a therapeutic agent is applied, while at the same time a highly flavored vehicle (e.g., toothpaste, mouthrinse, or gum) may temporarily promote salivary flow and enhance clearance. Development of methods to enhance the retention of fluoride in the mouth presents an ongoing challenge. Use of a small device, containing a reservoir of fluoride, that is attached to the tooth surface to constantly and slowly release fluoride has been shown to be highly effective in clinical trials (56,57), but has not yet found a place in the market.

Incorporation of fluoride into microcapsules that would adhere to the mucosa and mouth surface also appears to offer attractive possibilities. Theoretically, such capsules could be created from starch or similarly biodegradable substances, which could act as substrates for the multitude of enzymes found in saliva and dental plaque. Clearly the principle of encapsulation into biodegradable agents could be applied to a wide range of active agents, including, but not limited to, antimicrobial agents or enzyme inhibitors. While a number of supplier companies have expertise in encapsulation technologies, this approach has not yet been proven to be a practical route to deliver superior anticaries efficacy.

Antimicrobial Agents and the Prevention of Plaque and the Reduction of Gingivitis

In contrast to dental caries, where the major chemotherapeutic approach to prevention has been to reduce the consequences of dental plaque by modulating the host response, that is, tooth enamel, the primary mechanistic approach to prevention of gingivitis and more severe forms of periodontal disease has been to prevent and control dental plaque formation (47,48). Substantial effort has been made over the past 20 years to identify suitable antimicrobial agents and to validate them in proof-of-concept clinical research. However, remarkably few antimicrobial agents have been successfully formulated into commercial products and have been clinically proven to deliver efficacy in preventing plaque and reducing gingivitis (47,48). Among these are three mouth rinses—one containing chlorhexidine (CHX), the second containing cetylpyridinium chloride (CPC), and the third containing essential oils—and two toothpastes each containing triclosan, one in combination with a copolymer and the other with a second antimicrobial, zinc citrate. The efficacy and mode of action of these systems has been widely documented (48).

Enzyme Systems and Their Current Roles in Oral Care

Products containing enzymes or enzyme-based systems currently play a very minor role in oral health and in the prevention and control of the two key oral diseases. The most well recognized of the ten or so existing commercial brands are Rembrandt®, Biotene® and Zendium® toothpastes. Each of these occupies niche positioning in strictly limited geographies. While these brands have enjoyed some market success—notably Zendium has reached a 30% share in Denmark—together they have a very minor share (<1%) in the global oral care market.

Attributes claimed of the three top enzyme brands are briefly summarized in Table 1. It is noteworthy that the consumer benefits fall into the "pseudotherapeutic" area. Despite early academic interest in enzymes as natural plaque-dispersing agents and/or as natural antimicrobial agents, it is particularly interesting and important to note that current enzyme products have not been proven to prevent or reduce dental plaque formation and have not been shown to prevent or reduce dental caries and/or gingivitis or more advanced forms of periodontal disease (48,58).

Table 1 Main Toothpaste Brands Containing Enzymes in Current Global Oral Care Market

Toothpaste brand	Enzyme system	Claimed benefits
Rembrandt (US)	Papain plus citric acid	Cleaning, whitening and relief of canker sores
Biotene (US)	Lactoperoxidase, lactoferrin and lysozyme	Reduces bacteria, helps natural defense and prevents problems associated with dry mouth
Zendium (Eu)	Glucose oxidase, amylo-glucosidase, lactoperoxidase, and thiocyanate	Mild, supports natural defense and prevents problems associated with dry mouth

A BRIEF HISTORY OF THE DEVELOPMENT AND EVALUATION OF ENZYME SYSTEMS FOR ORAL CARE

Plaque-Dispersing Enzymes

The most widely studied class of enzymes is the glucanhydrases, or glucanases. This area of research and its potential application to plaque control was stimulated in the late '60s and early '70s by increased understanding of the composition of dental plaque and recognition of the importance of the glucan matrix. The majority of the early work focused on dextranase (US Patent 04115546, Ref. 58), which degrades the α-1,6-linkages in glucan, with some additional interest in mutanase (US Patent 04353891, Ref. 50) and amylase (60), which degrade the α-1,3- and α-1,4-linkages in glucan, respectively. Despite the apparent promise of the approach, and a number of encouraging laboratory (60,61) and animal studies (62,63) using the enzymes under ideal conditions, clinical studies showed little or no effect on plaque formation (64–66).

Among the suggested explanations for the lack of effectiveness of a single glucan-digesting enzyme in reducing plaque in human clinical studies was the need for broader enzyme specificity and enhanced or prolonged retention in the oral cavity. Little academic research followed to address these two issues.

Enzymes (US Patents 03855142, 04082841, and 04154815, and JP Patent application 2250816A2) and enzyme combinations (US Patent 04438093, and JP applications 57165312A2 and 4316511A2) have been disclosed to address enzyme specificity and activity. In the mid 70's, a new protease, and a combination of mutanase and the new protease, marketed in the denture cleanser Steradent®, were shown to prevent denture plaque formation in proof-of-concept human studies (67). However, it appeared that mature plaque may resist digestion by combinations of enzymes, such as dextranase and mutanase, even under ideal laboratory conditions (68), although dextranase was shown to effectively block adherence of *S. mutans* to a glucan surface (69) and both enzymes were shown to disrupt the formation of glucan if present during its synthesis in vivo, suggesting potential to reduce initial colonization and early plaque maturation (70). Both enzymes are produced in a range of fungi and dextranase is expressed in several oral bacteria. However, the potential of mixed plaque-digesting enzyme systems was not subject to broader clinical investigation at that time.

Likewise, limited attempts were made to enhance enzyme retention in the oral cavity. Noteworthy was the preliminary research that established the principle of using lectins as anchoring agents in the mouth. Specifically, dextranase was conjugated to concanavalin A and the enzyme was shown to retain its activity, while the lectin was shown to retain its ability to bind to saliva-coated surfaces (71). Unfortunately, this approach was not progressed through human clinical studies to validate the principle.

Antibacterial Enzyme Systems

The Zendium and Biotene toothpastes each contain oxidoreductase enzymes in combination with other enzymes that, in principle, could deliver antibacterial effects in vivo. There are a number of patents describing these and related systems (US Patents 4178362, 4269822, 4537764, 4564519, and 5270033, WO Patent 08802600). Although the delivery of antibacterial action through natural mechanisms is a highly attractive concept, there have been remarkably few clinical studies published on either of these systems. This is possibly a consequence of the lack of antibacterial effects seen in vivo (72,73), as well as the equivocal results found in short-term studies of plaque and gingivitis (48,58,74).

THE POTENTIAL OF BIOTECHNOLOGY TO DELIVER SIGNIFICANT ORAL HEALTH BENEFITS IN THE FUTURE

The extensive patent literature in this area, coupled with the dedicated academic research of a few notable individuals and groups in the field, underpins the belief that, ultimately, biotechnology, in one form or other, will deliver a breakthrough technology that can be exploited to deliver significant oral health benefits. While the academic research is largely focused on long-term development and validation of highly sophisticated approaches to disease prevention, the patent literature covers the area more broadly and includes numerous options for application of "next generation" enzyme systems for plaque removal and prevention.

Enzyme Systems

There are significant numbers of patents and patent applications that describe ways to overcome the apparent deficiencies of plaque-dispersing enzymes, noted in the previous section, in respect of substrate specificity and delivery and retention in the oral cavity. It is also apparent from a review of the patent literature that improved enzyme stability in product formulations and reduced enzyme allergenicity may be important in ensuring that enzyme-containing oral care products become a reality in the market place.

In respect of enhanced enzyme activity, the key approaches taken in the patents are: new recombinant polypeptides and/or enzymes with glucan or fructan hydrolase activity, dextranase or mutanase activity to reduce plaque; new combinations of plaque-disrupting enzymes for enhanced cleaning and reduced desquamation or for plaque and gingivitis control; new combinations of one or more plaque-disrupting enzymes and an antibacterial enzyme; new combinations of lactoperoxidase with a plaque-disrupting enzyme and/or an antibacterial enzyme; new combinations of plaque-disrupting enzymes with polycationics; new combinations of plaque-disrupting enzymes from new sources, especially krill enzymes. A summary of the patents is given in Table 2.

In addition to patent activity, there have been a number of reports on the cloning, sequencing, purification and characterization of new enzymes. As examples, a pullulanase has been described with wider substrate specificity (75), as well as an exo-1,3-glucanase (76). The relevance, if any, of such new enzymes to oral care has yet to be determined. In contrast, a new combination of protease enzymes extracted from Antarctic krill shrimp has shown promise in removing dental plaque formed in vitro and in situ, suggesting that these enzymes are worthy of formulation development and evaluation in clinical studies (77). Likewise, a novel glucanhydrolase with the combined activities of dextranase and amylase (DXAMase) has been purified and characterized (78) and simple mouthwash formulations have been reported to show potential to reduce plaque formation (79). Again, further research to formulate and clinically test this enzyme appears warranted. In a third development, a combination of oxidoreductases, glucose oxidase and lactoperoxidase, and polysaccharide-hydrolyzing enzymes, dextranase and mutanase, appears to deliver both bactericidal activity and removal of biofilm in vitro (80). Although the commercialization of such a complex enzyme mixture for plaque control may be difficult, further work to evaluate its full potential may be appropriate.

In respect of improving the delivery and retention of enzymes, the key approaches outlined in patents are: recombinant plaque dispersing or antibacterial enzymes with a binding domain comprising a mutan-binding domain, or a cellulose-binding domain, or a starch-binding domain, or a polyanionic domain; new enzyme anchor complexes; and polypeptides with glucan-binding capacity to Gtf and an antibacterial enzyme or peptide. Also disclosed are methods to enhance the delivery and retention by physicochemical means, including enrobed enzymes, inorganic particulate and organic carrier systems, and polymer "sandwich" systems. Details of the patents are given in Table 3.

One patent and one patent application disclose new enzymes with enhanced stability for use in commercial products (Table 4). Likewise, one patent and two patent applications describe methods to select enzymes with reduced allergenicity compared to the parent protein (Table 5).

Table 2 Patents on Enzyme Systems with Plaque-Dispersing Activity

Patent number	Assignee	Technology
WO 9533470A1	Hellgren et al.	Krill enzymes for the manufacture of a prophylactic composition for preventing dental plaque formation in humans
WO 9624371A1	Phairson Medical	Multifunctional enzyme homologous to krill; multifunctional hydrolase inactivates cell surface adhesion to prevent bacterial infections, including oral
WO 9920239A1, US 20020006385A1 US 6413501	Novozymes	Oral compositions with plaque-inhibiting or plaque-removing enzymes, one starch-hydrolyzing and one starch-modifying enzyme
US 5747005	Barels and Cohler	Composition with at least one enzyme, from proteases, lipases and saccharinases, plus vitamin E
WO 03043517A2 US20030003059A1	Dana	Oral composition containing colustrum and a plaque-dispersing and/or antibacterial enzyme
EP 0884950A1	Novozymes	A method of killing bacteria with one or more enzymes and a polycationic compound
EP 01449513A1	Sara Lee	A dental product comprising lactoperoxidase and zinc ions and a plaque-dispersing or antibacterial enzyme
EP 01011700B1	Novozymes	A composition comprising a pullulanase and a dextranase, plus one or more plaque-disrupting or antibacterial enzymes
US 5622689 US 5849271	P&G	Oral composition for improved cleansing and reduced desquamation containing a plaque-disrupting enzyme
US 5431903 US 5437856 US 5320830 US 5320831	P&G	Oral composition for preventing plaque and gingivitis containing one or more plaque-disrupting enzyme
WO 09800528A1	Novozymes	Recombinant enzyme with mutanase activity
WO 09531533A1	Novozymes	An enzyme with endo-beta-glucanase activity
WO 09729197A1	Novozymes	Polypeptides with mutanase activity
WO 09800529A1 US 6156553	Novozymes	Recombinant enzyme with dextranase activity
US 20020076790A1 WO 0017331A1	Novozymes	Polypeptides with fructan hydrolase activity
JP 8308559A2	Lion	New mutanase that suppress dental plaque formation and is stable
JP10201483A2	Lion	Gene encoding a mutanase enzyme for prevention and removal of dental plaque

Table 3 Patents on Enzyme Systems with Enhanced Delivery and Retention

Patent number	Assignee	Technology
US 6355228	Novozymes	Oral care product comprising a mutan-binding domain and a plaque-disrupting or antibacterial enzyme
US 2003118572A1 WO 9933957A1	Novozymes	Modified (recombinant) (oxidoreductase) enzymes with a polyanionic domain
US 6264925 WO 9816191	Novozymes	Cellulose-binding domains for oral care products and a plaque-disrupting enzyme
US 6207149 WO 9816190	Novozymes	Starch-binding domains for oral care products and a plaque-dispersing or antibacterial enzyme
WO 0047174A1 WO 0047175A1 US 2002037260A1 US 2002037259A1 US 5871714 US 6159447	Pharmacal Biotechnologies	New composition comprising a coupled enzyme–anchor complex for controlling bacterial colonization and reducing dental plaque
WO 9531556A1	Unilever	Polypeptide with specific binding affinity for the glucan-binding domain of glucosyltransferase and an antibacterial enzyme or peptide
WO 0211688A1	Unilever	Oral composition containing petroleum jelly in the form of droplets enrobing a particulate active, including enzymes
WO 09723241A1	Unilever	Composition for delivering an antibacterial enzyme; a positively charged inorganic carrier particle with one or more antimicrobial enzymes
JP 61186309A2	Toyobo	Composition having long duration time of effects, comprising a layer of polymer, a layer of a plaque-disrupting enzyme and a layer of the polymer with polyacrylic acid
US 4138476	U.S. Navy	Long-acting plaque-dispersing enzymes prepared by binding the enzyme to an ethyl chloroformate carrier for control of dental caries and periodontal disease

Table 4   Patents on Enzyme Systems Relating to Improved Product Stability

Patent number	Assignee	Technology
US 05741487	Lion	Oral composition containing mutanase (and dextranase) with commercially acceptable stability
JP 8308559A2	Lion	New mutanase that suppress dental plaque formation and is stable to form a product

Table 5   Patents on Enzyme Systems Relating to Reduced Allergenicity

Patent number	Assignee	Technology
WO 0183559A2	Novozymes	A method of selecting protein variants having modified immunogenicity
US 6686164	Novozymes	A method of selecting low allergenic protein variants
US 20040175757A1	Novozymes	A method of selecting a protein variant with reduced immunogenicity

Vaccines and Other Immunogenic Routes to Reduce Bacterial Infections and Prevent Oral Disease

The concept of developing a vaccine to prevent the two major diseases of the mouth has been promoted for many decades (81). Attention on developing an anticaries vaccine sharpened following identification of *S. mutans* as a prime etiological agent in the pathogenesis of the disease. Considerable difference of opinion exists on whether a systemic vaccine is appropriate for essentially a non-fatal disease (82). Controversy also abounds on whether the protection reported in animals resides in IgG or sIgA (83); identification of the most appropriate antigen and the optimum route and number of vaccinations are all issues awaiting resolution (83).

However, the use of antibodies applied topically remains a viable prospect, in particular, because it is not difficult to produce large amounts of antibody inexpensively. The most appropriate antigenor antigens to use remains controversial. The focus of many studies has been to target early events in infection, especially microbial adhesion. The principle of reducing bacterial virulence through adhesion-deficient micro-organisms has been demonstrated, for example in urinary tract infections. Passive immunization with antiadhesion antibodies offers the potential to reduce *S. mutans* to undetectable levels. Monoclonal antibodies (Mabs) and antibody fragments against antigen 1/11, which is associated with the adherence of *S. mutans* to saliva-coated surfaces (pellicle), have been reported to offer great promise (84). Further, it is evident both from the scientific (85,86) and patent literature (e.g., see Table 6 patent applications WO 0215931A1 and 02102975A2, and US 20020068066A1, as well as Table 10 patent applications WO 9425591A1 and 9424577A2) that developments in biotechnology for engineering and large-scale production of antibodies and antibody fragments offers increased availability of these novel therapeutics at much reduced cost.

Specifically, antibody to the *S. mutans* antigen 1/11 has been cloned into tobacco leaves and has led to large-scale production of antibody relatively inexpensively (87). This antibody has shown to prevent adherence of *S. mutans* to pellicle in vitro. However, results from clinical studies investigating the ability of the antibody to prevent colonization by *S. mutans* in the human mouth, following suppression or elimination by intense topical treatment with chlorhexidine, have been mixed. A study in a small group of subjects showed some effects (88): results from a study in a much larger group revealed no effects (89). It is interesting to note that deletion of the gene responsible for production of antigen 1/11 in *S. mutans* did not lead to the diminution in the virulence of the organism (90).

It is, of course, possible to use biotechnology to clone the genes encoding selective antibodies into appropriate genomes such that they are expressed in foods likely to be consumed in bulk. This approach would appear to be directly applicable to, for example, potatoes, and indirectly applicable to hens, where the antibody appears in eggs, and to cows, which result in milk containing antibody. Whole bacteria have been used to vaccinate cows and resulted in production of antibody to a range of antigens (91). Some success has been reported in animal models (92).

Recently, antibody produced in eggs to Gtfs successfully inhibited the activity of GtfB and GtfC (93). Topical application of this antibody in rats fed a cariogenic diet and infected by *S. mutans* resulted in significantly fewer carious lesions and less severe lesions than those observed in control animals (93).

The principle of blocking adhesion of a specific bacterium associated with periodontal disease has also been demonstrated using an adhesion-blocking monoclonal antibody to *P. gingivalis*. Following subgingival antibiotic treatment to suppress the organism, four treatments with Mab over ten days resulted in significant protection against *P. gingivalis* recolonization over a nine-month period (94). Given the complexity of the etiology and pathogenesis of periodontal disease, much research will likely be needed to demonstrate meaningful clinical benefits in humans over the long term.

The use of topical antibody is attractive because its action can be directed either toward a particular group of pathogens or virulence factors associated with disease, in contrast to the effects of broad-spectrum antimicrobial agents. The attraction of this approach is further illustrated in Table 6 by the number of patents and patent applications disclosing antibodies and other immunogenic compositions, such as small peptides, for the treatment of both dental caries

Table 6 Patents on Application of Biotechnology in Oral Care; Vaccines and Other Immunogenic Compositions

Patent number	Assignee	Technology
WO 0215931A1 US 20020068066A1	Shi and Anderson	Monoclonal antibodies to *S. mutans*, produced in edible plants, elicit a humoral response to prevent dental caries
WO 02102975A2	Washington Dental Service and Regents of University of California	DNA molecules and recombinant DNA molecules for producing humanized monoclonal antibodies to *S. mutans* in plants and that elicit immune response to destroy cariogenic organisms
WO 9322341AQ1	Forsyth Dental Infirmary	Synthetic glucosyltransferase peptides provoking T and B cell immune responses for the prevention of dental caries
US 20040127400A1	Smith and Taubman	Immunogenic compositions comprising peptide subunits of glucan-binding protein with/without peptide subunits of Gtf useful as vaccines for passive immunization against *S. mutans* and dental caries
WO 9952548C2	Smith	Immunogenic glucan-based compositions (conjugate vaccine) and method to stimulate the immune response against *S. mutans* for treatment and prevention of dental caries
US 24105824A1	Goodman and Kay	Composition comprising competence stimulating peptide to prevent dental caries and infective endocarditis
WO 9849192A1	CSL Limited	Synthetic peptide constructs for the diagnosis and treatment of periodontitis associated with *P. gingivalis* and an immunogenic composition thereof
WO 0052041A1	Victorian Dairy Industry Association	Synthetic peptides containing protective epitopes for the treatment and prevention of periodontitis associated with *P. gingivalis* and an immunogenic composition thereof
WO 04045499A2	University of Florida	Antibodies and novel *A actinomycetemcomitans* immunogenic polypeptides for detection, prevention, and treatment *A* a associated periodontitis

Abbreviations: S. mutans, Streptococcus mutans; P. gingivalis, Porphyromonas gingivalis, A actinomycetemcomitans, Actinobacillos actinomycemcomitans

and periodontal disease. For further information on this approach, the reader is referred to two recent reviews on this topic (84,95).

Replacement Therapy and the Use of Pro- and Prebiotics

The microbial ecology of the mouth varies from site to site and overall is quite distinct from that which occurs in other parts of the body. The concept of excluding pathogens from particular sites by "precolonizing" the site by a nonvirulent organism has been established. For example, eyes of newborn children were deliberately infected by a nonpathogenic *Staphylococcus* to prevent infection by a virulent strain. A similar approach has been adopted to prevent disease in livestock.

Application of the principle of replacing a pathogen by a benign organism to the mouth has been explored over many years through the dedicated efforts of a few individuals (96). Specifically, the approach of replacing *S. mutans* in the mouth by a genetically altered strain that is preferentially bound to the teeth but is deficient in lactic acid production has been investigated (97) and patented (Table 7). This strain of *S. mutans* has been successfully implanted in rodents and resulted in reduced levels of caries. The strain has also been implanted in

Table 7 Patents on Application of Biotechnology in Oral Care; Replacement Therapy and Pro- and Prebiotics

Patent number	Assignee	Technology
US 5607672 EP 0832186B1	University of Florida	Recombinant *S. mutans* strain with a deficiency in lactic acid production (and other defined characteristics) and oral pharmaceutical compositions thereof for preventing and treating dental caries
WO 9907826A1 US 20030077814A1	Oh	Compositions containing lactic acid bacteria that inhibit the production of water-insoluble glucan or inhibit Gtf in dental plaque to prevent caries or that inhibit the growth of anaerobic bacteria to reduce gingivitis, periodontitis, and halitosis
WO 0069890A1	Johansson	New oligopeptides ($N = 5-10$) protecting against dental caries containing two or more arginine residues; a method and composition thereof

Abbreviation: S. mutans, Streptococcus mutans.

a small number of humans and has remained as part of the flora for several years (97). Clinical trials in large populations are in progress to assess the potential of this approach to prevent or retard caries in normal and high-risk populations.

The possibility of supplanting harmful organisms by similar bacteria with reduced virulence is certainly attractive because theoretically, at least, the "normal ecology" would not be disrupted. Whether this particular approach will be successful remains to be elucidated. There are many micro-organisms present in plaque that are potent producers of acid from sugars.

An alternative approach to replacement therapy has been to replace *S. mutans* with a benign species, such as *Streptococcus salivarius*, that can additionally effectively exclude or prevent regrowth of *S. mutans* by producing and targeting antimicrobial moieties, such as bacteriocins or bacteriocin-like substances (BLIS) (98). Although this approach has potential application to the prevention of dental caries, the propensity of this organism to colonize the mucosal surfaces of the throat and the dorsum of the tongue has led these investigators to focus on application to prevent acute pharangeal infections, as well as to prevent oral malodor (99).

The extension of the concept of replacement therapy and permanent or long-term suppression of disease pathogenesis is the use of pro- and/or prebiotics. The principle of the use of probiotics to modify the flora and positively reinforce health has been first established in the area of gastrointestinal infection and the maintenance of a balanced intestinal flora. Specifically, regular ingestion of *Lactobacillus* species, in the form of a dietary supplement or through milk products, especially yoghurt, has been shown to reduce specific debilitating conditions, such as irritable bowel syndrome, as well as to enhance overall wellness.

The concept of regularly introducing innocuous bacterial species to the mouth to suppress the outgrowth of normal oral pathogens is also being considered. Compositions containing lactic acid bacteria for inhibiting the production of water-insoluble glucan and for inhibiting Gtf in dental plaque to prevent caries or for inhibiting the growth of anaerobic bacteria to reduce gingivitis, periodontitis, and halitosis have been disclosed in the patent literature (Table 7). It is possible that these lactic acid bacteria may find a niche in the oral cavity and, thereby, exert ecological pressure on *S. mutans* and other pathogenic species. More likely, however, is the notion that these bacteria produce peptides or other antimicrobial species, such as BLIS mentioned earlier, and that these suppress the outgrowth of *S. mutans* and other species. The ability of such probiotic compositions to suppress specific bacterial pathogens and, thereby, to reduce clinical indices of disease remains to be investigated.

The concept of using a prebiotic or bacterial nutrient to influence the development of the normal oral flora and to maintain oral health is also of some interest and appeal. It was noted earlier that the arginine deiminase system is well developed in *S. sanguis* and that this may serve to break down arginine to ammonia to neutralize the acid found in plaque. New oligopeptides containing two or more arginine residues and 5 to 10 amino acids in total have been disclosed to protect against dental caries (Table 7). Likewise, this concept needs to be investigated and shown to be feasible.

Interestingly, lactic acid bacteria are widely used in industrial food fermentations and are now receiving attention as "cell factories" for the production of pharmaceutical products (100).

Antimicrobial Peptides

The potential of natural and synthetic antimicrobial peptides to deliver bactericidal effects to a developing biofilm is of interest. Natural antimicrobial peptides, known as defensins, are produced by epithelial and related cells in many multicellular organisms. They kill a range of bacteria, fungi and viruses, but their exact function and mechanism of action is not known. While defensins are directly involved in killing oral bacteria in the mouth, they also appear to play a role in activating the host's immune response through multiple pathways (101). Although much remains to be learned, interest in using these peptides, their synthetic analogs and other antimicrobial peptides has increased as evidenced by disclosures in the patent literature (Table 8). Investigation of their potential to reduce plaque and to prevent or control oral disease is in its infancy. They are certainly worthy of further exploration, both in respect of their activity and selectivity in killing bacteria in dental plaque biofilms and of their wider role in directing or impacting the adaptive immune response (101).

Phage-Encoded Enzymes and Proteins

The introduction of phage display offers the exciting possibility of developing biotechnologies that will express enzyme- and protein-based therapeutic agents in the mouth and deliver them to specific sites to block bacterial adhesion or to kill specific oral bacteria. Many fungi and bacteria have had genes cloned into them for the express purpose of producing therapeutic or pharmacological active agents, cheaply and in bulk.

The concept of cloning genes into an oral microorganism to allow expression of an active agent and reimplanting the modified organism into the mouth has only recently attracted attention. It is noteworthy that vectors encoding for a single chain of an antibody fragment to antigen 1/11 have been constructed and expressed in *Lactobacillus zeae*. The antibody fragments were shown to be excreted into the medium and to be aggregated by *S. mutans* cells expressing antigen 1/11 on the surface. This example has established the principle that oral micro-organisms can be genetically manipulated to produce active antibodies (102). It remains to be seen whether this approach can be validated in human clinical trials and developed into a meaningful therapy.

Table 8 Patents on Application of Biotechnology in Oral Care; Antimicrobial Peptides

Patent number	Assignee	Technology
US 6475771	University of Florida	Antimicrobial polypeptides, nucleic acid sequences encoding them and Streptococcus host for use in an oral composition
US 20020128186A1	University of Florida	Antimicrobial peptides (including antibiotics) and pharmaceutical compositions thereof for the control of bacterial infections (including oral bacteria)
US 2003 0118590A1	University of Florida	Antimicrobial peptides (including antibiotics) and pharmaceutical compositions thereof for the control of bacterial infections (including oral bacteria)
WO 9301723A1	Magainin Pharmaceuticals	Ion channel-forming polypeptides, for preventing or treating adverse oral conditions, plaque, gingivitis, caries and periodontal disease, and compositions thereof
WO 9926971A1	Victorian Dairy Industry	Antimicrobial peptides for use in the treatment of dental caries and periodontal disease
WO 03030821A2	Human Genome Sciences	Fusion proteins of albumin with a therapeutic protein or peptide where the albumin confers stability to the therapeutic for treating or preventing multiple systemic disorders

Additional examples of the possibility of expressing therapeutic actives, such as plaque-dispersing and antibacterial enzymes, as well as agents to block bacterial adhesion, are found in the patent disclosures listed in Table 9.

Earlier we referred to the ability of plaque to produce alkali and, in addition, persons who have renal disease and who must undergo renal dialysis have much lower than anticipated caries experience. With these observations in mind, several investigators have cloned genes expressing urease into oral micro-organisms and have successfully implanted them into the oral cavity of

Table 9 Patents on Application of Biotechnology in Oral Care; Phage-Encoded Enzymes and Proteins

Patent number	Assignee	Technology
WO 09607329A1 US 2001001463A1 US 20020044911A1	University of Maryland	A method for treatment of dental caries and periodontal disease using bacteriophages and phage-encoded antibacterial enzymes, including dextranase and lysozyme
US 20030129146A1 US 20030129147A1	Fischetti and Loomis	A composition and method for treating dental caries by use of a bacterial phage coding a lytic enzyme specific for the bacteria causing caries (and other oral organisms associated with disease)
WO 04000222A2	New Horizons Diagnostics Corp	A method for treating dental caries comprising at least one lytic enzyme coded in a bacteriophage specific to bacteria-causing caries and others for treatment of periodontitis
WO 9206191A1	Protein Engineering Corporation	Bacterial/pellicle-binding proteins to block bacterial adhesion and/or inhibit glucosyltransferase activity generated by random mutagenesis and expressed in a phage or bacterial cell or spore

rats. When subjected to a carcinogenic challenge, the animals experience significantly less caries than uninfected controls (102).

Antibody and Other Biologically Targeted Actives

The use of antibodies and antibody fragments opens up several additional approaches to the targeted delivery of therapeutic agents. Antibodies are most frequently generated against infectious agents, such as specific plaque bacteria; however, they can also be formed against mammalian epitopes and used to deliver chemotherapeutic substances to particular host sites, that is, they can be used as homing agents. This property could be used to deliver agents specifically to the tooth surface and, possibly, to particular surfaces of the oral mucosa. The principle behind this concept was first established in the medical field by demonstrating that antibodies to tumor cells could target cell-killing enzymes and peptides (104). More recently, the principle of targeting plaque bacteria has been demonstrated in vitro (105).

Salivary glycoproteins adsorbed to tooth surfaces undergo conformational change, frequently providing binding sites for bacteria that do not interact with the same glycoproteins in solution. Furthermore, antibodies induced to salivary proteins adsorbed to hydroxyapatite (by injecting rabbits with hydroxyapatite (HA) powder coated by specific salivary proteins) may not react with the same salivary protein in solution. It is clear that specific binding sites (epitopes) or cryptotopes are exposed when salivary proteins are adsorbed to an insoluble surface. It is highly probable, although not yet demonstrated, that a similar phenomena may occur on the mucosa. Mucosal pellicle has a distinct composition from that which occurs on tooth surfaces.

Both academic and industrial interest has been demonstrated in the potential application of targeted approaches to plaque control and disease prevention as evidenced by the patent disclosures listed in Table 10.

Although antibodies, especially humanized antibody fragments, offer an interesting approach to the development of homing agents, there are additional possibilities, as has been mentioned previously. Specifically, plant lectins will bind to specific sites on glycoproteins and so have the potential to act as targeting entities.

CONCLUSIONS

Overall it is apparent that, in practical terms, there has been little application of biotechnology in disease diagnosis, understanding the etiology and pathogenesis of disease or as new therapeutic agents to treat or prevent dental caries or the periodontal diseases.

Completion of the Human Genome Project was a milestone that may, ultimately, lead to a change in paradigm in respect of disease diagnosis and assessment of individual risk. At this point, tools are available, but extensive work is required to collect genomic and proteomic data from healthy individuals, individuals at risk and individuals with specific disease states in order to provide a solid foundation for the development of new functional diagnostics. The shear complexity of the disease processes is a challenge, especially in periodontal disease, but perhaps the greatest challenge in the future will be in integrating and interpreting the vast amounts of acquired information. Assuming this is realized, the understanding gained on host factors in disease pathogenesis could lead to new tools for screening based on disease mechanisms and new approaches to host intervention.

Likewise, microbial genomics and proteomics will, ultimately, lead to better understanding of the bacterial aspects underlying disease pathogenesis. Application of state-of-the-art techniques, such as PCR, has already begun to expand our knowledge base. They will also add impetus to research into new

Table 10 Patents on Application of Biotechnology in Oral Care; Antibody and Other Biologically Targeted Actives

Patent number	Assignee	Technology
WO0009164A1 US 20020034508A1	Horbach et al.	Antibodies and antibody fragments with/without an active substance for diagnostic, therapeutic, or cosmetic treatment, including compositions for oral care. The active substance may be a plaque-dispersing or antibacterial enzyme
US 5490988	Unilever	A product to treat the mouth comprising an antibody/antibody fragment system to target dental plaque and an enzyme-based therapeutic agent
EP 0736544B1	Unilever	Antibodies to target salivary pellicle to deliver enzyme-based therapeutic or cosmetic agents
WO 9425591A1	Unilever	Production of antibodies or functionalized fragments in Camelidae
WO 9429457A2	Unilever	Process for producing fusion proteins comprising single chain fragment variable region (SCFV) fragments in a transformed mold; includes targeting caries, gingivitis, periodontal disease, and oral malodor
US 24137482A1	Shi et al.	Composition comprising a targeting peptide and an antimicrobial peptide (fusion protein) to treat microbial infections in the mouth, gastro intestinal tract, and esophageal tract
US 20040052814A1	Shi et al.	Fusion protein for targeted delivery of antimicrobial peptides to *S. mutans* (and others) for detection and treatment of dental caries
US 6231857	Shi and Hume	Monoclonal antibodies specific to *S. mutans* for the detection and quantification of bacterial infection in dental caries
WO 04034979A2	Regents of University of California	Monoclonal antibodies recognizing surface antigens of *Actinomyces* and *Lactobacillus* for targeting an active agent for treating dental caries

Abbreviation: S. mutans, Streptococcus mutans.

therapeutics, especially into such areas as cloning genes into oral bacteria to express molecules with novel functionality at the site of interest.

Whilst none of the potential applications of biotechnology in oral care, discussed in this chapter, have been fully validated, there are several promising avenues for future application in professional, as well as consumer over-the-counter products.

REFERENCES

1. NCHS—Healthy People 2000. Oral Health Progress Review. National Center for Chronic Disease Prevention and Health Promotion. Available online at www.cdc.gov/OralHealth/factsheets/sgr2000-fsl.htm.
2. Brown LJ, Loe H. Prevalence, extent, severity and progression of periodontal disease. Periodontol 2000 1993; 27(2):57–71.
3. Axelsson P, Lindhe J. Effect of controlled oral procedures on caries and periodontal disease in adults. J Clin Periodontol 1990; 17:729–733.
4. Albandar JM, Brunell JA, Kingman A. Destructive periodontal disease in adults 30 years of age and older in the United States, 1988–1994. J Periodontol 1999; 70:13–29.
5. Pitts NB. Clinical diagnosis of dental caries: a European perspective. J Dent Educ 2001; 65:972–978.
6. Dove SB. Radiographic diagnosis of dental caries. J Dent Educ 2001; 65:985–990.
7. Stookey GK, Gonzalez-Cabezas C. Emerging methods of caries diagnosis. J Dent Educ 2001; 65:1001–1006.
8. Tanzer JM, Livingston J, Thomson A. The microbiology of primary dental caries in humans. J Dent Educ 2001; 65:1029–1037.
9. Saxton CA, van der Ouderaa FJG. The effect of a dentifrice containing zinc citrate and triclosan on developing gingivitis. J Periodontol Res 1989; 24:75–80.
10. Rosling B, Wannfors B, Volpe AR, Furuichi Y, Ramberg P, Lindhe J. The use of a triclosan/copolymer dentifrice may retard the progression of periodontitis. J Clin Periodontol 1997; 24:873–880.
11. Socransky SS, Haffajee AD, Cugini MA. Microbial complexes in subginvigal plaque. J Clin Periodontol 1998; 25:134–144.
12. Page RC, Offenbacher S, Schroeder HE. Advances in the pathogenesis of periodontitis:summary of developments, clinical implications and future directions. Periodontol 2000 1997; 14:216–248.
13. Costerton JW, Lewandowski Z, DeBeer D, Caldwell D, Korber D, James G. Biofilms, the customized microniche. J Bacteriol 1994; 176(8):2137–2142.
14. Marsh PD. Dental plaque as a microbial biofilm. Caries Res 2004; 38:204–211.
15. Paster BJ, Boches SK, Galvin JL. Bacterial diversity in human subgingivial plaque. J Bacteriol 2001; 183:3770–3783.
16. Critchley P, Wood JM, Saxton CA, Leach SA. The polymerization of dietary sugars by dental plaque. Caries Res 1967; 1:112–129.
17. Bowen WH, Velez H, Aquila M, Velasquez H, Sierra LI, Gillespie G. The microbiology and biochemistry of plaque, saliva and drinking water from two communities with contrasting levels of caries in Columbia, SA. J Dent Res 1977; 56:C32–C39.

18. Hotz P, Guggenheim B, Schmid R. Carbohydrates in pooled dental plaque. Caries Res 1972; 6:103–121.
19. Vacca-Smith AM, Bowen WH. In situ studies of pellicle formation on hydroxy-apatite discs. Arch Oral Biol 2000; 45:277–291.
20. Al-Hashimi I, Levine MJ. Characterization of in vivo saliva-derived enamel pellicle. Arch Oral Biol 1989; 34:289–295.
21. Schilling KM, Blitzer MH, Bowen WH. Adherence of *Streptococcus mutans* to glucans formed in situ in salivary pellicle. J Dent Res 1989; 68:1678–1680.
22. Clark WB, Bammann LL, Gibbons RJ. Comparative estimated bacterial affinities and adsorption sites on hydroxyapatite surfaces. Infect Immun 1978; 19:846–853.
23. Busscher HJ, van der Mei JC. Physico-chemical interactions in initial microbial adhesion and relevance for biofilm formation. Adv Dent Res 1997; 11(1):24–32.
24. Jenkinson HF, Lamont RJ. Streptococcal adhesion and colonization. Crit Rev Oral Biol Med 1997; 8:175–200.
25. Kolenbrander PE. Oral microbial communities: biofilms, interactions, and genetic systems. Ann Rev Microbiol 2000; 54:413–437.
26. Vacca-Smith A, Bowen WH. Binding properties of streptococcal glucosyltransferases for hydroxyapatite and bacterial surfaces. Arch Oral Biol 1998; 43:103–110.
27. McCabe RM, Denkerstoat JA. Adherence of *Veillonella* species mediated by extracellular glucosyltransferase from *Streptococcus salivarius*. Infect Immun 1977; 18:726–734.
28. Yamashita Y, Bowen W, Burne RA, Kuramitsu H. Role of *Streptococcus mutans* glucosyltransferase genes in caries induction in the specific-pathogen-free rat model. Infect Immun 1993; 61:3811–3817.
29. Listgarten M. Formation of dental plaque and other biofilms. In: Newman HN, Wilson M, eds. Dental Plaque Revisited: Oral Biofilms in Health and Disease. Cardiff: Biocure 1999:187–210.
30. Auschill TM, Arweiler NB, Natuschel L, Brecx M, Reich E, Sculean A. Spatial distribution of vital and dead organisms in dental biofilms. Arch Oral Biol 2001; 46:471–476.
31. Bowen WH. Food components and caries. Adv Dent Res 1994; 8:215–220.
32. Geddes DAM. Acids produced by human dental plaque metabolism in situ. Caries Res 1975; 9:98–109.
33. Quivey RG, Kuhnert WL, Hahn K. Adaptation of oral streptococci to low pH. Adv Micro Physiol 2000; 42:239–274.
34. Sturr MG, Marquis RE. Inhibition of proton-translocating ATPases of *Streptococcus mutans* and *Lactobacillus casei* by fluoride and aluminum. Arch Microbiol 1990; 155:22–27.
35. Bender GR, Sutton SV, Marquis RF. Acid tolerance, proton permeabilities and membrane ATPases of oral streptococci. Infect Immun 1986; 53:331–338.
36. Marquis R, Bender GR, Murray DR, Wong A. Arginine deiminase system and bacterial adaptation to acid environments. Appl Environ Microbial 1987; 53: 198–200.
37. Meyerowitz C. Caries in renal dialysis patients. In: Bowen WH, Tabak LA, eds. Cariology for the Nineties. Rochester, NY: University of Rochester Press, 1993: 249–260.
38. Stickland LH. Studies on the metabolism of the strict anaerobes (Genus *Clostridium*). I. The chemical reactions by which *Cl. sporogenes* obtains its energy. Biochem J 1934; 28:1746–1759.

39. Curtis M, Eastoe J. Comparison of free amino acid pools in dental plaque fluid from monkeys (Macaca fascicularis) fed on high and low sugar diets. Arch Oral Biol 1978; 23:989–992.

40. Haffajee AD, Socransky SS. Microbial etiologic agents of destructive periodontal diseases. Periodontology 2000 1994; 5:78–111.

41. Listgarten M. The structure of dental plaque. Periodontology 2000 1994; 5:52–62.

42. Darveau R, Tanner A. The microbial challenge in periodontitis. Periodontology 2000 1997; 14:24–32.

43. Page RC. The etiology and pathogenesis of periodontitis. Compendium 2002; 23(suppl 5):11–14.

44. Scannapieco FA. Periodontal inflammation: from gingivitis to systemic disease? Compend Contin Educ Dent 2004; 25(7 suppl 1):16–25.

45. Grossi SG, Genco RJ. Periodontal disease and diabetes mellitus: a two-way relationship. Ann Periodontol 1998; 3:51–61.

46. van der Ouderaa FJG, Cummins D. Delivery systems for supra- and sub-gingival plaque control. J Dent Res 1989; 68:1617–1624.

47. Newman HN. The rationale for chemical adjuncts in plaque control. Int Dent J 1998; 48(suppl 1):298–304.

48. Cummins D. Mechanisms of action of clinically proven antiplaque agents. In: Embery G, Rolla G, eds. Clinical and Biological Aspects of Dentifrices. Oxford: Oxford University Press, 1992:205–228.

49. 21 CFR 355; Anti-caries Drug Products for Over-the-Counter Human Use; www.accessdata.fda.gov/scripts/cdrh/cfdocs/cf CFR/CFR search.cfm?CFRpatr_355 sources 60FR52507, Oa 1995.

50. Lynch RJM, Navada K, Walia R. Low levels of fluoride in plaque and saliva and their effects on de-mineralization and re-mineralization of enamel. Int Dent J 2004; 5:310–314.

51. Sutton SV, Bender GR, Marquis RE. Fluoride inhibition of proton-translocating ATPases of oral bacteria. Infect Immun 1987; 55:2597–2603.

52. Marquis RF. Antimicrobial actions of fluoride for oral bacteria. Can J Microbiol 1995; 41:955–964.

53. Bowen WH, Hewitt MJ. Effect of fluoride on extracellular polysaccharide production by *Streptococcus mutans*. J Dent Res 1974; 53:331–338.

54. Edgar WM, Ingram GS, Morgan SN. Fluoride in saliva and plaque in relation to fluoride in drinking water and in dentifrice. In: Embery G, Rolla G, eds. Clinical and Biological Aspects of Dentifrices. Oxford University Press, 1992:145–156.

55. Scheie AA. Dentifries in the control of dental caries. In: Embery G, Rolla G, eds. Clinical and Biological Aspects of Dentifrices. Oxford University Press, 1992: 29–40.

56. Mirth D, Adderly DD, Amsbaugh SM, Monell-Torrens E, Li SH, Bowen WH. Inhibition of experimental dental caries using an intraoral fluoride-releasing device. J Am Dent Assoc 1983; 107:55–58.

57. Meyerowitz C, Watson GE. The efficacy of an intraoral fluoride-releasing system in irradiated head and neck cancer patients; a preliminary study. J Am Dent Assoc 1998; 129:1252–1259.

58. Moran J, Addy M, Newcombe R. Comparison of the effect of toothpastes containing enzymes or antimicrobial compounds with a conventional fluoride toothpaste

on the development of plaque and gingivitis. J Clin Periodontol 1989; 16:295–299.

59. Inoue M, Yakushiji T, Mizuno T, Yamamoto J, Tanii S. Inhibition of dental plaque formation by mouthwash containing an endo-alpha-1,3 glucanase. Clin Prev Dent 1990; 12:10–14.

60. Fitzgerald RJ, Spinell DM, Stoudt TH. Enzymatic removal of artificial plaques. Arch Oral Biol 1968; 13:125–128.

61. Goldstein-Lifschitz B, Bauer S. Comparison of dextranases for their possible use in eliminating dental plaque. J Dent Res 1976; 55(5):886–892.

62. Bowen WH. The effect of dextranase on caries activity in monkeys (Macaca inus). Br Dent J 1971; 131:445–449.

63. Guggenheim B, Regolati B, Schmid R, Meeklemann R. Effects of the topical application of mutanase on rat caries. Caries Res 1980; 14:128–135.

64. Caldwell RC, Sandham HJ, Mann WV Jr, Finn SB, Formicola AJ. 1. The effect of a dextranase mouthwash on dental plaque in young adults and children. J Am Dent Assoc 1971; 82:124–131.

65. Lobene RR. 2. A clinical study of the effect of dextranase on human dental plaque. J Am Dent Assoc 1971; 82:132–135.

66. Keyes PH, Hicks MA, Goldman BM, McCabe RM, Fitzgerald RJ. 3. Dispersion of dextranous bacterial plaques on human teeth with dextranase. J Am Dent Assoc 1971; 82:136–141.

67. Budtz-Jörgensen E. Prevention of denture plaque formation by an enzyme denture cleanser. J Biol Buccale 1977; 5:239–244.

68. Bowen WH. Unpublished data, 2005.

69. Schilling KM, Blitzer MH, Bowen WH. Adherence of *Streptococcus mutans* to glucans formed in situ in salivary pellicle. J Dent Res 1989; 68:1678–1680.

70. Marotta M, Martino A, De Rosa A, Farina E, Carteni M, De Rosa M. Degradation of dental plaque glucans and prevention of glucan formation using commercial enzymes. Process Biochem 2002; 38:101–108.

71. Barker SA, Giblin AG, Gray CJ, Bowen WH. Preparation and properties of a conjugate containing dextranase and concanavalin A. Carbohyd Res 1974; 36:23–33.

72. Lenander-Lumikari M, Tenovuo J, Mikola H. Effects of a lactoperoxidase system-containing toothpaste on levels of hypothiocyanite and bacteria in saliva. Caries Res 1993; 27:285–291.

73. Modesto A, Lima KC, de Uzeda M. Effects of three different infant dentifrices on biofilms and oral microorganisms. J Clin Pediatr Dent 2000; 24(3):237–243.

74. Addy M. Chlorhexidine compared to other locally delivered antimicrobials. J Clin Periodontol 1986; 13:957–964.

75. Duffner F, Bertoldo C, Andersen JT, Wagner K, Antranikian G. A new thermoactive pullulanase from *Desulfurococcus mucosus*: cloning, sequencing, purification, and characterization of the recombinant enzyme after expression in bacillus subtilis. J Bacteriol 2000; 182(22):6331–6338.

76. Kulminskaya AA, Thomsen KK, Shabalin KA, Sidorenko IA, Eneyskaya EV, Savel'ev AN, Neustroev KN. Isolation, enzymatic properties, and mode of action of an exo-1,3-β-glucanase from *Trichoderma viride*. Eur J Biochem 2001; 268:6123–6131.

77. Hahn Berg IC, Kalfas S, Malmsten M, Arnebrant T. Proteolytic degradation of oral biofilms in vitro and in vivo: potential of proteases originating from *Euphausia superba* for plaque control. Eur J Oral Sci 2001; 109:316–324.

78. Ryu SJ, Kim D, Ryu HJ, Chiba S, Kimura A, Day DF. Purification and partial characterization of a novel glucanhydrolase from *Lipomyces starkeyi* KSM 22 and its use of inhibition of insoluble glucan formation. Biosci Biotechnol Biochem 2000; 64(2):223–228.

79. Kim D, Ryu SJ, Heo SJ, Kim DW, Kim HS. Characterization of a novel carbohydrase from *Lipomyces starkeyi* KSM 22 for dental applications. J Microbiol Biotechnol 1999; 9:260–264.

80. Johansen C, Falholt P, Gram L. Enzymatic removal and disinfection of bacterial biofilms. Appl Environ Microbio 1997; 63(9):3724–3728.

81. Taubman MA, Smith DJ. Vaccination: a cariostatic option? In: Bowen WH, Tabak LA, eds. Cariology for the Nineties. Rochester, NY: University of Rochester Press, 1993:441–457.

82. Bowen WH. Relevance of caries vaccine investigations in rodents, primates and human: critical assessment. In: Bowen WH, Genco RJ, O'Brien TC, eds. Immunologic Aspects of Dental Caries. Spec. Suppl., Immunol. Abstr. Washington DC: Information Retrieval Inc., 1976:11–20.

83. Bowen WH. Vaccine against dental caries—a personal view. J Dent Res 1996; 75:1530–1533.

84. Kelly CG, Medaglini D, Younson JS, Pozzi G. Biotechnological approaches to fight pathogens at mucosal sites. Biotechnol Gene Eng Rev 2001; 18:329–347.

85. Winter G. Synthetic human antibodies and a strategy for protein engineering. FEBS Lett 1998; 30:92–94.

86. Larrick JW, Yu L, Chen J, Jaiswal S, Wycoff K. Production of antibodies in transgenic plants. Res Immunol 1998; 149(6):603–608.

87. Ma JK, Lehner T, Stabila P, Fax CT, Hiatt A. Assembly of monoclonal antibodies with IgG1 and IgA heavy chain domains in transgenic tobacco plants. Eur J Immunol 1994; 24:131–138.

88. Ma JK, Hikmat BY, Wycoff K, Vine ND, Chargelegue D, Yu L, Hein MB, Lehner T. Characterization of a recombinant plant monoclonal secretory antibody and preventive immunotherapy in humans. Nat Med 1998; 4(5):601–606.

89. Weintraub JA, Hilton FF, White JM, Hoover CL, Wycoff K, Wu L, Larrick J, Featherstone JDB. A plant derived mutans streptococci antibody clinical trial. Caries Res. In press, 2005.

90. Bowen WH, Schilling K, Giertsen E, Pearson S, Lee SF, Bleiweis A, Beeman D. Role of a cell surface-associated protein in adherence and dental caries. Infect Immun 1991; 59:4606–4609.

91. Shimazakik Y, Mitoma M, Oho T, Nakano Y, Yamashita Y, Okano K, Nakano Y, Fukuyana M, Fijihara N, Nada Y, Koga T. Passive immunization with milk produced from an immunized cow prevents oral recolonization by *Streptococcus mutans*. Clin Diagn Lab Immunol 2001; 8:1136–1139.

92. Mitoma M, Oho T, Michibata N, Okano K, Nakano Y, Fukyuwama M, Koga T. Passive immunization with bovine milk containing antibodies to a cell surface protein antigen-glucosyltransferase fusion protein protects rats against dental caries. Infect Immun 2002; 70:2721–2724.

93. Kruger C, Pearson SK, Kodama Y, Vacca-Smith A, Bowen WH, Hamanstrom L. The effects of egg-derived antibodies to glucosyltransferases on dental caries in rats. Caries Res 2004; 38:9–14.

94. Booth V, Ashley FP, Lehner T. Passive immunization with monoclonal antibodies against *Porphyromonas gingivitis* in patients with periodontitis. Infect Immun 1996; 64:422–427.

95. Abiko Y. Passive immunization against dental caries and periodontal disease: development of recombinant and human monoclonal antibodies. Crit Rev Oral Biol Med 2000; 11(2):140–158.

96. Hillman JD, Socransky SS. Replacement therapy of the prevention of dental disease. Adv Dent Res 1987; 1:119–125.

97. Hillman JD, Principles of microbial ecology and their application to xerostomia-associated opportunistic infections of the oral cavity. Adv Dent Res 1996; 10(1): 66–68.

98. Tagg JR, Dierksen KP. Bacterial replacement therapy: adapting "germ warfare" to infection prevention. Trends Biotechnol 2003; 21(5):217–223.

99. BLIS K12 Throat guard lozenges markted by BLIS Technologies Limited, Wellington, New Zealand. Access: www.blis.co.nz.

100. de Vos WM, Hugenholtz J. Engineering metabolic highways in Lactocci and other lactic acid bacteria. Trends Biotechnol 2004; 22(2):72–79.

101. Marshall RI. Gingival defensins: linking the innate and adaptive immune responses to dental plaque. Periodontol 2000, 2004; 35:14–20.

102. Kuepper MB, Huhn M, Spiegel H, Ma J, Barth S, Fischer R, Finnern R. Generation of human antibody fragments against *Streptococcus mutans* using a phage display chain shuffling approach. BMC Biotechnol 2005; 5:4.

103. Clancy K, Pearson S, Bowen WH, Burne RA. Characteriation of recombinant urealytic *Streptococcus mutans* demonstrates an inverse relationship between dental plaque, urealytic capacity, and cariogenicity. Infect Immun 2000; 68:2621–2629.

SUPPLEMENTARY PATENT REFERENCES

US 0411546	Oral compositions containing dextranase and a manganese activator
	Assignee: Colgate-Palmolive
US 04353891	Mutanase enzyme which breaks down dental tartar and plaque
	Assignee: Guggenheim and Muhlemann
US 03855142	Enzymatic denture cleaner containing lipase, instead of proteolytic enzymes
	Assignee: Lever Bros
US 04082841	Antiplaque and anticalculus dentifrice with zinc ions and hydrolytic dentifrice
	Assignee: Lever Bros
US 04154815	Zinc and enzyme dentifrice: with hydrolytic enzyme
	Assignee: Lever Bros

JP 225081642   Composition for preventing tooth decay with alkali protease and alkaline agent to prevent caries and periodontitis
Assignee: Kao

US 04438093   Oral composition containing dextranase and α-1,3 glucanase and a method for preventing and suppressing oral diseases using the same
Assignee: Research Foundation for Microbial Diseases, Osaka University

JP 5716531ZAZ   Production of oral compositions: dextranase and α-1,3 glucanate to prevent dental plaque, caries, gingivitis and other
Assignee: Nandai Bisei Butsubiyou Kenkyukai

JP 4316511AZ   Composition for the oral cavity containing enzyme with macerating activity and use of protease, β-1,3 glucanase, dextranase, or mutanase
Assignee: Sunstar

US 4178362   Toothpaste with hydrogen peroxide-generating enzymes: glucose oxidase and glucose
Assignee: Telec

US 4269822   Antiseptic dentifrice: containing amino acid, oxidoreductase enzyme
Assignee: Laclede Professional Products

US 4537764   Stabilized enzyme dentifrice containing β glucose and glucose acidase
Assignee: Laclede Professional Products

US 4564519   Dienzymatic chewable dentifrice: oxidizable substrate, oxidoreductase enzyme, thiocyanate, and lactoperoxidase
Assignee: Laclede Pharmaceutical Products

US 5270033   Antimicrobial composition and method of making same: oxidoreductase/substate
Assignee: RE Montgomery

WO 08802600   Enzyme containing bactericidal composition and dental wound treatment preparations comprising this composition: containing oxidase, peroxidase, thiocynate, and lysozyme
Assignee: OM Poulson

14

Biotechnology in Perfumery

Anthony J. Clark, Michel Schalk, and Fredi Brühlmann
*Department of Biotechnology, Corporate R&D, Firmenich SA,
Geneva, Switzerland*

INTRODUCTION

This chapter provides a summary of the main areas in which biotechnology has had, and will in the future have, an impact on the fragrance industry. The implications of knowledge gained from biotechnology are clear to the perfume industry and provide much excitement over the potential applications. Here we will outline three subject areas that relate to both the perfumery industry and to biotechnology.

First, our current understanding of the sense of smell owes much to studies in molecular biology. Molecular biology has permitted the cloning and identification of all the odorant receptors in humans, and it continues to be used to reveal new insights into the mechanisms of chemosensation in humans and other creatures. Application of this knowledge may eventually lead to new technologies relevant to our industry.

Second, corporal and other malodors are key to perfumery because many fragranced products are designed to neutralise them. Advances in biochemical studies supported by recombinant DNA technology have greatly helped our understanding of the generation and perception of such odors. The role of steroid, fatty acid, amino acid metabolism, and the composition of apocrine sweat have all been implicated in body odor formation, resulting in clear understanding of the biology of this system. Subsequently, our understanding of this area has been used to formulate more efficient cosmetic products.

Third, the impact of recombinant DNA technology in understanding secondary plant metabolism cannot be overestimated. Recombinant DNA technology has, therefore, provided the impetus for generating new organic molecules for use in perfumery. Clearly, plants provide the raw material for the vast majority of perfumes and is where biotechnological leverage may provide the best results. From this standpoint, many biotechnological studies have established the framework from which the flavor and fragrance industry can work toward biocatalytic routes to new raw materials. However, the translation of what we have learned into new products lies some way in the future. It is important to realize just what the impact areas are and the future challenges we face.

MECHANISMS OF OLFACTORY PERCEPTION

Smell is a primary sense enabling the detection of airborne low molecular weight molecules. The discriminatory power of our nose is remarkable: Humans are capable of distinguishing thousands of different odors. Although the perception of smell is well understood at the anatomical level, many questions remain, particularly in the area of molecular recognition and on how sensory signal processing in higher brain areas translates into odor perception. Thus far, molecular biology has heavily contributed to the better understanding of smell detection at the molecular level (receptors) and interestingly also on the anatomy allowing signal-specific dissection of the neural network at an unprecedented resolution.

A better understanding of smell perception could aid in the rational design of novel perfumes and likely will lead to technical devices allowing a more meaningful detection of odorants. Although "artificial noses" have already reached the market, their applications seem confined to small odor spaces. Indeed, the discriminatory capability of artificial noses has remained far behind the performance of the human nose, which enables not only discrimination but also hedonic evaluation of odors.

The Anatomy of Smell

Volatile molecules reach the nasal cavity containing the olfactory epithelium, a sensory tissue, that harbors olfactory sensory neurons expressing odorant receptors. It now seems well established that each olfactory sensory neuron produces only one specific type of odorant receptor (1). Interestingly, a given olfactory sensory neuron responds to different odorant molecules (receptive range), whereas a given odorant molecule can be sensed by different olfactory sensory neurons (2). Olfactory sensory neurons project their axons into the main olfactory bulb, which is the brain's first relay station of smell perception (3). The axons of olfactory sensory neurons establish synaptic connections with mitral and tufted neurons of the olfactory bulb within structures called glomeruli. Thus, every odorous chemical produces a specific map of glomerular activation in the bulb (4). The specificity of axon projection is tightly linked to the type of receptor produced because receptor gene swapping in olfactory sensory neurons lead to different axonal projections (5,6). Mitral and tufted cells interact with different glomeruli via short axon cells as well as with granule cells located in the deeper layers of the bulb through their secondary dendrites. The processed sensory information is then projected by the bulb mitral and tufted cells to the primary olfactory cortex, where further signal processing occurs. From there information is forwarded to subcortical, thalamic, and cortical regions (7). Gene targeting technologies in transgenic animals have allowed the tracing of axon projections of individual olfactory sensory neurons into the olfactory bulb and via transneuronal transfer of a tracer into olfactory cortical areas at unprecedented resolutions (8–10). Interestingly, the same olfactory sensory neurons project via the olfactory bulb into multiple olfactory cortical areas, thus revealing parallel and perhaps differentiated signal processing (Fig. 1). These findings are, in part, further supported by noninvasive brain imaging techniques, such as functional magnetic resonance imaging (fMRI), that can also be applied to humans. The combined use of these techniques will help to gain a deeper understanding of the neuronal network for odor perception. In many mammals, there is an accessory olfactory organ, called the vomeronasal organ, that is distinct from the main olfactory epithelium. The vomeronasal organ harbors vomeronasal sensory

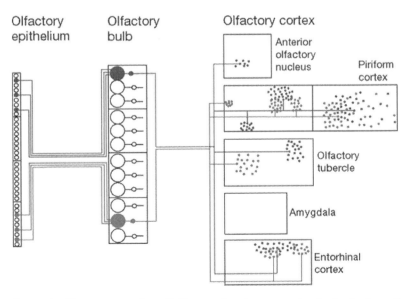

Figure 1 The anatomy of smell. Transgenic mice expressing barley lectin as the transneuronal tracer in specific olfactory sensory neurons were used to identify areas of the olfactory cortex receiving input from a particular odorant receptor. Different olfactory cortical areas receive inputs from olfactory sensory neurons expressing the same receptor. *Source*: From Ref. 10.

neurons expressing pheromone receptors. Although there is some evidence available on the presence of the vomeronasal organ in humans, the accessory olfactory bulb seems missing in adults. Our understanding on the functionality of such a sensory system in humans has remained nonconclusive (11).

Molecular Olfaction

In 1991, Linda Buck and Richard Axel published a milestone paper describing a novel multigene family of putative odorant receptor genes expressed in the olfactory epithelium of rats (12). That work triggered a plethora of research activities mainly in academia aimed at the interpretation of olfaction in molecular terms.

Olfactory receptors belong to the G-protein-coupled-seven-transmembrane-domain-receptors (GPCRs). They constitute the largest multigene family in multicellular organisms. Interestingly, a given vertebrate olfactory sensory neuron expresses only one type of odorant receptor gene (6). The underlying genetic mechanism of this exclusivity has been at least in part unveiled recently (1).

Odorant receptor genes are intronless with about 310 codons. Hypervariability in sequence among different odorant receptors mainly occurs in the third, fourth, and fifth transmembrane region, which is assumed to harbor at least part of the binding site for odorant molecules. This observation is further supported by site-directed mutagenesis (13). Binding of an odorant molecule activates a G-protein, which leads to rapid stimulation of the adenylyl cyclase and subsequent increase in cyclic adenosine monophosphate (cAMP). Elevation of cAMP levels triggers depolarisation of olfactory sensory neurons by activation of cyclic nucleotide gated cation channels. Once a threshold potential is reached, the cell generates an action potential, thus translating the chemical into an electrical signal, which is sent to the olfactory bulb, from where it is relayed into higher areas of the brain.

Since the pioneering work of Buck and Axel, many more groups have succeeded in identifying odorant receptor genes in vertebrates—most notably humans—and invertebrates. With the completion of the human genome project, odorant receptor genes could be rapidly identified (14,15). According to a recent report 388 potentially functional olfactory genes and 414 apparent pseudogenes have been identified in humans (16). The remarkably large portion of pseudogenes likely reflects our reduced dependence on the sense of smell for survival and reproduction. Intriguingly, olfactory receptor genes are also expressed in nonolfactory tissues such as sperm where they might play a role in chemotaxis (17).

Characterization of the receptive range has been achieved for a few odorant receptors only, such as the rat I7 odorant receptor. One major bottleneck is the difficulty in getting recombinant receptor genes functionally expressed in heterologous systems, despite the first report more than a decade ago. A functional expression system for odorant receptors requires proper folding, targeting to the plasma membrane, and the efficient coupling with a second messenger system that produces a measurable signal upon binding of a ligand. Various expression systems have been described, including, among others, the baculovirus system (18), infection of olfactory sensory neuron cells of the rat epithelia with an engineered adenovirus (19), or creating a fusion protein with a membrane import protein for functional expression in human embryonic kidney (HEK) 293 cells (20). In HEK 293 cells, coupling is achieved with the promiscuous G protein ($G_{\alpha 15}$). Detection of calcium or cAMP can then be used to study the interaction between odorant and receptor. Such interactions were studied after infecting rat nasal eptithelia in vivo with a recombinant adenovirus providing the I7 receptor from rat. The accessible range of the I7 receptor was explored by electrophysiological recording upon exposure of the epithelium of infected animals to various odorants (19,21). The receptor was tested against nearly 200 individual chemicals and was found to have a strong preference for short chain aldehydes. In fact, the I7 receptor from rat has a strong requirement for an aldehyde carbonyl with strict prerequisites around the carbonyl. In contrast, the I7 receptor appears to only poorly discriminate structural variations at the tail of the molecule. The laboratory of Hanns Hatt expressed and characterized the first odorant receptor from human relying on transient expression in HEK 293 cells (20).

The prediction of the receptive range for a given odorant receptor has been attempted by homology modeling, using the crystal structure of bacteriorhodopsin and more recently bovine rhodopsin as the template (22,23). The structure-function predictions are in good agreement with experimental data, although bacteriorhodopsin (no GPCR) and bovine rhodopsin (currently the only known structure of a GPCR) exhibit only low sequence homologies with odorant receptors. Such predictions should become even more accurate once high-resolution structural maps for odorant receptors become available.

Application of Molecular Olfaction

Despite the remarkable discriminatory power of the human nose, this powerful organ is not without limitations. Although adaptation to odors might be useful for our daily life, it is not a desired feature whenever the nose has to be used, for example, for analytical work over a prolonged time. Furthermore, apart from individual variations, our nose does not easily allow quantitative measurements and is insensitive to certain volatiles. Many attempts have been made to develop artificial noses for process control and monitoring, control of raw materials, intermediates, and final products, for screening purposes, etc. Chemical "noses" are often based on the physical monitoring of sensing surfaces during adsorption of volatiles (24–26). Sensing surface arrays of different specificities can be monitored during exposure to odorants via one or more detection principles (e.g., capacitance, mass-sensitive frequency changes of oscillating coated cantilevers, color, surface plasmon resonance, etc.). The recorded physical responses from these sensors may then be correlated with a perceived odor. Progress in the field has allowed improvement in signal stability and reduction of the influence of humidity and temperature on the signal. Additionally, the use of fast gas chromatography (GC) or mass spectrometry can in some cases offer a valuable alternative.

Could odorant receptors find applications as chemical sensors? Data mining of the human genome allowed rapid identification of the human odorant receptor repertoire. However, odorant receptor genes have remained difficult to express in heterologous systems, which limits efforts in developing robust chemical sensors based on odorant receptors (27). On the one hand, odorant receptors could offer an interesting alternative to existing sensing surfaces because of the sensitivity (signal amplification) and the significant selectivity. Alternatively, functional odorant receptors could be immobilized on microfabricated cantilevers to detect nanochemical responses upon binding of odorants. Indeed, membrane protein micro-arrays have been recently fabricated for GPCRs (28). On the other hand, the large number of different odorant receptors responding to any particular odorant, albeit with different affinities, poses a challenging task. Deciphering the "receptor code" for an extended odor space could require the handling of a large portion of the odorant receptor repertoire—if not the entirety. However, with the rapidly increasing know-how in the use of recombinant odorant receptors and a deeper understanding in odor perception, such a task might well become feasible in the near future.

San Diego-based Senomyx has acquired licenses on most human and non-human chemosensory receptors. The start-up wants to exploit these receptors for the discovery of novel molecules from combinatorial libraries of chemicals. In the field of odors, the use of odorant receptors seems most promising for applications, which may require only a limited set of odorant receptors. First proof of principles relevant to odors will likely originate from the work on modulators and antagonists (e.g., blockers of specific malodors), which *per se* are difficult to identify in repetitive tasks by the human nose.

CORPORAL BODY ODOR

It is often desirable to reduce malodors in many environments, and masking bad odors forms a fundamental part of the perfumery business. The perfumer's art encompasses the ability to complement a malodor with a fragrance composed in such a way as to counter the bad odor. For example, indole is a component of toilet odor and possesses a characteristic faecal note. However, at low concentrations, this molecule takes on a jasminelike identity, reminiscent of white flowers. A capable perfumer can therefore harness elements of a malodor and create around them in order to almost instantaneously transform a perceived off-odor into something much more agreeable. Biotechnology and molecular biology have helped greatly in our understanding of volatile odor chemistry assigned to the human body and in particular the underarm area. Here we need to look at what exactly sweat malodor is and what technologies are being considered for perfuming cosmetic products. A major impact area for perfumery will be in masking and inhibition of malodor generation.

Axillary vaults possess specialized apocrine sweat glands at high density. The localized nature of body odor generation can be attributed to a range of metabolic activities at work on these apocrine secretions. In summary, these glands secrete a highly proteinaceous, although odorless cocktail, very different from normal (eccrine) sweat. The gland contracts and squeezes the secretion through the duct in order to be deposited on the skin surface. Elucidation of this mechanism has been aided by a recent report suggesting that transepithelial Cl$^-$ efflux in sweat ducts is regulated by the gene product of WNK4, a serine-threonine kinase. WNK4 expression was localized to the cuboidal cells lining sweat duct lumens. Inhibition of this process may lead to new cosmetic products that could provide longer lasting antiperspirants (29).

Lipase and protease activities, as part of essential cutaneous metabolism, can be readily detected on the human skin surface. However, a wide range of other enzymatic activities can also be induced, for example, by xenobiotic application. The resulting cascade of complex metabolic pathways involve steroid oxidising P450 monooxygenases, as well as aryl sulphatases, esterases, reductases, and hydrolases. In addition, steroid 5α-reductase activity has also been reported from within the apocrine glands themselves (30). Many of the above enzyme activities have been reported in relation to steroid biosynthesis and secretion. Many molecular studies have centred on the endocrine control of apocrine glands and have greatly helped our understanding of the sweat process. This mechanism appears important in the very rapid induction of odor from people under stress. There is evidence that even subtle changes in mood can alter axillary odor profiles (31). From the first indications thirty years ago, it is clear that bacteria are necessary to generate human body odor. The volatile metabolism that occurs under the arm appears to be due to a complex degradative process. *Corynebacterium* species are often associated with the clinical condition of *plantar bromidrosis* (acute offensive body odor). It comes as no surprise then that this genus of organisms possess all the enzymatic machinery to carry out all of the biochemical conversions described earlier.

What Is the Composition of Body Odor?

Steroids

Cholesterol, androgens, and other steroids have been extensively investigated and their biochemical pathways elucidated (32). Key to our understanding of the function of androgens has been the cloning and molecular studies of the androgen receptors. Interestingly, androgen receptor levels have been shown to be elevated in patients with the clinical condition osnidrosis (excessive sweating) and suggests that androgen activity is directly involved in apocrine gland function (33–35).

It has been assumed that the sterols commonly found in sweat are derived from a similar biochemical route to androgens found in other tissues, such as the testis. For example, androst-16-enes can be formed from pregnenolone in testes of pigs and man. It has long been assumed that a similar mechanism exists in axillae and accounts for 16-androstene deposition in apocrine secretions.

The four very odorous steroids; 5-α-androst-16-ene-3-one, androsta-4,16-diene-3-one and their respective alcohols (5-α-androst-16-ene-3α-ol and androsta-4,16-diene-3α-ol) have all been found in male sweat (36). The exact identity of the steroid precursors remain unclear. However, it is known that several strains of *Corynebacterium* possess the ability to reduce androst 4/5-ene to the 5α-androstenes with the aid of a 5α-reductase. Recently, Austin and Ellis reported a detailed mechanism by which *Corynebacterium* strains are able to interconvert steroids. This represents the first clear evidence of molecular precursors of volatile odorous steroids in sweat (37). Molecular studies of these enzymatic activities and genetic regulation will greatly aid our understanding of this extremely complex biological phenomenon.

Steroids of this type have been found in apocrine secretions in the form of glycosides and sulphates. The enzymes necessary to liberate the free steroid from conjugates are common in bacteria but are also indigenous to human skin. Reports on inhibiting β-glucuronidase and aryl-sulphatase activity have demonstrated a correlative relationship between the odor formed from apocrine sweat and subsequent enzyme inhibition (38,39). It has been clearly demonstrated that some aerobic coryneforms (designated underarm odor-forming bacteria) can convert glycosyl and sulphate conjugates to adrost-16-one/ols. The enzymatic nature of these conversions was confirmed by Gower and coworkers. Interestingly *Staphylococci* species could also convert the conjugates to odorous forms (36).

Volatile Fatty Acids

Certain coryneform bacteria have been implicated in fatty acid degradation and the generation of volatile fatty acids (VFAs) (C_{6-11} acids). The *Corynebacterium* subgroup A do not appear to be able to fully catabolise long chain fatty acids (LCFAs), instead partial degradation products are formed. Taking into account the very high lipase activity reported for group A *Corynebacterium* strains, it seems reasonable to assume that these organisms are primarily responsible for the generation of the VFA component of the human axillary malodor. The subsequent VFA accumulation in apocrine sweat will then depend on the relative activities of subgroup A bacteria versus VFA degrading bacteria, such as *Micrococcus luteus* or *Brevibacterium epidermidis* (40).

(E)-3-Methyl-2-Hexenoic Acid

The predominant olfactory contributor-compound in axillary sweat is most likely to be (E)-3-methyl-2-hexenoic acid (3M2HA), discovered by Preti and coworkers (41). Interestingly, as this compound was first isolated from patients suffering from schizophrenia, it was proposed as an indicator for this psychological profile for some time. A comparison of the relative quantities in male sweat estimated 3M2HA at more than 700-fold higher concentration than the volatile odorous steroid androstenone (42). The release of 3M2HA was studied, and it was subsequently reported that the release kinetics of this compound was too rapid to be due to putative catabolic metabolism of axillary associated bacteria, for example, fatty acid degradation. It transpired that this acid was bound to proteins secreted from the apocrine glands called Apocrine Secretion Odor-Binding proteins (ASOBs) (43,44). These proteins were immuno-reactively identical to apolipoprotein D (apoD), a well-characterized member of the lipocalin carrier protein superfamily. Interestingly, this family of proteins also mediates odor binding to receptors in the ofactory epithelium. Release of the bound 3M2HA appears to rely principally on the metabolism of lipophilic *Corynebacterium* spp.

Recently Acuna and coworkers cloned the gene for the enzyme responsible for the liberation of 3M2HA from *Corynebacterium striatum*. In fact, they identified that the chemically related acid 3-hydroxy-3-methylhexanoic acid represents the protein-bound form. It appears that ligand acid is bound to the carrier protein in the form of a conjugate with a glutamine residue. By synthesising the precursors, these workers identified a Zn^{2+} dependent aminoacylase that effectively mediated the cleavage of both acids from the bound substrate. Analysis of the coding region of the cloned gene revealed four conserved amino acid motifs common to a number of zinc-dependent metalloproteases (45,46). It would seem that human bacterial flora has coevolved with the host to the extent where they present enzymes with unique substrate profiles in tune with the host secretions and chemosensory signaling.

Volatile Sulphur Compounds

Amino acid degradation appears also to be associated with malodor generation. It is known that sulphur containing amino acids are secreted in sweat. It is well reported that leucine can act as a potential substrate for isovaleric acid generation. Other reports have centered on a pyridoxal phosphate-dependent β-lyase, which was characterised as being responsible for the generation of axillary malodor from apocrine secretions (47). This represents one of the few examples where thiols and other volatile sulphur compounds (VSCs) are indicated as key components of the human axillary malodor. It also highlights an obvious area where perhaps biotechnology will help illucidate the pathways and mechanisms by which VSCs are generated (48,49).

Developments in Personal Care and Hygiene Products

Clearly, researchers into axillary malodor have realised that considerable financial benefits were possible by harnessing knowledge gained from their studies into inhibition of odor generation. Consequently, many patents have been deposed on active ingredients for deo/antiperspirant and laundry products. These include: enzyme inhibitors, inhibitors, of steroid metabolism, fatty acid inhibitors, and masking agents (50,51).

One research area that could be exploited is the enzymatic release of compounds in order to mask bad odors. In fact, several recent patents describe precursors of fragrance raw materials that, when acted upon by one or more of the enzyme activities identified on the skin surface, liberate fragrance molecules that mask or inhibit malodor (52,53). Hygiene and personal care products have benefited from many ingredients designed to kill or inhibit corynebacterial growth. More recently, formulators have tried to specifically inhibit areas of corynebacterial metabolism with varying degrees of success.

Another biotechnological approach, using recombinant enzyme systems as screening tools may lead to new fragrance molecules with enhanced properties of masking or inhibition of malodor.

As we understand more about how volatile molecules are used by biological systems, then biotechnology can be applied to deliver previously unforeseen product ranges and open up new markets (54).

The picture is fundamentally complex, but the image appears to be coming into focus!

BIOTECHNOLOGICAL ROUTES TO PERFUMERY RAW MATERIALS

Plants produce a large number of secondary metabolites that serve for defense, reproduction, and interaction with other organisms. Firmenich, among others, have built their business around the identification of the main impact chemicals found in the extracts and essential oils of plants, followed by the chemical synthesis in purer form, at higher volumes, and of course more cheaply. Plant secondary metabolism, of course, provides many areas of interest to researchers within the perfumery industry. For example, hydroperoxide cleavage of lipids can generate many oxylipin structures that currently are used extensively in fragrance creation. However, research into biotechnological routes to perfumery raw material production is expensive, and the return on such an investment leads inevitably to the conclusion that commercial success will rely on engineering pathways to families of structures. Here, we describe research into such a family, the isoprenoids.

Isoprenoids (or terpenoids), also named terpenes, almost certainly represent the most structurally diverse family of secondary metabolites. Plants accumulating large amounts of monoterpenes and sesquiterpenes have been of interest for thousands of years because of their flavor and fragrance properties and their cosmetic, medicinal, and antimicrobial effects. The perfume industry has largely exploited the natural diversity of terpene composition of plants. Complex mixture of ingredients rich in terpenes, generally obtained by distillation or extraction of plant leaves, root, wood or flowers, have become important ingredients of perfume compositions. Classical examples include: sandalwood oil, vetiver oil, patchouli oil, citrus oils, or mint oils. Perfumers are continuously in search of new compounds. Great effort has therefore been made to discover new odors by analyzing plants from all origins to discover new terpene molecules or by fractionating or purifying terpenes from complex mixtures.

Tens of thousands of isoprenoid compounds have been characterized, and many new compounds are continuously discovered. From a biosynthetic point of view, they are made up of five carbon units called isoprene units and can be classified by the number of isoprene units present in their structure. The monoterpenes (C10) and sesquiterpenes (C15) have attracted the most attention from the perfume and flavor industry because of their volatility and their vast spectrum of olfactory characteristics.

During the past decades, many researchers, mainly in academic laboratories, have investigated the biosynthesis of terpenes in plants and microorganisms with the objective to elucidate the pathway and understand its regulation and to study the functioning of each enzyme individually. The recent progress in biotechnology and particularly in gene technology has been of great help

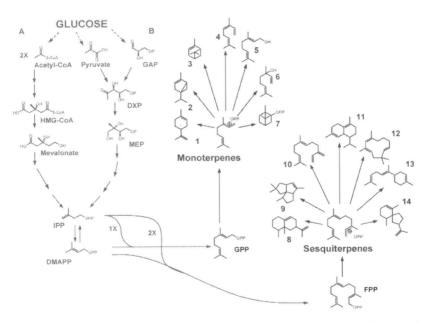

Figure 2 Monoterpene and sesquiterpene biosynthetic pathway. The mevalonate pathway (**A**) and the MEP (or DXP) pathway (**B**) for the biosynthesis of IPP and DMAPP and the prenyltransferase condensation of IPP and GPP and FPP are indicated in gray. Examples of monoterpene and sesquiterpenes produced by different terpene synthases are also indicated (1–14). Limomene (1), thujene (2), α-pinene (3), β-ocimene (4), geraniol (5), linalool (6), bornyl diphosphate (7), valencene (8), pentalenene (9), farnesene (10), cadinene (11), α-humulene (12), bisabolene (13), premnaspirodiene (14). *Abbreviations*: HMG-CoA, 3-hydroxy-3-methylglutaryl coenzyme A; GAP, D-glyceraldehyde-3-phosphate; DXP, 1-deoxy-D-xylulose-5-phosphate; MEP, 2-C-Methyl-D-erythritol-4-phosphate; IPP, isopentenyl pyrophosphate; DMAPP, dimethylallyl pyrophosphate; GPP, geranyl pyrophosphate; FPP, farnesyl pyrophosphate.

and has considerably accelerated discoveries in the terpene field. The knowledge has now reached a stage were industry could benefit.

The biosynthesis of mono- and sesquiterpene in all organisms can arbitrarily be divided into two stages: (*i*) the synthesis of the universal precursors, geranyl pyrophosphate, and farnesyl pyrophosphate, respectively, for the monoterpenes and the sesquiterpenes (*ii*) utilisation of these precursors by specific enzymes to elaborate the carbon skeleton and subsequently oxido/reduction modifications by specific enzymes (Fig. 2).

In all organisms, two distinct pathways (the mevalonate pathway and the methylerythritol phosphate pathway) control the carbon flux to the universal precursor of all monoterpenes and sesquiterpenes. Both pathways were recently elucidated in microorganisms and plants, and this was achieved particularly with the use of genetic and genomic techniques (55,56). It is now possible to study in detail the enzymology and regulation of each enzyme of the pathway and to identify key steps controlling the carbon flux to final terpene structures.

Terpene synthases are key enzymes in the terpenoid pathway. They allow the formation of the complex carbon skeletons by catalysing the cyclisation of the acyclic pyrophosphate precursors. Each plant contains a specific set of terpene synthases responsible for the terpene profile observed. Until recently, studies on terpene synthases were carried out using enzymes partially purified from natural extracts. The use of molecular biology to isolate genes encoding for terpene synthases and the heterologous expression in a recombinant organism has been crucial to aiding our understanding of the mechanism of enzyme reaction involved. During the past 15 years, tens of monoterpene and sesquiterpene synthases encoding genes have been isolated, and the enzyme heterologously expressed in a microorganism and functionally characterized (57). The number of genes isolated is growing continuously, and this is considerably accelerated by the increasing DNA sequence information provided by the genomic projects.

The isolation of DNA molecules encoding for terpene synthases permits the heterologous expression of the enzymes in recombinant microorganisms, and, as a consequence, a relatively large quantity production and easy purification of the enzymes has been achieved. To date, the structure of four sesquiterpene synthases (58–61) and one monoterpene synthase (62) has been determined, providing an insight into the enzyme's mechanism. Researchers have shown that it is possible to alter the activity of terpene synthases (i.e., changing the product profile) by exchanging amino-acid domains between different enzymes (63,64) or by directed mutatagenesis or deletion of specific amino acids (65).

Using the molecular biology techniques it is now routine work to transfer genes from one organism to another and to upregulate, downregulate or suppress the expression of endogenous genes. Recent publications have proven the feasibility of manipulating terpene biosynthesis in plants or microorganisms for different purposes. For instance, it is now possible to alter the terpene productivity or profile in plants. Croteau and collaborators have manipulated the production of monoterpenes in the oil glands of peppermint by up- or downregulating key genes in the pathway. They were able to increase the yield and the quality of the oil produced by the modified plants (66). Other laboratories have expressed heterologous terpene synthases in plants and showed that these resulted in production of novel terpenes (67–69). It has also been shown that manipulation of terpene synthase can enhance the aroma or scent of plants by increasing the production of key terpenes (70). A similar approach has been applied to microorganisms, and it has been reported that bacteria and yeast can be engineered to produce mono and sesquiterpenes. This has been achieved by increasing the carbon flux into the terpene pathway by genetically engineering key regulatory enzymes and by introducing genes coding for enzymes catalysing the synthesis of targeted terpenes. Thus monoterpenes and sesquiterpenes were produced in bacteria and yeast, although only at low levels (71–74).

In conclusion, the recent progresses in biotechnology and the elucidation at the molecular level of many key steps in the terpenoid pathways in plants and microorganisms has opened up the route to the engineering of the isoprenoid pathway in plants or microorganisms for applications, such as modification of the composition of existing oils, production of new or rare terpene molecules, or construction of new systems for production of terpenes (75–77). It can be predicted that perfumery industry will benefit from these new technologies in the near future.

OUTLOOK AND FUTURE PROSPECTS

In the foreseeable future recombinant DNA technology will become a fundamental part of the process for discovery and production of new fragrance raw materials that will be cheaper or, more likely, novel in character.

- Diagnostics application for the detection of trace quantities of volatiles should be possible in the future, although it seems unrealistic that the creation of a true artificial nose will be possible at this point. This is due mainly to the complexity of the cognitive process where translation and interpretation of the stimuli in the brain have still to be elucidated.
- Manipulation of enzyme functions present within the axillary vault should lead to the design of functional and innovative slow release profragrances.
- New mechanisms of fragrance release in the future may well hinge upon studies into biological processes involving recombinant enzyme technology and there exists the potential to use immobilised recombinant proteins and cells in allergenicity, toxicity, and carcinogenicity testing as substitutes for animal testing programmes.

REFERENCES

1. Serizawa S, Miyamichi K, Nakatani H, Suzuki M, Saito M, Yoshihara Y, Sakano H. Negative feedback regulation ensures the one receptor-one olfactory neuron rule in mouse. Science 2003; 302:2088–2094.

2. Malnic B, Hirono J, Sato T, Buck LB. Combinatorial receptor codes for odors. Cell 1999; 96:713–723.
3. Firestein S. How the olfactory system makes sense of scents. Nature 2001; 413:211–218.
4. Rubin BD, Katz LC. Optical Imaging of odorant representations in the mammalian olfactory bulb. Neuron 1999; 23:499–511.
5. Singer MS, Shepherd GM, Greer CA. Olfactory receptors guide axons. Nature 1995; 377:19–20.
6. Mombaerts P, Wang F, Dulac C, Chao SK, Nemes A, Mendelsohn M, Edmondson J, Axel R. Visualizing an olfactory sensory map. Cell 1996; 87:675–686.
7. Shepherd GM. From odor molecules to odor images: Towards a molecular psychology of smell. In: Salvadori G, ed. Olfaction and Taste. Carol Stream, IL: Allured Publishing Corporation, 1997:204–222.
8. Horowitz LF, Montmayeur J-P, Echelard Y, Buck LB. A genetic approach to trac neural circuits. Proc Natl Acad Sci USA 1999; 96:3194–3199.
9. Mombaerts P. Seven-transmembrane proteins as odorant and chemosensory receptors. Science 1999; 286:707–711.
10. Zou Z, Horowitz LF, Montmayeur J-P, Snapper S, Buck LB. Genetic tracing reveals a stereotyped sensory map in the olfactory cortex. Nature 2001; 418:173–179.
11. Meredith M. Human vomeronasal organ function: a critical review of best and worst cases. Chem Senses 2001; 26:433–445.
12. Buck L, Axel R. A novel multigene family may encode odorant receptors: a molecular basis for odor recognition. Cell 1991; 65:175–187.
13. Krautwurst D, Yau KW, Reed RR. Identification of ligands for olfactory receptors for functional expression of a receptor library. Cell 1998; 95:917–926.
14. Zozulya S, Echeverri F, Nguyen T. The human olfactory receptor repertoire. Available online at http://genomebiology.com/2001/2/6/research/0018.1.
15. Crasto C, Singer MS, Shepherd GM. The olfactory receptor family album. Available online at http:// genomebiology.com/2001/2/10/reviews/1027.1
16. Niimura Y, Nei M. Evolution of olfactory receptor genes in the human genome. Proc Natl Acad Sci USA 2003; 100:12235–12240.
17. Spehr M, Gisselmann G, Poplawski A, Riffell JA, Wetzel CH, Zimmer RK, Hatt H. Identification of a testicular odorant receptor mediating human sperm chemotaxis. Science 2003; 299:2054–2058.
18. Raming K, Krieger J, Strotmann J, Boekhoff I, Kubick S, Baumstark C, Breer H. Cloning and expression of odorant receptors. Nature 1993; 361:353–356.
19. Zhao H, Ivic L, Otaki JM, Hashimoto M, Mikoshiba K, Firestein S. Functional expression of a mammalian odorant receptor. Science 1998; 279:237–242.
20. Hatt H, Geisselmann G, Wetzel C. Cloning, functional expression and characterization of a human olfactory receptor. Cell Mol Biol 1999; 45:285–291.
21. Araneda RC, Kini AD, Firestein S. The molecular receptive range of an odorant receptor. Nat Neurosci 2000; 3:1248–1255.
22. Singer MS. Analysis of the molecular basis for octanal interactions in the expressed rat I7 olfactory receptor. Chem Senses 2000; 25:155–165.
23. Vaidehi N, Floriano WB, Trabanino R, Hall SE, Freddolino P, Choi EJ, Zamanakos G, Goddard WA III. Prediction of structure and function of G protein-coupled receptors. Proc Natl Acad Sci USA 2002; 99:12622–12627.

24. Ampuero S, Bosset JO. The electronic nose applied to dairy products: a review. Sens Actuators B 2003; 94:1–12.
25. Hagleitner C, Hierlemann A, Lange D, Kummer A, Kerness N, Brand O, Baltes H. Smart single-chip gas sensor system. Nature 2001; 414:293–296.
26. Rakov NA, Suslick K. A colorimetric sensor array for odour visualization. Nature 2001; 406:710–712.
27. Gilbert AN, Firestein S. Dollars and scents: commercial opportunities in olfaction and taste. Nat Neurosci 2002; 5:1043–1045.
28. Fang Y, Frutos AG, Lahiri J. Membrane protein microarrays. J Am Chem Soc 2002; 124:2394–2395.
29. Kahle KT, Gimenez IG, Hassan H, Wilson FH, Wong RD, Forbush B, Aronson PS, Lifton RP. WNK4 regulates apical and basolateral Cl⁻ Flux in extrarenal epithelia. Proc Natl Acad Sci USA 2004; 101:2064–2069.
30. Hotchkiss SAM. Skin as a xenobiotic metabolising organ. Prog Drug Metabol 1992; 13:218–253.
31. Chen D, Haviland-Jones J. Rapid mood change and human odors. Physiol Behav 1999; 68(1–2):241–250.
32. Andersson S, Bishhop RW, Russell DW. Expression cloning and regulation of steroid 5α-reductase, an enzyme essential for male sexual differentiation. J Biol Chem 1989; 264:16249–16255.
33. Blauer M, Vaalasti A, Pauli SL, Ylikomi T, Joensuu T, Tuohimaa P. Location of androgen receptor in human skin. J Invest Dermatol 1991; 97(2):264–268.
34. Choudhry R, Hodgins MB, Van der Kwast TH, Brinkmann AO, Boersma WJ. Localization of androgen receptors in human skin by immunohistochemistry: implications for the hormonal regulation of hair growth, sebaceous glands, and sweat glands. J Endocrinol 1992; 133(3):467–475.
35. Li W, Liu M. Method and composition for preventing sweat-related odor. United States Patent 6,426,061. 2002.
36. Gower DB, Mallet AI, Watkins WJ, Wallace LM, Calame J-P. Capillary gas chromatography with chemical ionisation negative ion mass spectrometry in the identification of odorous steroids formed in metabolic studies of the sulphates of androsterone, DHA and 5α-androst-16-en-3β-ol with human axillary bacterial isolates. J Steroid Biochem Molec Biol 1997; 63:81–89.
37. Austin C, Ellis J. Microbial pathways leading to steroidal malodour in the axilla. J Steroid Biochem Molec Biol 2003; 87:105–110.
38. Foebe C, Simone A, Charig A, Eigen E. Axillary malodour production a new mechanism. J Soc Cosmet Chem 1990; 41:173–185.
39. Eigen E, Froebe C. Deodorant compositions comprising inhibitors of odour producing axillary bacterial enzymes. United States Patent 5,676,937. 1997.
40. James AG, Casey J, Hylands D, Johnston H, Mycock G. Generation and tunover of volatile fatty acids by axillary bacteria. 22nd IFSCC Congress Edinburgh, 2002.
41. Zeng X-N, Leyden JJ, Brand J, Spielman AI, McGinley K, Preti G. An investigation of human apocrine gland secretion for axillary odor precursors. J Chem Ecol 1992; 18:1039–1055.
42. Spielman A, Zeng X-N, Leyden JJ, Preti G. Proteinaceous precurors of human axillary odor: isolation of two novel odor-binding proteins. Experimentia 1995; 51:40–47.

43. Zeng X-N, Spielman A, Vowels BR, Leyden JJ, Biemann K, Preti G. A human axillary odourant is carried by apolipoprotein. Proc Natl Acad Sci USA 1996; 93:6626–6630.
44. Spielman, et al. Identification and immunohistochemical localisation of protein precursors to human axillary odors in apocrine glands and secretions. Arch Dermatol 1998; 134:813–818.
45. Natsch A, Gfeller H, Gygax P, Schmid J, Acuna G. A specific bacterial aminoacylase cleaves odorant precursors secreted in the human axilla. J Biol Chem 2003; 278:5718–5727.
46. Natsch A, Acuna G, Fournie-Zaluski M-C, Gfeller H. Compounds and methods for inhibiting axillary malodour. International Patent N° WO 02/092024 A2. 2002.
47. Lyon S, O'Neal C, Van Der Lee H, Rogers B. Amino acid beta lyase enzyme inhibitors as deodorants. International Patent No WO 91/05541, 1991.
48. Forestier S, Courbiere C. Deodorant cosmetic composition. International Patent No. WO 00/33787. 2000.
49. Brockett S, O'Neal C,Van der Lee H, Rogers B. Amino acid beta-lyase enzyme inhibitors as deodorants. United States Patent 5,595,728. 1997.
50. Acuna G, Georg F, Urech P. Malodour preventing agents. European Patent Application EP 0 815 833, 1998.
51. Preti G, Spielman AI, Zeng X-N, Leyden JJ, Leftheris K, McGinley K. Inhibition of odor formation and bacterial growth. International Patent N° WO 93/07853. 1993.
52. Ikemoto T, Okabe B-I, Minura K, Kitahara T. Formation of fragrance materials from odourless glycosidically-bound volatiles by skin microflora (Part I). Flavour Fragr J 2002; 17:452–455.
53. Ikemoto T, Minura K, Kitahara T. Formation of fragrance materials from odourless glycosidically-bound volatiles by skin microflora (Part II). Flavour Fragr J 2002; 17:45–47.
54. Cork A, Park KC. Identification of electophysiologically-active compounds for the malaria mosquito, Anopheles gambiae, in human sweat extracts. Med Vet Entomol 1996; 10:269–276.
55. Rodrigues-Conception M, Boronat A. Elucidation of the Methylerythritol Phosphate Pathway for Isoprenoid Biosynthesis in Bacteria and Plastids. A Metabolic Milestone Achieved Through Genomics. Plant Physiol 2002; 130:1079–1089.
56. Lange MB, Ghassemian M. Genome organization in Arabidopsis thaliana: a survey for genes involved in isoprenoid and chlorophyll metabolism. Plant Mol Boil 2003; 51:925–948.
57. Bohlmann J, Meyer-Gauen G, Croteau R. Plant terpenoid synthases: molecular biology and phylogenetic analysis. Proc Natl Acad Sci USA 1998; 95:4126–4133.
58. Lesburg CA, Zhai G, Cane DE, Christianson DW. Crystal structure of pentalenene synthase: mechanistic insights on terpenoid cyclization reactions in biology. Science 1997; 277:1820–1824.
59. Starks CM, Back K, Chappell J, Noel JP. Structural basis for cyclic terpene biosynthesis by tobacco 5-epi-aristolochene synthase. Science 1997; 277:1815–1820.
60. Caruthers JM, Kang I, Rynkiewicz MJ, Cane DE, Christianson DW. Crystal structure determination of aristolochene synthase from the blue cheese mold, Penicillium roqueforti. J Biol Chem 2000; 275:25533–25539.

61. Rynkiewicz MJ, Cane DE, Christianson DW. Structure of trichodiene synthase from *Fusarium sporotrichioides* provides mechanistic inferences on the terpene cyclization cascade. Proc Natl Acad Sci USA 2001; 98:13543–13548.
62. Whittington DA, Wise ML, Urbansky M, Coates RM, Croteau RB, Christianson DW. Bornyl diphosphate synthase: structure and strategy for carbocation manipulation by a terpenoid cyclase. Proc Natl Acad Sci USA 2002; 99:15375–15380.
63. Back K, Chappell J. Identifying functional domains within terpene cyclases using a domain-swapping strategy. Proc Natl Acad Sci USA 1996; 93:6841–6845.
64. El Tamer MK, Lucker J, Bosch D, Verhoeven HA, Verstappen FW, Schwab W, van Tunen AJ, Voragen AG, de Maagd RA, Bouwmeester HJ. Domain swapping of Citrus limon monoterpene synthases: impact on enzymatic activity and product specificity. Arch Biochem Biophys 2003; 411:196–203.
65. Little DB, Croteau RB. Alteration of product formation by directed mutagenesis and truncation of the multiple-product sesquiterpene synthases delta-selinene synthase and gamma-humulene synthase. Arch Biochem Biophys 2002; 402:120–135.
66. Mahmoud SS, Croteau RB. Metabolic engineering of essential oil yield and composition in mint by altering expression of deoxyxylulose phosphate reductoisomerase and menthofuran synthase. Proc Natl Acad Sci USA 2001; 98:8915–8920.
67. Hohn TM, Ohlrogge JB. Expression of a fungal sesquiterpene cyclase gene in transgenic tobacco. Plant Physiol 1991; 97:460–462.
68. Zook M, Hohn T, Bonnen A, Tsuji J, Hammerschmidt R. Characterization of Novel Sesquiterpenoid Biosynthesis in Tobacco Expressing a Fungal Sesquiterpene Synthase. Plant Physiol 1996; 112:311–318.
69. Lucker J, Schwab W, van Hautum B, Blaas J, van der Plas LH, Bouwmeester HJ, Verhoeven HA. Increased and altered fragrance of tobacco plants after metabolic engineering using three monoterpene synthases from lemon. Plant Physiol 2004; 134:510–519.
70. Lewinsohn E, Schalechet F, Wilkinson J, Matsui K, Tadmor Y, Nam K-H, Amar O, Lastochkin E, Larkov O, Ravid U, et al. Enhanced levels of the aroma and flavor compound S-linalool by metabolic engineering of the terpenoid pathway in tomato fruits. Plant Physiol 2001; 127:1256–1265.
71. Martin VJ, Pitera DJ, Withers ST, Newman JD, Keasling JD. Engineering a mevalonate pathway in Escherichia coli for production of terpenoids. Nat Biotechnol 2003; 21:796–802.
72. Martin VJ, Yoshikuni Y, Keasling JD. The in vivo synthesis of plant sesquiterpenes by Escherichia coli. Biotechnol Bioeng 2001; 75:497–503.
73. Carter OA, Peters RJ, Croteau R. Monoterpene biosynthesis pathway construction in *Escherichia coli*. Pytochemistry 2003; 64:425–433.
74. Jackson BE, Hart-Wells EA, Matsuda SPT. Metabolic engineering to produce sesquiterpenes in yeast. Org Lett 2003; 5:1629–1632.
75. Schoenbeck M, Chappell J. Engineering isoprenoid metabolism and biochemistry in plants. In recent adv Photochem 2001; 35:171–203.
76. Haudenschild C, Croteau RB. Molecular engineering of monoterpene production. Genet Eng 1998; 20:267–280.
77. Lange MB, Croteau R. Genetic engineering of essential oil production in mint. Curr Opin Plant Biol 1999; 2:139–144.

15

Safety and Regulatory Perspectives

Helmut Greim

Technical University of Munich, Institute of Toxicology and Environmental Hygiene, Freising-Weihenstephan, Germany

INTRODUCTION

Products for personal care are unique in that there is direct and long-term human dermal and possibly inhalation exposure. The specific aspect of ingredients that are produced by using recombinant organisms is that they comprise peptides, proteins, and enzymes. According to a few reports, the major concern of human exposure seems to be sensitization after long-term dermal contact or exposure via inhalation. Basically, the same criteria as those for other chemicals apply for hazard identification and risk assessment, and consumer and workplace exposure. Because there are no specific regulations for personal care products obtained from recombinant organisms, it is the aim of this chapter to evaluate which data are necessary for hazard identification and risk assessment and to conclude which experimental and human studies are considered necessary for risk assessment and regulation of such materials. This chapter provides a toxicologist's view on the safety assessment of such material.

GENERAL CONSIDERATIONS FOR HAZARD IDENTIFICATION AND RISK ASSESSMENT

All chemicals and proteins have the intrinsic potential to induce adverse effects, such as irritation, inflammation, sensitization, genotoxicity, or carcinogenicity. The potencies necessary to induce these effects vary widely among the different substances. However, according to Paracelsus's paradigm "all things are poisons except the dose makes that a thing is not a poison." Toxicological risk assessment has to consider the intrinsic toxic (hazardous) properties of an agent and the dose response of the toxic effects to identify the no-observed-effect level (NOEL) and the extent of human exposure. Consequently, risk characterization comprises the following elements:

> Hazard identification describing the intrinsic toxic potential, including toxicokinetics, toxic mechanisms, and identification of the most sensitive target,
>
> Dose response, including the information about the NOEL of the most sensitive effect and the extent by which the effects increase with increasing exposure,
>
> Exposure assessment evaluating duration and concentration of exposure,

Risk characterization describing the difference between human exposure and the NOEL or, in case of nonthreshold carcinogenesis, the risk at a given exposure.

As the dose makes the poison, effects are not to be expected when human exposure does not exceed the NOEL, provided that mechanistic information permits assumption of a NOEL. In case of primary genotoxicity in association with carcinogenicity, mechanistic consideration does not allow definition of a NOEL because any exposure is associated with a specific risk. In such cases, the risk at a certain human exposure level needs to be quantified from dose-response information, either from epidemiological data or from animal studies and their extrapolation to humans. Similarly, it is difficult to identify a NOEL for sensitizing agents unless precise data are obtained from studies in humans. In contrast to the NOEL, the term threshold describes any point at the dose-response curve where the slope changes. This may be a steep increase when inactivating mechanisms become overwhelmed or a reduced slope when activating mechanisms are saturated: In spite of increasing doses the amount of toxic reactants formed from the parent compound does not increase.

INFORMATION REQUIRED FOR RISK ASSESSMENT

Hazard Identification

Intrinsic (Hazardous) Properties

Compounds exert a large variety of toxic effects. Acids or alkaline agents induce local effects, for example, corrosions or irritation at the area of exposure. Most chemicals induce specific systemic effects, for example, hepatotoxicity, neurotoxicity, embryotoxicity, or they are sensitizers, mutagens, or carcinogens. Depending on route, concentration, and time of exposure, acute or chronic effects may result. Acute effects usually occur after accidental or deliberate high exposures. Chronic effects in humans are seen after continuous exposure to compounds that accumulate at the critical target or after short-term high exposure resulting in persistent damage due to slow elimination. In laboratory animals and humans, 2,3,7,8-tetrachlorodibenzo-p-dioxin (TCDD) induces tumors at various organs. Due to its high persistence, one sufficiently high accidental exposure can result in long-lasting body burden with the consequence of long-lasting effects leading to carcinogenicity.

Reactive metabolites of compounds interact with tissue components and induce cellular damage. The concentration of the compound or its reactive metabolite at the sensitive target over a given time ("target dose") is an important parameter to understand the relation between internal exposure and external exposure, the targets' response to toxic insults, and the toxic mechanisms involved.

Of utmost importance for risk assessment is the evaluation of whether the toxic effects are reversible. When effects are repaired during and after exposure and disappear after cessation of exposure, a NOEL can be defined. If damage is not sufficiently repaired, the effect persists and accumulates upon repeated exposure. In such cases a NOEL cannot be determined. Reversibility depends on the regenerative capacity of cells, subcellular structures and macromolecules, and the lifetime of the cells.

Primary genotoxic mutagens and carcinogens (or their metabolites) that interact with the DNA are considered irreversible. There is increasing knowledge about DNA repair mechanisms, the function of tumor-suppressor genes, and apoptosis, which repair or eliminate genetically damaged cells. However, the effectiveness and the dose response are not sufficiently understood to conclude whether NOELs can be determined for genotoxic effects. There is still the paradigm that in case of primary genotoxicity a linear increase of carcinogenic potency with increasing dose has to be anticipated. The dose response may show a threshold that is a deviation from linearity, for example, when inactivating mechanisms become overwhelmed and the slope steeply increases or the slope decreases when activating mechanisms are saturated: In spite of increasing doses the amount of toxic reactants formed from the parent compound does not further increase. (For dose response and NOEL of sensitizing agents, see the section on Exposure Assessment.)

Toxicokinetics

Information on toxicokinetics is relevant, especially for accumulating compounds with relatively long half-lives of elimination, to define the internal exposure at which no effects are observed under steady state conditions.

Toxicokinetics of a compound comprise uptake, distribution, degradation, and excretion. After entering the organism the compound or its degradation products (metabolites) distribute to the target organs, where they can accumulate, for example, in fat or bones, or be further degraded and eliminated. The toxic potential and the intensity of effects (potency) are determined by the concentration of the compound or its toxic degradation product at the critical target (internal or target dose). The latter is affected by several parameters: the external dose (concentration of the compound, e.g., in air), duration and route of external exposure, rates of degradation and elimination, the dose response, and the susceptibility of the exposed. TCDD is lipophilic and accumulates in fat tissue. According to general toxicokinetic principles, steady state concentrations at the target organ are reached after four half-lives. TCCD is poorly metabolized, being very slowly eliminated in humans with a half-life of about eight years. Consequently, the TCDD contamination of food results in a continuous increase of TCDD concentrations in human fat tissues over at least 32 years. Similarly, man-made mineral fibers accumulate in the lung due to their relatively high half-lives of weeks to months.

Due to its lipophilic and poorly perfused structure the skin retains chemicals and releases them to the body compartments for a certain time, even when dermal exposure has ended. Previously, this skin reservoir had been considered as a relatively stable compartment. However, kinetic considerations indicate that the reservoir is in a dynamic equilibrium with other compartments of the body. As indicated in Figure 1, several parameters, such as evaporation, desquamation, metabolism, and skin perfusion, affect this equilibrium. Considering the different kinetics of parameters given in Figure 1, several authors

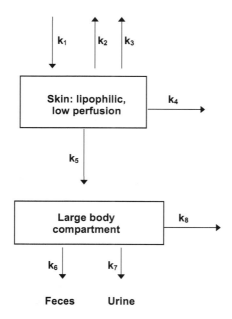

k_1: Dermal uptake k_2: Evaporation
k_3: Desquamation k_4: Skin metabolism
k_5: Uptake into blood k_6: Excretion via feces
k_7: Excretion via urine k_8: Metabolism/degradation

Figure 1   Pharmacokinetic considerations of skin penetration and parameters that determine uptake through the skin.

concluded that lipid solubility of a compound is the rate-limiting factor that determines skin penetration, whereas others contribute less to the process. Consequently, information from such simple tests as the octanol/water distribution coefficient permits estimation of the skin penetration rate using available toxicokinetic models (1).

Dose Response of Effects

Occurrence and intensity of toxic effects are dose dependent, which has already been described by Paracelsus (1493–1541). His paradigm addresses the concept of threshold effects, which implies information of the dose response of the effects.

Animal or human exposure is usually defined by mg of the chemical/kg body weight per day or in the case of inhaled material by mg/m^3. This external exposure leads to a specific internal dose, which depends on the amount absorbed via the different routes or deposited on the skin or in the lung. Absorption rates via the different routes can vary significantly, although oral exposure and inhalation usually lead to higher internal exposure than dermal exposure. Exposure results in specific target doses, which are the concentrations at the critical targets over a given time.

The dose responses of the external and internal exposure (target dose) define the toxic potency of a compound and the NOEL. Consequently, no effects will be seen if the dose is below the NOEL. Usually the dose response curves are of sigmoid shape, but the slopes may vary significantly, resulting in different increases in the intensity of effects when the dose increases.

Of utmost importance is the understanding of the pharmacokinetics of a compound to evaluate whether there is accumulation during repeated exposure or a steady state concentration is reached during repeated exposure. When elimination is rapid with a half-life of hours or a few days, the steady state concentration in the animal organism will be reached within a short-term exposure study. Prolonged exposure will not result in further increases of the target doses.

Exposure Assessment

Exposure defines the amount of a chemical to which a population or specific individuals are exposed via inhalation, oral, and dermal routes. Animal or human exposure is commonly defined by mg of the chemical/kg body weight per day. For estimation of the exposure of consumers to personal cleansing products, sufficient data on frequency, duration and site of product use, concentration and weight of substance in the product, and the amount of product used per contact surface needs to be available. Otherwise unrealistically high exposure data will result from application of conservative exposure estimates.

Risk Assessment

To evaluate the risk of a substance for human health, the exposure levels to which the consumer is exposed are compared with the exposure levels or concentrations at which no toxic effects have been found to occur. The latter should be the NOEL of the most sensitive targets or at least the lowest-observed-effect level (LOEL). By comparing the exposure level with the NOEL or LOEL the margin of safety can be defined. In the case of effects that do not permit identification of a NOEL, such as carcinogenicity of genotoxic agents, the risk, for example, incidence per number of exposed persons, can be determined. This usually requires extrapolation from animals to humans and from high- to low-dose exposure when results from animal experiments have to be used.

POTENTIAL TOXICITY OF INGREDIENTS DERIVED FROM RECOMBINANT ORGANISMS

Ingredients that are produced by recombinant organisms comprise peptides, proteins, and enzymes. There is sufficient evidence that the most relevant adverse effect of proteins, such as enzymes, used in personal cleansing products is sensitization.

Originally, certain enzymes were identified as eliciting type I hypersensitivity responses (2). When enzyme powders containing the proteolytic enzymes subtilisins were incorporated into laundry detergents in the late 1960s, workers' exposure during detergent manufacturing resulted in immunoglobinE (IgE)-mediated hypersensitivity reactions (3,4). After appropriate measures were taken to reduce exposure during production, reports of adverse health effects and development of IgE antibodies in workers have been greatly reduced. Subtilisins are a group of proteolytic enzymes derived from *Bacillus subtilis*. These proteins are known primarily as dermal and respiratory tract irritants and have caused bronchoconstriction and respiratory allergies. Especially workers who manufactured a laundry detergent became sensitized, suffering from dyspnea associated at times with wheezing or other signs of respiratory obstruction. A survey of 121 workers exposed to subtilisin dusts revealed that sensitization as determined by skin patch tests was higher in atopic individuals than among workers considered normally sensitive (5).

Because of consideration to incorporate subtilisin into personal care products, Kelling et al. (6) evaluated the sensitizing potential for inhalation of the proteolytic enzyme during showering when it was present in a personal cleansing product. In addition, a clinical trial was conducted to determine whether the level, duration, and routes of exposure during the use of the product would induce a type I sensitization response. Exposure assessment revealed that airborne enzyme levels were primarily dependent on the concentration of the enzyme in the personal cleansing product. The mean values for total airborne enzyme protein during showering ranged from 5.7 to 11.8 ng/m^3, which is in the range of the Procter & Gamble occupational exposure guideline of 15 ng/m^3 but below the threshold limit value of 60 ng/m^3 (7). Concentrations in the room outside the shower were about 2.5-fold lower. After six months of using the product, four of the 61 test subjects had positive skin prick test responses when tested with the enzyme. Serological analyses detected IgE specific for the enzyme. None of the subjects showed any clinical symptoms indicative for allergic reaction. The finding resulted in the decision to halt further development of the product. The likelihood of both induction of an immunologic response and subsequent elicitation of allergy symptoms of the user population was considered high.

Another enzyme known to induce IgE-mediated disease is papain, a high molecular weight sulfhydryl protease obtained from the fruit of the papaya tree. Allergy has developed when this enzyme was used in such formulations as lens cleaning solutions that came in close contact with mucous membranes (8,9). A cosmetologist who handled papain powder in cosmetics also developed an allergy (10).

These examples show that the major routes of exposure are the skin, mucous membranes, and the lung via inhalation and that evaluation of sensitizing potential of these products is of high priority for identification of intrinsic toxic properties.

STUDIES TO ASSESS THE POTENTIAL RISK OF BIOLOGICALLY DERIVED MATERIALS

Hazard Identification

Intrinsic (Hazardous) Properties

In general, the following studies should be considered:

Acute toxicity (dermal)
Irritation including phototoxicity
Sensitization including photosensitization
Repeated dose toxicity
Genotoxicity (carcinogenicity)
Toxicity for reproduction

Acute toxicity: The need to determine acute toxicity of chemicals that are considered for human exposure is obvious. It is necessary to describe toxic effects and symptoms of acute intoxication and to label as toxicants. As proteins derived from recombinant organisms are most likely of low toxicity and exposure is low, determination of acute toxicity does not add to the information required for risk assessment of such material.

Irritation including phototoxicity: Dermal irritation of compounds is evaluated by studies in animals and humans prior to testing for sensitization. These are usually performed by using a single occluded patch under the same conditions as applied when testing skin sensitization (11).

Phototoxicity and photoallergic reactions have to be expected when compounds show significant absorption in the ultraviolet range (290–400 nm). According to the test strategy for irritation, an additional patch site is irradiated immediately after application of the test substance or after patch removal. For details see Sams and Epstein (12) and Morikawa et al. (13). If lack of phototoxicity has been demonstrated by appropriately validated in vitro tests, such as uptake of Neutral Red by 3T3 cells (14), in vivo testing may not be necessary.

Sensitizing potential including photosensitization: Due to the inherent sensitizing potential of proteins, special emphasis should be given to evaluating the sensitizing potential. For detection of the sensitizing potential of products obtained from recombinant organisms, the choice of a relevant animal is crucial. However, in many cases animal models may be inappropriate for detection of a sensitizing potential so that several dermatologists prefer studies in humans. Christ (15) recommends studies with nonhuman primate species, such as cynomolgus or rhesus monkeys, as an acceptable alternative because at least human proteins might have cross-reactivity in such species. Christ also recommends detection of antibodies in the serum during the studies using specific enzyme-linked immunosorbent assay (ELISA) methods or bioassays to measure neutralizing antibodies.

Animal test methods. Generally, the Buehler guinea pig test and the mouse local lymph node assay are used in the preclinical testing program (16–18). From the guinea pig tests the Research Institute for Fragrance Materials selected a modified Buehler technique that is assumed not to overestimate the potency of weak, mild, and moderate human sensitizers (17). This test includes 20 guinea pigs in the test group and 10 control animals, including naïve and vehicle controls. Applications to the skin are made via 25 mm Hill Top Chambers® throughout the study. The induction phase consists of three 6-hour induction occluded applications for three weeks, using the minimum irritating concentration of one application per week. To identify a NOEL, the challenge applications are made after a 2-week rest period at three different concentrations, the maximal nonirritating concentration as well as 0.3% and 0.1% of this concentration. Rechallenges are conducted as needed on naïve sites.

Procter & Gamble uses the mouse local lymph node assay as first choice for preclinical assessment of new ingredients (16). For details of the test see Basketter et al. (19). According to Gerberick and Robinson (16) this test provides an objective endpoint, requires less time for completion with approximately half the number of animals, and is less costly than most currently used guinea pig assays. So far the test has been successfully applied to determine relative potencies of contact allergens and has been reported to closely correlate with NOELs established from human repeat patch testing (20).

Due to low skin penetration of proteins and possible hydrolysis, tests that use topical application may not be suitable to detect sensitizing effects of proteins. Recently, the popliteal lymph node assay (PLNA) received considerable attention because it is the only reliable test for screening compounds that cause sensitization via routes other than the skin. Instead of being applied topically, the test substance is injected subcutaneously into one hind footpad of mice or rats. Usually six days after treatment, the draining (popliteal) lymph node is isolated and analyzed for weight and cellularity and compared with the corresponding parameters of the untreated contralateral lymph node. For details and criticism see Descotes (21) and Tuschl et al. (22), who also discuss the disadvantage of false positive results induced by irritants. So far, the PLNA has not been applied for proteins particularly enzymes. Subcutaneous rather than topical application may be better suited to detect sensitizing potential of proteins, so that this test should be evaluated for its sensitivity in screening for sensitizing proteins.

Human test methods. When the animal data indicate a weak contact sensitizing potential, human skin sensitizing testing is conducted usually by a human repeated-insult patch test (HRIPT) (16–18). For testing chemicals Api (17) recommends that in case of negative animal data a ten-fold higher than the average maximum use level should be applied. When the compound is found positive in animal testing a ten-fold lower concentration should be applied. (16,17). The NOEL of the contact sensitizing potential can be identified by applying several concentrations of the test compound.

On the other hand, the report by Kelling et al. (6) indicates that the commonly applied assays in humans may not be sufficiently sensitive to detect the sensitizing potential of a protein. Positive prick test responses to the protease enzyme were observed in four out of 61 healthy volunteers who used the shower bath product containing a proteolytic enzyme after only six months of continuous use. None of these subjects developed clinical symptoms indicative of allergic reactions.

Unfortunately, a "diagnostic" HRIPT was used to exclude a contact dermatitis in a person who developed dermatitis approximately two months after the start of the study. Results from other participants who may have been tested are not provided. Serological analysis of the four subjects with positive prick tests detected IgE specific for the enzyme.

The late responses to enzyme exposure may be due to the relatively low airborne exposure of 5.7 to 11.8 ng/m^3 during showering; there were no dermal reactions in these subjects. Therefore the authors concluded that sensitization was the result of inhalation and/or mucous membrane exposure rather than dermal exposure.

The publication does not provide information whether higher exposure to the enzyme would have resulted in earlier appearance of positive prick tests, nor is there information whether the regular HRIPT using tenfold the estimated use levels was positive. However, Greenberg et al. (5) did find positive patch tests in subjects sensitized to subtilisins who had developed allergic respiratory illness after exposures to dusts. This permits the conclusion that patch testing may not only detect contact allergens but respiratory allergens as well. The study also demonstrates the need to confirm information from preclinical testing by an appropriate clinical study, which should cover months of low exposure.

Repeated dose toxicity: The specific use patterns of personal care products imply that the major routes of exposure are skin, mucous membranes, or the lung via inhalation. Considering this, the necessary preclinical studies should be preferentially performed by dermal exposure, and if the product might be inhaled, for example, as an ingredient of a shower bath formulation, an inhalation study becomes necessary.

Although it seems obvious that repeated dose toxicity tests should be performed preferentially via dermal exposure, there is no final conclusion which route should be used to obtain optimal information on the long-term effects of a material preferentially used for personal care products applied to the skin. Whereas the dermal route represents the most common exposure in humans, animal studies via dermal application may not provide sufficient information on all endpoints, especially when the test compound is poorly absorbed through the skin (18). The oral route provides more reliable information on all endpoints, although it may overestimate the hazard. In such cases subacute studies (28 days repeated exposure) or subchronic studies (90 days) via oral application should be supplemented by dermal absorption studies. In case of low-toxicity and low-dermal absorption, no further repeated dose studies are required. In case of high toxicity and relevant dermal absorption, the test program should be extended to include chronic and reproduction toxicity studies. The decision concerning which route of exposure to choose for the repeated dose studies can only be made on the basis of a careful case-by-case evaluation of all available information. If there is evidence of systemic toxicity, then an oral study is indicated. If human exposure is exclusively via the skin, then a dermal repeated dose study is more appropriate for proteins, especially when there is indication of irritation. The study should provide a NOEL for irritation during long-term exposure.

Genotoxicity (carcinogenicity):   Although proteins are unlikely to be genotoxic, there are arguments that they might contain mutagenic impurities so that genotoxicity testing will be required for these products for the time being. Special considerations for conducting genotoxicity tests with protein materials have been discussed by Kirkland and Kim (23). In vitro tests to detect mutagenicity in bacteria and chromosomal aberrations in mammalian cells demand special approaches to produce acceptable results. The potential adsorption of the protein to glass and plastics has to be considered as well as degradation of the protein by the medium, for example, serum proteases. As an in vivo test model, the mouse bone marrow micronucleus test is preferred. It is the best validated, most widely used test system; it detects aneugens as well as clastogens, and the test protein is likely to circulate freely in the blood. It will reach the bone marrow as well as the liver and other organs where it might be degraded. The latter will lead to relatively short half-lives so that determination of the area under the plasma concentration curve might be needed to provide an adequate exposure. This will also allow better comparison of the dose response in the animal as compared to man.

Toxicity for reproduction and development: Studies to evaluate reproductive and developmental effects may be needed only if there is indication that the protein is absorbed and becomes systemically available. In such cases either a reproduction/developmental toxicity screening test (OECD 421), the combined repeated dose toxicity study with the reproduction/developmental toxicity screening test (OECD 422), or the appropriate standard tests to evaluate effects on reproduction (One-generation reproduction toxicity, OECD 415) and prenatal developmental (OECD 414) should be selected. For further details, advantages, and disadvantages of the tests, see Reuter et al. (24).

EXPOSURE ASSESSMENT

Precise data on exposure to a fragrance ingredient is essential for the safety evaluation process (18). This requires information on the extent of workplace exposure, the concentration of the compound in the consumer product, the amount of product applied or used daily, and the amount washed off or retained on the skin. These data allow estimation of daily dermal exposure for comparison with amounts that induce dermal or systemic toxicity including sensitization. Assuming 100% transdermal penetration, such information also allows determination of the margin of exposure and the difference between systemic exposure and the NOEL of systemic effects.

Data for developing estimates of dermal and systemic exposures from different consumer products have been published by Ford et al. (25) and are given in Table 1.

Table 1 Calculation of Dermal and Systemic Exposures of a 60 kg Person to a Specific Fragrance Ingredient in Cosmetic Products

Type of product	Grams applied	Applications per day	Retention factor	Ingredient per product	Ingredient exposure (mg/day)	Systemic exposure (mg/kg per day)
Body lotion	8.00	0.71	1.00	0.004	27.7	0.38
Face cream	0.80	2.00	1.00	0.003	4.8	0.08
Eau de toilette	0.75	1.00	1.00	0.08	60	1.0
Fragrance cream	5.00	0.03	1.00	0.04	58	0.1
Antiperspirant	0.50	1.00	1.00	0.01	5.0	0.08
Shampoo	8.00	1.00	0.01	0.005	0.04	0.007
Bath products	17.00	0.29	0.001	0.02	0.01	0.0016
Shower gel	5.00	1.00	0.01	0.012	0.64	0.011
Toilet soap	0.80	6.00	0.01	0.015	0.72	0.012
Hair spray	5.00	2.00	0.01	0.005	0.5	0.008

Source: From Refs. 18, 26.

NO-OBSERVED-EFFECT LEVELS FOR SENSITIZERS?

There is general agreement that an exposure response relationship exists for occupational inhalation allergens. Although there are difficulties in identifying dose-response relationships because exposure is usually determined by measuring dust that may contain different levels of allergens, Baur et al. (26) state in their review on occupational allergens: "in general an increased exposure to dust is related to an increased level of allergens." For flour dust, they note that a number of investigators have found that dust concentrations of 1 to 2.4 mg/m^3 were associated with a significantly elevated risk of sensitization to wheat antigens. A similar conclusion for respiratory allergy in bakery workers has been drawn by Houba et al. (27). More recently, Kimber et al. (28) have discussed the theoretical and practical perspectives of thresholds for both the induction and elicitation of contact sensitization. The sensitizing chemical must penetrate into the viable layers of the epidermis and the various cells therein, where the chemical must react with carrier protein or peptide to form a complete antigen. Langerhans cells and cutaneous dendritic cells interact with and internalize the antigen, are mobilized, and travel via the afferent lymphatics to the draining lymph nodes. There the antigen is presented to T lymphocytes, which are activated, resulting in selective clonal expansion of allergen-specific T lymphocytes. This represents the cellular basis for the elicitation of more vigorous immune responses following subsequent exposure to the allergen. The differentiation and stimulation of T lymphocytes and the vigor of these responses is modulated by epidermal cytokines that are upregulated or induced by the chemical allergen and other forms of epidermal traumalike inflammation. It may be assumed that a certain level of local cytokine production is necessary to initiate the process of skin sensitization. These mechanistic considerations are supported by observations in experimental animals and in humans. Referring to the work of Friedmann (29), who demonstrated dose response and "thresholds" in the induction and elicitation by DNCB (2,4-dinitrochlorobenzene) in humans, Kimber et al. (28) conclude several important points:

- The induction of clinical skin sensitization by chemical allergens is dose dependent. Although the dose required for sensitization may vary between individuals, there are concentrations that do not induce relevant clinical sensitization.
- The critical determinant of exposure is the concentration of a chemical per unit area of skin, not the total dose delivered.
- At lower concentrations, contact allergens may provoke immune responses that are of insufficient magnitude to induce clinically detectable skin sensitization. If exposure is even below this level the individual would never become sensitized.

Two levels of thresholds exist for skin sensitizers: "The first is the amount of chemical, or more accurately, the dose of chemical per unit area of skin that is required to stimulate an immune response (which may result in sensitization). The second is the concentration of chemical that is necessary to induce clinically relevant skin sensitization such that subsequent challenge will provoke a dermatitic reaction."

Doubtlessly, these considerations are plausible and should be further evaluated. From a toxicological point of view special emphasis should be laid on the threshold versus NOEL concept and the inclusion of time in the definition of dose.

As indicated in section II the NOEL defines the highest dose without observable effects, which should not be compromised with the term threshold. It may well be that the mechanistic considerations described above justify assumption of a NOEL. However, they can also be interpreted as evidence for threshold effects. The relatively flat dose-response curve resulting from reaction of the allergen with carrier protein and presentation of the hapten to the draining lymph nodes steeply increases when additional stimulation-like irritation enhances this process.

Defining dose exposure as concentration of a chemical per unit area of skin is of great advantage and may allow better comparison of the outcomes of different studies. However, as seen from the study of Kelling et al. (6), exposure to a proteolytic enzyme required six months of continuous use before there was indication for sensitization; higher doses may have shortened the time required. This is consistent with the toxicological definition of dose: exposure per time. This should also be applied for definition of exposure to sensitizing agents: concentration per unit of skin x time.

CONCLUSION

There are no regulations for the experimental approach to evaluate potentially adverse effects of ingredients in personal care products that are produced by using recombinant organisms. These ingredients are usually proteins (peptides or proteins with specific enzyme activities). Evaluation of the risks to human health when used in personal care products should consider extent and routes of human exposure to the well-defined material and the relevant toxic effects of such proteins. Thus, when establishing design of the study program to identify the hazards and risks of the material, one should consider the following aspects and if possible discuss them with the regulatory agency:

> The protein needs to be specified, including information on molecular weight, stability in the consumer product, and on the skin.
> To evaluate exposure concentration in the consumer product, routes of exposure and frequency and duration of intended use need to be known.

Due to the inherent sensitizing potential of proteins, special emphasis should be given to evaluate this adverse effect. One of the standard animal models using topical application may be used, although the results are debatable due to the poor skin penetration of proteins. A promising alternative is the PLNA because the test substance is injected subcutaneously into one footpad of mice or rats.

However, in many cases animal models may not be appropriate for detection of a sensitizing potential, so the outcome of animal studies should be verified by studies in humans. As an alternative, Christ (15) recommends studies with nonhuman primate species, such as cynomolgus or rhesus monkeys, because at least human proteins might have cross-reactivity in such species. Christ also recommends detection of antibodies in the serum during the studies using specific ELISA methods or bioassays to measure neutralizing antibodies.

Although there is no final conclusion whether low exposure to sensitizers do not induce allergic reactions at prolonged exposure, the dose response of effects should be accomplished and the apparent NOEL identified in all animal and human studies. This permits definition of the relative sensitizing potency of the material and identification of a "pragmatic" NOEL for use as a starting point to determine an acceptable concentration in a consumer product.

Special consideration should be given to the time of exposure. The study of Kelling et al. (6) revealed that repeated but short-term, very low inhalation exposures and dermal exposures resulted in elevated indicators for sensitization after six months of exposure only. Therefore, in addition to the amount of a material per unit area of skin, definition of dose should include time of exposure (concentration per unit skin area x time of exposure). Because irritation might enhance the induction of allergy, evaluation of the potential for irritation, its dose response, and identification of the NOEL are essential to define the acceptable concentration of a material in the consumer product by using an appropriate safety factor.

The need for 28- or 90-day repeated-dose studies in rodents, usually rats, depends on the evaluation of all available information (18). As indicated earlier, the route of exposure depends on the intended use of the material and the likelihood of systemic effects. For proteins dermal application might be preferable to define a long-term irritation NOEL in a 28-day study and other potential topical or systemic effects. Studies to determine developmental and reproduction toxicity seem to be unnecessary for proteins assuming that bioavailability of the protein after oral or topical application is low or absent. They might become necessary if there is the (unlikely) indication that the protein degrades into toxic derivatives.

REFERENCES

1. Pirot F, Kalia YN, Stinchcomb AL, Keating G, Bunge A, Guy RH. Characterization of the permeability barrier of human skin in vitro. Proc Natl Acad Sci 1997; 94: 1562–1567.
2. Gutman AA. Allergens and other factors important in apoptotic disease. In: Patterson R, ed. Allergic Diseases, Diagnosis and Management. Philadelphia, PA: Lippincott, 1985:123–175.
3. Filndt MLH. Pulmonary disease due to inhalation of derivatives of Bacillus subtilis containing proteolytic enzyme. Lancet 1969; 1:1177–1181.

4. Pepys J, Longbottom JL, Hargreave FE, Faux J. Allergic reactions of the lungs to enzymes of Bacillus subtilis. Lancet 1969; 1:1181–1184.
5. Greenberg M, Milne JF, Watt A. Survey of workers exposed to dusts containing derivatives of Bacillus subtilis. Br Med J 1970; 2:629–633.
6. Kelling CK, Bartolo RG, Ertel KD, Smith LA, Watson DD, Sarlo K. Safety assessment of enzyme-containing personal cleansing products: exposure characterization and development of IgE antibody to enzymes after a 6-month use test. J Allergy Clin Immunol 1998; 101:179–187.
7. American Conference of Governmental Industrial Hygienists. (ACGIH) Threshold limit values for chemical substances and physical agents & biological exposure indices (TLVs and BEIs) 2004. See also Documentations. www.acgih.org
8. Bernstein DI, Gallagher JS, Grad M, Bernstein IL. Local ocular anaphylaxis to papain enzyme contained in a contact lens cleansing solution. J Allergy Clin Immunol 1984; 74:258–260.
9. Fisher AA. Allergic reactions to contact lens solutions. Cutis 1985; 36:209–211.
10. Ninimaki A, Reijula K, Pirila T, Koistinen AM. Papain-induced rhino-conjunctivitis in a cosmetologist. J Allergy Clin Immunol 1992; 92:492–493.
11. Kligman AM, Epstein W. Updating the maximization test for identifying contact allergens. Contact Dermatitis 1975; 1:231–239.
12. Sams Jr NM, Epstein JH. Experimental production of drug phototoxicity in guinea pigs, using sunlight. J Invest Dermatol 1967; 48:89–94.
13. Morikawa F, Nakayama Y, Fukuda M, Hamano M, Yokoyama Y, Ishihara M, Toda K. Techniques for the evaluation of phototoxicity and photoallergy in laboratory animals and man. In: Fitzpatrick TB, Pathak MA, Harber LC, Seiji M, Kukita A, eds. Sunlight and Man. Normal and Abnormal Photobiologic Responses. Tokyo: University Tokyo Press, 1974:529–557.
14. Spielmann H, Balls M, Dupuis J, Pape WJ, Pechovity G, DeSilva O, Holzhutter HG, Clothier R, Desole P, Gerberick F, et al. The international EU/COLIPA in vitro phototoxicity validation study: results of phase II (Blind Trial). Part 1. The 3T3 phototoxicity test. Toxicol In Vitro 1998; 12:305–327.
15. Christ M. Preclinical safety evaluation strategies of gene transfer products: regulatory and technical considerations. Comp Clin Path 2002; 11:38–43.
16. Gerberick GF, Robinson MK. A skin sensitization risk assessment approach for the evaluation of new ingredients and products. Am J Cont Dermatol 2000; 11:65–73.
17. Api AM. Sensitization methodology and primary prevention of the Research Institute for Fragrance Materials. Dermatol 2002; 205:84–87.
18. Bickers D, Calow P, Greim H, Hanifin JM, Rogers AE, Saurat J-H, Sipes IG, Smith RL, Tagami H. The safety assessment of fragrance materials. Reg Toxicol Pharmacol 2003; 37:218–273.
19. Basketter DA, Blaikie L, Dearman RJ, Kimber I, Ryan CA, Gerberick GF, Harey R, Evans P, White IR, Rycroft RJG. Use of the local lymph node assay for the estimation of relative contact allergenic potency. Contact Dermatitis 2000; 42:344–348.
20. Gerberick GF, Robinson MK, Ryan CA, Dearman RJ, Kimber J, Basketter DA, Wright Z, Marks JG. Contact allergenic potency: correlation of human and local lymph node assay data. Am J Contact Dermatol 2001; 12:156–161.
21. Descotes J. The popliteal lymph node assay: a tool for studying the mechanisms of drug-induced autoimmune disorders. Toxicol Lett 1992; 64/65:101–107.

22. Tuschl H, Landsteiner H, Kovac R. Application of the popliteal lymph node assay in immunotoxicity testing: complementation of the direct popliteal lymph node assay with flow cytometric analysis. Toxicology 2002; 172:35–48.
23. Kirkland DJ, Kim NN. Special consideration for conducting genotoxicity tests with protein materials. Mutagenesis 1995; 10:393–398.
24. Reuter U, Hirsch-Heinrich B, Hellwig J, Hollum B, Welsch F. Evaluation of OECD screening tests 421 (reproduction/developmental toxicity screening test) and 422 (combined repeated dose toxicity study with the reproduction/developmental screening test). Regul Toxicol Pharmacol 2003; 38:17–26.
25. Ford RA, Domeyer B, Easterday O, Maier K, Middleton J. Criteria for development of a database for safety evaluation of fragrance ingredients. Regul Toxicol Pharmacol 2000; 31:155–181.
26. Baur X, Chen Z, Liebers V. Exposure-response relationships of occupational inhalative allergens. Clin Exp Allergy 1998; 28:537–544.
27. Houba R, Heederik D, Doekes G. Wheat sensitization and work-related symptoms in the baking industry are preventable: an epidemiologic study. Am J Respir Crit Care Med 1998; 158(5.1):1499–1503.
28. Kimber I, Gerberick GF, Basketter DA. Thresholds in contact sensitization: theoretical and practical considerations. Fd Chem Toxicol 1999; 37:553–560.
29. Friedmann PS. The immunology of allergic contact dermatitis: the DNCB story. Adv Dermatol 1990; 5:175–196.

16

Intellectual Property Perspective

Louis C. Paul

Louis C. Paul & Associates, PLLC, New York, New York, U.S.A.

INTRODUCTION

The pace of innovation in what some call a "mature" biotechnology industry, now in its third decade, shows no signs of slowing. Biotechnological advances are increasingly reflected in commercial products, including in the personal care sector. This rapid growth has forced an equally dramatic evolution in the patent law. Patents are now an essential feature of the biotech and high-tech landscape (1). The primary objective of this chapter is to provide a practical introduction to key concepts of U.S. patent law for scientists in the cosmetic and personal care industry.

Patents—What Are They?

Patents are often viewed, wrongly, as the right to market a product. Rather, patents give inventors (or their assignees) the right to exclude others from making, using, selling or offering for sale, or importing a patented invention in the United States without permission (i.e., a license) for the term of the patent. In other words, a patent confers a monopoly on an inventor. Patents are therefore sometimes described as acting as both a sword and shield. For newly filed patent applications, the monopoly is 20 years, beginning on the date the application is filed.

There are three types of patents. Utility patents are the most common in the field of cosmetics and personal care products. There are also design patents (i.e., for containers and applicators) as well as patents for certain types of plants that impact botanical and herbal products. This chapter, however, will focus on utility patents—those covering finished products, ingredients, processes for making finished products and ingredients, and methods for treating skin conditions or delivering active ingredients.

Patents are made up of several parts, the most important of which are the claims. It is the claim that provides the legal rights to exclude others. A patent claim comprises individual elements. Claim construction—how to read and understand a patent claim—will be treated in depth later. For purposes of this introduction, one point needs to be clear—each and every element in a patent claim is of critical importance. If at the time a patent application was filed, each and every element of a patent claim was publicly known (e.g., in a printed publication) or was in public use, the claim is not novel and should not be granted. Likewise, if a patent does issue, but a product, process, or method of use is missing a single element of a patent claim, a properly informed court should find no patent infringement.

Why Worry About Patents?

Patents have become increasingly important business documents in the personal care and biotech industry. Patents are more than a right to exclude. Patent rights are commercially valuable because they can be sold or licensed. In addition, "patented" and "patent pending" connote newer, better, or improved products; these labels have a strong impact on consumers—helping to keep existing customers and attracting new ones.

A company that chooses not to take patents seriously does so at its peril. Without patent protection, competitors are free to copy an unpatented idea. Worse still, another company can patent your idea and then sue both you and your customers for infringement of patent.

From a purely defensive standpoint, discovering another's "blocking patent" late in the product development lifecycle, but prior to actual launch, can result in losing months, possibly years, of R&D and marketing efforts. A company accused of patent infringement can become embroiled in years of costly patent infringement litigation, disrupting not only its operations but also that of its customers. A finding by a judge that patent infringement has occurred will result in a company being enjoined from selling its products for the life of the patent. Additionally, the infringer may be ordered to pay the patent holder up to three times the monetary damages.

Promoting Progress in Science

Patents are one of the very few monopolies permitted by U.S. law. The concept of patent rights goes back to the Constitution. The Founding Fathers recognized that a free market economy must also "promote progress in science and the useful arts by securing for limited times to authors and inventors the exclusive right to their respective writings and discoveries." From these broad principles, the U.S. patent laws are set out in statute (Title 35 of the U.S. Code) and implemented in regulations [Title 37 of the Code of Federal Regulations (CFR)] issued by the U.S. Department of Commerce, through the U.S. Patent and Trademark Office (USPTO). The ultimate arbiter of the meaning of these statutes and regulations are the federal courts.

INVENTORSHIP

Inventive Contribution

Under U.S. patent law, there is no requirement to produce a commercial product; instead an idea may be "reduced to practice" by one or more inventors filing for a patent application. In the United States (unlike, e.g., Europe), individuals, not companies, are the inventors on patents. Inventorship is of critical business importance because each inventor has an equal right to the issued patent. Each inventor has the right to manufacture or sell the claimed invention. Likewise, each inventor has the right to license others to manufacture or sell the claimed invention. In the personal care field, there is an emerging trend for companies to "outsource" R&D or formulation to consultants. These consultants often have inventive contribution. Indeed, in many instances, consultants are the only properly named inventors. For these reasons, care must be given to obtaining assignments from all properly listed inventors.

The statutory standards for inventorship in the United States are set out in Sections 102(f) and 102(g) of Title 35 of the U.S. Code. Section 102 (f) provides that a person shall be entitled to a patent unless he/she did not himself/herself invent the subject matter sought to be patented. In other words, only true inventors are entitled to receive patent rights. Section 102(g) provides that patents are awarded to the first person to invent, not the first to file a patent application. This is a defining feature of U.S. patent law, which distinguishes it from the majority of the industrialized world (e.g., Europe and Japan). More specifically, Section 102(g) is divided into two subsections. Section 102(g)(1) provides that a person shall be entitled to a patent unless an earlier invention date for the same invention is established in an interference. The second party to file a patent application may nonetheless obtain a patent over the party who was first to file if the second party can demonstrate an earlier date of invention or can demonstrate an earlier date of conception plus diligence in reducing the invention to practice. Section 102(g)(2) requires that an earlier invention was not suppressed, concealed, or abandoned. Inventorship disputes based on priority of invention are discussed later in this section.

Determining Joint Inventorship

The standard for inventorship is contribution to the subject matter of at least one patent claim. Given the complexities of biotechnology, it is common for teams to work on projects. Different researchers may work at different places, at different times, on different aspects of a project. The question thus becomes which team member or members are properly considered to be inventors.

There is no inventive contribution if a team member merely acted under direction or supervision of the person or persons who conceived of the idea to be patented. However, a team leader who maintains intellectual domination over the invention is properly considered an inventor. For purposes of U.S. patent law, intellectual domination is the power to adopt or reject the suggestions of employees or consultants.

As stated earlier, the sole legal criterion is contribution to at least one claim in the issued patent. If, for example, a researcher made a contribution to only one claim in a patent application that later was rejected by the Patent Office examiner and cancelled (see section "Patentability," for a discussion of the patent application process) that researcher would no longer be properly listed as an inventor. The following examples are illustrative and provide guidance on determining inventorship.

Inventorship Example 1—The marketing group of a finished goods company is looking for a new moisturizing eye cream that reduces the appearance of fine lines and wrinkles. The company has heard that short chain peptides are a hot topic among beauty editors and consumers and wants to include at least one such peptide. The company assigns a project leader who, in turn, hires a Ph.D. in biochemistry, specializing in short chain peptides. The project leader communicates the product concept to the biochemist but thereafter does nothing more than monitor progress, approve budgets, and arrange for clinical testing. The biochemist develops a prototype containing what is considered to be a novel short chain peptide. Under these facts, the biochemist and not the project leader would be the inventor.

Inventorship Example 2—The project leader on the same moisturizing eye cream reviews industry and scientific journal articles as well as trade literature from raw materials suppliers. The project leader arrives at the concept that the eye cream should upregulate the expression of five specific genes. With this idea in mind, the project leader contacts the Ph.D. biochemist. After considering the product concept, the biochemist suggests to the project leader that upregulating the expression of one of the selected genes could inhibit the expression of another gene known to be important in wound healing. The Ph.D. biochemist suggests instead upregulating the expression of a different gene that would not have the unintended effect on wound healing. The biochemist creates what is considered to be a novel pentapeptide.

The biochemist also notes that the peptide is somewhat easily denatured by synthetic surfactants commonly used in cosmetic emulsions. The project leader, in turn, retains a private label cosmetic formulator, explains the problem, and asks the formulator to develop an extremely mild topical delivery system based on natural (i.e., nonsynthetic) emulsifiers. The formulator develops what is considered to be a novel emulsion system.

A patent is later filed for a topical system comprising a novel pentapeptide for diminishing the appearance of fine lines and wrinkles and a natural emulsifier system that does not denature the polypeptide. As the project leader maintained intellectual domination over the final formulation and contributed the idea of four of the five peptides, the project leader is properly listed as an inventor. The Ph.D. biochemist's idea to change one peptide should be viewed as an inventive contribution. Likewise, the formulator's emulsifier system—which could be patentable in its own right—would properly be considered as an inventor. In order to secure the exclusive rights to market and sell the moisturizing eye cream, the finished goods company should have each of the listed inventors—its own employee (the project manager) as well as the two hired consultants (the Ph.D. biochemist and the private label formulator)—execute an assignment.

ANATOMY OF A PATENT

Before examining what is patentable, it is helpful to quickly review the anatomy of a patent. The parts of a U.S. patent application are set out in Table 1.

Specification

The Specification provides a description in "full, clear, concise, and exact terms [so] as to enable any person skilled in the art . . . to make and use . . ." the claimed invention. A nonprovisional patent must "conclude with a claim particularly pointing out and distinctly claiming the subject matter which the applicant regards as his invention or discovery."

The Background of Invention section contains a description of relevant information known to the applicants, including, for example, references to scientific articles and commercial products—so-called prior art. As this prior art is the background against which the patentability of the claimed invention will be judged, patent applicants commonly describe problems in the prior art that are solved by their invention. Relatedly, the background section often speaks in terms of how the invention meets a long-felt but as yet unmet need.

Table 1 Parts of a U.S. Patent

Title of invention	Summary of invention
Cross-reference to related applications	Brief description drawing(s)
Federally sponsored R&D	Detailed description of the invention
Background	Claim(s)
Drawing(s)	Abstract
Nucleotide and/or amino acid sequence	

Claims

As discussed in the introduction, claims—which alone create the legal right to exclude others—are of three general types (utility, design, and plant) and take one of two forms (independent or dependent). If there is more than one claim, the claims may be independent or dependent upon other claims in the Specification.

Dependent claims refer back to, and further limit, the subject matter of the independent claim on which they depend. They are construed to include all of the limitations of the independent claim incorporated by reference. Independent and dependent claims are best explained through examples. Three claims—one independent and two dependent—from a recently filed biotechnology patent application in the personal care field follow:

US Patent Application Serial No. 10/696,536 entitled "Compositions containing peptide copper complexes and metalloproteinase inhibitors and methods related thereto" and assigned to the ProCyte Corporation was published on July 15, 2004. Claim 1 is the broadest independent claim and reads as follows:

1. A composition comprising at least one peptide copper complex and at least one metalloproteinase inhibitor.

Claims 2 and 3, both of which are dependent on Claim 1, further limit the claimed metalloproteinase inhibitor:

2. The composition of Claim 1 wherein at least one metalloproteinase inhibitor is a matrix metalloproteinase inhibitor.
3. The composition of Claim 2 wherein the matrix metalloproteinase inhibitor is a naturally produced tissue inhibitor of metalloproteinase, a recombinant tissue inhibitor of metalloproteinase, or a mutant thereof.

Claims are typically drafted from broad to narrow, encompassing both a genus and a species in that genus, as well as preferred embodiments of the claimed invention. Another common feature of claims is the inclusion of ranges—for example, "from about 0.1% to about 5%" or "at least about 10%." The broadest claims are those written in the open-ended "comprising" format. In comprising claims, such as Claim 1 of the ProCyte patent example cited earlier, at least one copper peptide and at least one metalloproteinase inhibitor are required or are essential elements. Other elements, such as for example, a wound healing protein or a sunscreen, may also be present.

In contrast, "consisting of" claims are the narrowest claims. They are said to be written in a closed format that excludes unrecited elements, steps, or ingredients. There is, however, a middle ground between "comprising" and "consisting of"—"consisting essentially of." "Consisting essentially of" claims, which are common in biotech patents, must contain specified materials or steps. In addition, such claims cover unrecited materials or steps "that do not materially affect the basic and novel characteristics" of the claimed invention. An example of a "consisting essentially of" claim is discussed in the Section Patent Litigation, Litigation Case Study 3.

Sequence Listings

Biotech patents frequently disclose and claim amino acid and/or nucleotide sequences. The mandatory rules for the presentation of sequence data are set out in 37 CFR §§1.822 to 1.824. The sequence rules cover all unbranched nucleotide sequences with 10 or more bases and all unbranched, non-D (i.e., nondextrorotatory) amino acid sequences with four or more amino acids, provided that there are at least four "specifically defined" nucleotides or amino acids. The sequence rules apply to all sequences disclosed in a patent application, whether claimed or not. Compliance with these rules is required for most disclosures of sequence data in new applications filed on or after October 1, 1990.

37 CFR §1.821(e) further requires that the sequence listing be submitted in computer readable form. This is not only to enable the USPTO to enter the sequence into its databases (e.g., for prior art searching) but also to facilitate the electronic exchange of sequence data with the Japanese Patent Office and the European Patent Office. Sequences in pending, unpublished applications are maintained in a separate database; this maintains the confidentiality of the sequence until the patent application containing that information is published or matures into a patent.

Deposit of Biological Materials

Another unique aspect of biotech patent applications relates to the deposit of biological materials. As discussed in section *Enzo v. Gen-Probe*, page 398, a requirement for patentability is that the application provides a written description of the invention sufficient to enable a person skilled in the art to which the invention pertains to make and use the invention. Where the invention involves a biological material and words alone cannot sufficiently describe how to make and use the invention, deposit of biological material in a specified manner can satisfy this statutory requirement. The deposit rules are set out in 37 CFR §§1.801 to 1.809.

PATENTABILITY

Everything Under the Sun

What is patentable? Nearly 25 years ago, Chief Justice Warren Burger, in writing the majority opinion for the U.S. Supreme Court in the *Diamond v. Chakrabarty* case, answered the question "Everything under the sun made by man." The Court ruled that a genetically modified microorganism—more specifically *Pseudomonas bacterium* capable of breaking down crude oil spills—was patentable matter. The quoted language was a paraphrase of the legislative history of the Patent Act of 1952 (which recodified the original Patent Act of 1793 authored by Thomas Jefferson): "... Congress intended statutory subject matter to include 'anything under the sun that is made by man'." With this evidence of Congressional intent in mind, the Supreme Court ruled that Chakrabarty's discovery was "not nature's handiwork, but his own."

Prior to the Chakrabarty decision, an organism itself was not patentable. It was, however, possible to patent the use of an organism (e.g., use of bacteria to make antibiotics) as well as methods for making antibiotics (e.g., fermentation). The reach of Chakrabarty was expressly extended to plants in 1987 when the Patent and Trademark Office (PTO) issued a pronouncement that "non-naturally occurring, non-human, multicellular living organisms, including animals [are] patentable subject matter." Thus, "anything under the sun" meant all forms of life—except humans.

Novelty

By statute, in order for an invention to receive a patent and with it, freedom from competition for the life of the patent, the invention must be (*i*) useful, (*ii*) novel, and (*iii*) nonobvious. Utility is often not an issue; after all, why would someone take the trouble to patent a nonuseful idea? The heart of patent law is novelty.

Two statutory provisions deal with novelty—Sections 102(a) and (b) of Title 35 of the U.S. Code. Section 102 (a) is keyed to the inventive idea itself. An idea is not novel if it was known or used by another in the United States. An idea can be publicly known through journal articles, brochures, tradeshow displays, seminars, or conferences. However, information disclosed under a confidentiality agreement ("CDA") is not considered to be publicly known. It is for this reason that new technologies and products are often introduced commercially under a CDA.

In addition, an invention is not considered to be novel under Section 102 (a) if it has been patented or described in writing in the "prior art." Prior art, as the term suggests, is the body of knowledge that existed before the invention was conceived and reduced to practice. Prior art includes issued patents, published patent applications, journal articles, conference abstracts, trade brochures, advertisements, and even internet postings.

Section 102(b) defines novelty differently. An idea is not novel if 12 months earlier than the filing of a U.S. patent application the idea was claimed in an issued patent or published anywhere in any language. Also, an idea that was publicly used or embodied in a product sold in the United States is not novel for patentability purposes under 102(b).

Sections 102(a) and (b) differ in several respects; the most important, from a practical standpoint, is that a patent applicant can swear behind a 102(a) reference. In other words, the applicant can claim that the idea was conceived prior to the date of the 102(a) reference. In contrast, Section 102(b), which imposes a 12-month limit, is an absolute statutory bar. An inventor cannot swear behind a 102(b) reference and claim an early date of invention. It is for this reason that 102(b) prior art is relied upon by those questioning the novelty of an idea, for example, a Patent Office examiner when rejecting an application or the defendant in a patent infringement lawsuit.

In summary, Sections 102(a) and (b) require that a novel, patentable idea not be anticipated. Each and every element of a patent claim must not be disclosed within the four corners of a single prior art reference. If most, but not all, of the elements of the putatively patentable idea are disclosed in a single reference, the idea may still not be patentable due to obviousness.

Nonobviousness

In the personal care field, challenges to the novelty of ideas based on obviousness are far more common than anticipation. Under Section 103 of Title 35, an idea that would have been obvious to a person of ordinary skill in the art is not patentable when the teachings of one prior art reference are viewed in combination with the teachings of one (or more) different prior art references.

The person of ordinary skill in the art is the key player in the world of patents. This person is a legal fiction, not an expert, but a person of ordinary skill in a particular field with a solid foundational training and limitless access to relevant books and articles, in all languages. The person of ordinary skill is capable of understanding scientific and engineering principles applicable to the pertinent art. Pertinent does not necessarily mean within a precise field of science. For example, articles on molecular biology and genomics as well as polymer or organic chemistry would be pertinent to personal care inventions. It is through the eyes of this person that patent claims are read and understood and from this vantage point obviousness determinations are made.

Obviousness is judged at the time of invention, not in hindsight. It is based on two or more references that, when combined, disclose each and every element of the patent claim. The standard is not one that would have been obvious to try. Rather, there must have been a motivation or suggestion to combine the references. Motivation to combine references can come from the references themselves or the fund of knowledge of the person of ordinary skill in the art. One caveat—there must be no teaching away from the combination. That is to say, there must not be a statement or suggestion in an obviousness reference that a particular approach has not worked or is not likely to work.

To recap, an obviousness inquiry has three parts: (*i*) determining the level of ordinary skill in the art, (*ii*) identifying the scope and content of the prior art, and (*iii*) establishing a motivation to combine two or more prior art references.

Secondary Considerations Showing Nonobviousness

Obviousness, unlike anticipation, can be rebutted. When present, objective indicia of nonobviousness must be considered by the PTO when evaluating a patent application or by a court when hearing arguments that an allegedly accused patent claim is invalid as obvious.

An increasingly common and powerful way to demonstrate nonobviousness is to show unexpected results. Such results can be in terms of a new, unexpected property, the absence of an expected property, or the superiority of a property. For example, a claimed invention could be found unexpectedly and surprisingly to have better feel or stability, increased potency, decreased time for onset of action, so on. Evidence of unexpected results based on comparative testing is submitted in the form of an inventor's declaration.

Other objective indicia of nonobviousness include: (*i*) meeting a long-felt but unmet need or, put differently, failure of others to solve the problem that the inventor solved, (*ii*) skepticism voiced by experts, (*iii*) copying by others in the field, or (*iv*) commercial acquiescence in the form of licenses. For a claimed invention's commercial success to be given substantial weight, a nexus must be established between the merits of the claimed invention and the commercial success.

Prior Invention by Another

A distinguishing feature of the U.S. patent law is that the right to patent an idea belongs to the first to invent, not the first to file a patent application. Unlike most of the industrialized world, U.S. patent law does not base patent rights on who wins the race to the patent office. In the United States, first-to-file does not necessarily win. Section 102(g) of Title 35 of the U.S. Code provides that an idea is not patentable if another person invented the idea earlier. This statutory rule has three components—conception, diligence, and reduction to practice.

Date of invention is measured from conception—the flash of creative brilliance or, more commonly, the non-Eureka moment where a new and useful idea is first formed—through reduction to practice. As discussed earlier, an inventor need not necessarily make a working prototype to have reduced an idea to practice; filing a patent application is considered constructive reduction to practice.

Section 102(g) has a third requirement—diligence. In order to secure allowance of a patent or avoid infringement based on a 102 (g) prior invention, an inventor must have been diligent during the period from conception to reduction. For the cosmetic chemist, this means that from the time an inventor conceives of the novel, patentable idea, he or she must regularly work to refine the idea either by formulating a final prototype or by filing a patent application. Putting the back-of-the-envelope scribblings in the bottom of a pile for months or taking an extended break after work has begun (e.g., because of a shift in work priorities) will likely indicate lack of diligence.

The "first to invent" rule is easiest to understand with an example. As shown in Figure 1, X and Y both claim to have the same invention. In April 2000, X conceived of the idea. Although X worked diligently, X did not file for a patent until January 2002. In May 2001, Y came up with the same idea

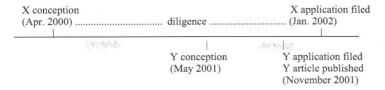

X conception   X application filed
(Apr. 2000) .... diligence .... (Jan. 2002)

                                    Y conception   Y application filed
                                    (May 2001)   Y article published
                                                            (November 2001)

Figure 1   First to invent.

and in November 2001 filed for a provisional patent application published an
the idea in a short communication to a scientific journal. Despite the fact that
Y's patent application was filed prior to X's—preceding it by two months—
if X can show diligence, X, not Y, should receive the patent. Likewise,
because Y's article was not published more than one year before X's application,
Y's article is not 102(b) prior art; X can swear behind it to establish an earlier date
of invention.

Resolving Inventorship Disputes—Interference

Inventorship disputes are heard in two different procedural settings. Section
102(g)(1) interferences are heard by a panel of three administrative patent
judges in the Board of Patent Appeals and Interferences in the USPTO.
Section 102(g)(2) issues can be raised in both the PTO and before a federal district court judge in a civil lawsuit.

In the biotech arena, disputes over who was first to invent—in patent law
parlance, "priority of invention"—are often decided in an interference. These
highly specialized, administrative trial-like proceedings are brought after a
claim to an invention is determined to have satisfied the requirements for patentability—utility, novelty, nonobviousness, written description, enablement, and
best mode, each of which is discussed in detail later. An interference can be
between two co-pending patent applications as well as between a pending
application and unexpired patent claiming the same or substantially the same
subject matter.

By statute, an interference brought by a third party must be made within
one year of either (*i*) publication of the challenged patent application, or (*ii*) issuance of the challenged patent. An interference may be triggered by a patent
examiner or by a request from a third party. In both cases, the decision of
whether to "declare" an interference is made by the Board of Patent Appeals
and Interferences.

Procedurally, the Board mails a notice declaring the interference in which it
identifies one "senior" party and one or more "junior" parties. The senior party,
based on the earliest filing date, is presumed to be the first inventor. This presumption is rebuttable by evidence, most commonly by laboratory notebook
records, showing that a junior party was the first to conceive of the idea and
diligently worked on reducing the idea to practice. Reduction to practice can

be an actual physical embodiment that works for its intended purpose. Alternatively, there can be constructive reduction to practice, where the inventor files a patent application.

Initially, the parties compile documentary evidence, including invention disclosures, laboratory notebooks, correspondence, analysis, and other test data. Further evidence of inventorship is submitted in the form of sworn written affidavits. The inventors and others who provided sworn affidavits may later be orally cross-examined in a deposition. Inventor testimony must be independently corroborated, for example, through the written and oral testimony and records of others (e.g., lab technicians) who did not contribute to the conception of the claimed invention.

Diligence must be proven from just prior to the date of conception of the competing claimant through reduction to practice. Reasonable delays—to obtain reagents, tissue cultures, or other testing materials; to enter into a confidentiality agreement and retain an independent testing laboratory; to secure institutional review board or other required approvals—should not create a lack of diligence. However, business reasons—such as reallocating research priorities or budget reallocations—do not excuse diligence.

Even if the an inventor shows diligence, an invention may not be patentable for failure to comply with the requirements of Section 102(g)(2), which requires that an invention has not been abandoned, suppressed, or concealed. Abandonment, suppression, or concealment occur where the inventors failed to make the invention public within a reasonable time. This does not require actual commercialization. Filing a patent application within a reasonable time also satisfies Section 102(g)(2).

Section 112—Written Description, Best Mode, and Enablement

There are other requirements for patentability—written description, enablement, and best mode. These requirements can best be understood in the broader context of the purpose for creating patent rights in the Constitution. By ensuring that patent applicants fully disclose the best way for making a working version of the claimed invention, the patentee has kept their side of bargain. In exchange for the grant of a monopoly, the patentee has clearly described the invention so that science and the arts could advance.

Written Description

Early U.S. biotech patents frequently included broad "prophetic" claims to inventions that the inventor had not actually tested. So-called paper patents are proper, provided the requirements of the Patent Act are satisfied; in other words, the inventor must provide sufficient written description to enable a person of ordinary skill in the art to practice the invention (enablement) and use it for its intended purpose (utility).

Amgen v. Chugai: For the biotech industry, the written description requirement has been shaped in a series of judicial decisions. One of the most important early cases was the 1991 decision in *Amgen Inc. v. Chugai Pharmaceutical Co. Ltd. and Genetics Institute* (2). There, Amgen brought a lawsuit alleging infringement of a claim to a DNA sequence consisting essentially of a DNA sequence encoding human erythropoietin (EPO). The Court of Appeals for the Federal Circuit held that simply knowing how to isolate a compound of unknown structure (i.e., the EPO gene) would not suffice; rather an inventor must actually isolate the gene being claimed: "It is not sufficient to define (a gene) solely by its principal biological property, for example, encoding human erythropoietin. . . . When an inventor is unable to envision the detailed construction of a gene so as to distinguish it from other materials, as well as a method for obtaining it, conception has not been achieved until reduction to practice has occurred, that is, until after the gene has been isolated."

Fiers v. Revel: Two years later, in *Fiers v. Revel*, the Federal Circuit heard a three-party inventorship dispute (an interference) between (*i*) Fiers and Tiollais, (*ii*) Revel, and (*iii*) Sugano over who was the first to conceive and reduce to practice the nucleotide sequence that codes for human fibroblast beta-interferon (3). The three parties had initially filed patent applications outside the United States and later filed applications in the United States claiming priority to the foreign filings.[a] The issue before the PTO and the Federal Circuit (on appeal from the PTO) was who was the first to invent. Both concurred and found Sugano to have been the first to satisfy the written description requirement by setting out the complete and correct nucleotide sequence of a DNA coding for beta-interferon.

According to the Court, "an adequate written description of a DNA requires more than a mere statement that it is part of the invention and reference to a potential method for isolating it; what is required is a description of the DNA itself." The holding of *Fiers*—in order to patent a protein, the sequence itself must be patented—had wide-ranging implications on the race to code and patent the human genome. Was it proper to grant a patent on a sequence without identifying what the claimed sequence did?

UC v. Lilly: Perhaps the seminal biotech written description case involved a suit brought by the Regents of the University of California (UC) against Eli Lilly relating to Lilly's process for producing human proinsulin (4). The patent at issue claimed a method for isolating cDNA encoding rat insulin as well as the cDNA itself. The patent also described methods for encoding for

---

[a]Sugano filed a U.S. application in October 1980 claiming priority to a March 1980 Japanese filing. Fiers filed in the United States in April 1981 and claimed priority to an April 1980 British application. Revel and Tiollais filed first in Israel in November 1979 and subsequently filed in the United States in September 1982.

other vertebrate insulins, including human insulin; however, the patent did not describe the nucleotide sequence of cDNA encoding for these other insulins.

The Federal Circuit found for Lilly, holding that the specification failed to provide an adequate written description of human insulin cDNA: "Describing a method of preparing a cDNA or even describing the protein that the cDNA encodes . . . does not necessarily describe the cDNA itself," The Court continued, "In claims to genetic material . . . a generic statement such as 'vertebrate insulin cDNA' or 'mammalian insulin cDNA,' without more, is not an adequate written description of the invention because it does not distinguish the claimed genus from others, except by function . . . [which] is only an indication of what the gene does, rather than what it is."

Enzo v. Gen-Probe: *UC v. Lilly* signaled a shift in biotech patent jurisprudence—a heightened written description standard would be applied in biotech cases, one requiring "a kind of specificity usually achieved by means of the recitation of the sequence of nucleotides that make up the DNA." In 2002, this strict standard was relaxed in another Federal Circuit decision, *Enzo Biochem v. Gen-Probe (Enzo II)* (5,6). There, the court held that public deposit of biological specimens satisfied the written description requirement.

The patent at issue *in Enzo II* claimed nucleic acid probes capable of selectively binding to the DNA of the bacteria that cause gonorrhea and thereby distinguishing those bacteria from other closely related and highly homologous bacteria. The patentee, Enzo, had isolated three DNA probes, inserted them into *Escherichia Coli*, which, in turn, were deposited at the American Type Culture Collection (ATCC). The ATCC deposit was referenced in the patent specification.

In the first two rounds—before the District Court and then on appeal to the Federal Circuit—Gen-Probe won by arguing that describing the claimed DNA probes by function (the ability to bind selectively to a particular bacterial stain) was not sufficient to satisfy Section 112, 1st Paragraph. Enzo petitioned for rehearing and prevailed. In siding with Enzo, the Federal Circuit followed the PTO Written Description Guidelines:[b] "In light of the history of biological deposits for patent purposes, the goals of the patent law, and the practical difficulties of describing unique biological materials in a written description, we hold that reference in the specification to a deposit in a public depository, which makes its contents accessible to the public when it is not otherwise available in written form, constitutes an adequate description of the deposited material sufficient to comply with the written description requirement of §112, ¶1." The case was then sent back to the district court to determine whether in light of the specification as a whole (including information obtainable from the deposits of the claimed sequences) the inventors were in "possession" of what they claimed.

---

[b]Guidelines for Examination of Patent Applications Under the 35 U.S.C. § 112, 1st Paragraph, 66 Fed. Reg. 1009 (Jan. 5, 2001).

In summary, inventions must be particularly and distinctly claimed for two reasons. First, by defining the metes and bounds of the claimed invention, again in the eyes of the person of ordinary skill in the art, the public is put on notice of what is patented. This enables others to avoid patent infringement. Second, clear written description allows others to improve upon patented ideas and promotes the advancement of science.

Best Mode

A separate requirement for patentability relates to best mode. If an inventor has a best way of manufacturing at the time of the invention, it must be disclosed. This is part of the bargain for receiving a monopoly. Others must be taught the inventor's best ideas so they can dissect and improve upon them, thereby advancing science.

Enablement

Written description is distinct from enablement. The purpose of the written description requirement is broader than to merely explain how to make and use; the applicant must convey with reasonable clarity to those skilled in the art that, as of the filing date sought, the applicant was in possession of the invention. Enablement is the requirement that a patent provide sufficient information for a person of ordinary skill in the art to practice the invention without undue experimentation.

A leading biotech patent case on enablement is *Enzo Biochem v. Calgene.* Enzo licensed three patents relating to the use of antisense technology in regulating three genes in the prokaryote *E. coli.*[c] Calgene patented the use of antisense technology in regulating gene expression in plants. Using that eukaryote technology, Calgene developed and marketed the Flavr Savr tomato. Enzo sued Calgene, claiming the Flavr Savr tomato infringed Enzo's antisense patents. In finding for Calgene, the Federal Circuit noted that virtually no guidance, direction, or working examples were provided for practicing the invention in eukaryotes, or even any prokaryote other than *E. coli.* According to the Court, "Tossing out the mere germ of an idea does not constitute enabling disclosure." The Court further explained, "While every aspect of a [broad] generic claim certainly need not have been carried out by an inventor, or exemplified in the specification, reasonable detail must be provided in order to enable members of the public to understand and carry out the invention."

The key to determining whether a disclosure is enabling is undue experimentation. Recognizing that this is a fact-specific inquiry, eight criteria, the so-called *Wands* factors, are considered by federal courts: (*i*) the quantity of experimentation necessary, (*ii*) the amount of direction or guidance presented,

---

[c]Antisense technology inhibits production of targeted proteins. A nucleotide sequence that is complementary to a sequence of mRNA, binds to the mRNA molecule and prevents translation into a protein.

(*iii*) the presence or absence of working examples, (*iv*) the nature of the invention, (*v*) the state of the prior art, (*vi*) the relative skill of those in the art, (*vii*) the predictability or unpredictability of the art, and (*viii*) the breadth of the claims.

In *Enzo v. Calgene*, the Court found that undue experimentation would be required to practice the invention claimed in the Enzo patents in eukaryotes because the number of working examples provided in the specifications were "very narrow" in comparison to the wide breadth of the claims that were alleged to be infringed. As further support for this conclusion, the Court commented that antisense technology is generally unpredictable.

PATENT INFRINGEMENT

Infringement of valid patent claim is decided not by the PTO but exclusively by federal courts. Patent infringement involves a two-step analysis. First, the scope and meaning of the claims must be determined without reference to the accused infringing product. That claim construction, in turn, is then applied and an evaluation made whether each and every element of a claim are present literally or by equivalents. Claim construction and infringement, both literal and under the doctrine of equivalents, are addressed, in turn, in the following subsections.

Claim Construction

Claim construction is the analysis performed by a judge, not a jury, to determine what a claim means. As interpretative tools, judges first rely on "intrinsic evidence"—the text of the patent itself as well as the back-and-forth between the patent applicant and the patent examiner. The publicly available, back-and-forth between the applicant and the PTO is referred to as the prosecution history, also known by the shorthand "file wrapper." Judges rely on intrinsic evidence because it is the same public record that will be relied upon by competitors to determine whether their activities infringe a valid patent claim.

In considering the intrinsic evidence, a judge first looks to the language of the claims. Next, the judge considers the remainder of the Specification—the detailed description and examples—as well as the prosecution history. Dictionaries and encyclopedias are also considered to be part of the intrinsic evidence. Judges must be careful, however, not to read limitations from examples into claims. A claim, if broadly drafted, must stand on its own and should not be narrowed to cover only those embodiments of the invention that are taught in the examples.

Where the scope of the claims is ambiguous from public record or where the technology at issue is complex, judges may look to extrinsic evidence. This includes the testimony of both experts and the inventors. An emerging trend in biotechnology cases is for judges to request a technology tutorial by a court-appointed expert. Another source of extrinsic evidence is prior art scientific articles.

There are rules followed by judges in interpreting claims. Three of the most important canons of construction are discussed here. First, patentees act as their "own lexicographers." In other words, they may define claim terms as they wish, provided the description is clear and is used consistently. A second, and related canon, is the plain meaning rule. Unless defined otherwise (i.e., in the specification or file wrapper), claim terms are given their plain meaning. Ordinary terms are given a dictionary definition. Technical terms are given a plain meaning as defined by person of ordinary skill in the art.

A third set of rules for interpretation views patents like contracts. Each and every claim element must be given meaning. A claim element cannot be "read out" or discarded. As we will see, this rule is of considerable importance when considering whether there is infringement under the doctrine of equivalents. Further, when a term has alternate meanings, interpretation should be avoided that would invalidate the claim (i.e., in light of what is in the prior art).

Claim Construction Example—Stem Cells

A breakthrough development in biotechnology was the discovery by Curt Civin of an antibody (anti-My-10) that selectively binds to an antigen (CD34) on the surface of immature stem cells but not on more differentiated cells. He also discovered a monoclonal antibody that recognizes the CD34 antigen and is useful in separating stem cells from mature cells. Civin filed for and was awarded patents for his discoveries. The patents were assigned to his employer, Johns Hopkins University, which, in turn, granted licenses to Baxter Healthcare Corporation and Becton, Dickinson & Co. to commercialize the Civin inventions. Several years later, Seattle-based CellPro began marketing its own stem cell separation technology and was sued for infringing the Civin patents.

One of the claims that CellPro was accused of infringing recited "a suspension of human cells comprising pluripotent lympho-hemapoietic stem cells substantially free of mature lymphoid and myeloid cells." Among the first questions to be decided by the court was what is meant by the claim element "substantially free of." CellPro's response was typical of many accused infringers—the claim is narrow and did not cover its products. CellPro argued that "substantially free of" meant an immeasurable amount of mature cells, whereas CellPro's suspensions contained measurable amounts of mature cells numbering in the "millions." Hopkins countered, arguing that the claim covered a cell suspension of "at least 90% purity" (i.e., no more than 10% mature lymphoid and myeloid cells).

The district court sided with Hopkins. On appeal, the Federal Circuit agreed. Both courts pointed to a table in the specification that described the only embodiment of the Civin invention. The table disclosed a cell suspension containing 3% mature neutrophils, 6% mature monocytes, and 1% mature lymphocytes, all of which constituted measurable quantities of mature lymphoid cells. The courts thus properly looked to the intrinsic evidence in order to determine the scope of the claims. Moreover, their interpretations were consistent with another tenet of patent law, namely, a patent claim should be construed to encompass at least one disclosed embodiment in the written description.

Determining Infringement

In the Introduction, briefly mentioned was the all elements rule—that each element must be present literally or by equivalents. Literal infringement means what it says. Each claim element is literally present in the accused infringing product or method. The doctrine of equivalents was created by courts to prevent unscrupulous copyists from committing a "fraud on the patent" by making products with insubstantial differences to avoid coming within the literal language of a patent claim. Insubstantial differences are considered to be generally recognized substitutions for the literal claim element that is missing from the accused product or process or an alternative that provides substantially the same function, in substantially the same way, to achieve substantially the same result as the literal claim element. Courts refer to this as the "triple identity" or "function-way-result" test: Does the missing component in the accused subject matter perform substantially the same function as the claimed limitation in substantially the same way to achieve substantially the same result.

There are important limitations on asserting infringement by equivalents. First, no equivalent can be claimed for something that was in, or an obvious variation on, the prior art. Second, could the patent applicant at the time the application was filed reasonably have claimed the equivalent? If so, under the hypothetical claim test, there should be no infringement by equivalents. Third, an equivalent can be surrendered during prosecution (i.e., by amending the filed claim or conceding the examiner's argument). Lastly, subject matter that is disclosed in specification, but not claimed, is considered to have been dedicated to the public and cannot later be reclaimed by asserting infringement by equivalents. The doctrine of equivalents is discussed in further detail in section "Biotech Patent Prosecution."

One final but very important rule of infringement—if an independent claim is not infringed, neither are its dependent claims.

SIX STEPS TO PATENT PEACE OF MIND

Step 1. Patent Clearance Search

As early as possible in new product development, a chemist should ask, "Has my idea been patented by another person?" To answer this question, the core element(s) of the product idea must be identified. A search is then conducted to determine whether each of these elements is recited in a claim of an unexpired patent. In searching for potential "blocking" patent claims, care must be taken to consider whether an element is present literally or equivalently because both can give rise to a claim of patent infringement.

With approximately 6.7 million patents issued in the United States alone, finding whether an idea has been claimed in an unexpired patent may seem daunting. To simplify this task, the USPTO has devised a scheme for classifying inventions based both on individual chemical constituents in a final product and by end use of the product. Many inventions in the field of cosmetics and personal care products belong to Class 424—Drug, Bio-Affecting and Body-Treating Compositions. These subclasses are summarized in the Table 2.

A chemist can conduct individual research (e.g., at www.uspto.gov) and arrive at important technical conclusions. However, even the most thorough and scientifically sound analysis may not be enough. A "freedom to operate" opinion from a patent attorney (see Step 4) can offer a company patent peace of mind. For this reason, a clearance search is conducted under the direction of, and reviewed by, a patent attorney.

Classification systems are, by their nature, imperfect. Therefore, classification-based searching is often supplemented by Boolean word searches using synonyms for the key individual ingredients in the new product formulation [e.g., International Union of Pure and Applied Chemistry (IUPAC) and International Nomenclature of Cosmetic Ingredients (INCI) names] as well as broader, more generalized, descriptors (e.g., transdermal delivery, oil-in-water emulsion). In the case of biotechnology inventions, sequences must be searched. Amino acid should also be searched by alphabetical abbreviations. For example, the palmitoyl pentapeptide, Lys-Thr-Thr-Lys-Ser, marketed under the tradename Matrixyl, should also be searched as Pal-KTTKS, representing palmitic acid attached to the peptide.

If there is a single, substantial point of difference between the product or process under development and the patent claim, the idea can be refined further

Table 2 Class 424 Personal Care Products: Drug, Bio-Affecting, and Body-Treating Compositions

Class	Description
424/49	Dentifrices, mouthwashes
424/59	Topical sun or radiation screening or tanning preparations
424/61	Manicure or pedicure compositions
424/62	Bleach for live hair or skin (peroxides)
424/63	Color makeup—live skin colorant applied topically for coloring the skin in either a limited or overall area (e.g., blemish cover, cheek rouge, eye shadow)
424/64	Lip (e.g., lip rouge, lipstick)
424/65	Antiperspirants or perspiration deodorant
424/69	Face or body powders for grooming, adorning, or absorbing
424/70	Shampoo

and finally cleared as "noninfringing" in a "freedom to operate" opinion letter. Otherwise, modifications to the formula, so-called "design arounds" can be explored.

Step 2. Design Around

A patent clearance search could save R&D months of following a path that would have led to a lawsuit and an injunction against selling your product. Knowing what already has been patented at the beginning of the product development life-cycle permits changes to be made to a prototype so that it differs from claims in a blocking patent in at least one important respect. The modified formula then can be cleared as noninfringing. If, however, a "design around" is not possible, and an allegation of patent infringement could be made, there may be options short of starting from scratch at the lab bench.

Step 3. Consider the Prior Art

As discussed in section "Patentability," by statute, a patentable invention must be both novel and nonobvious; in other words, a patent may be granted for ideas that have been neither publicly taught nor suggested at the time of invention. To determine whether a patent claim is truly novel and nonobvious, the relevant prior art needs to be identified and searched. In an industry with an ever-expanding knowledge base, this is easier said than done.

A common, and sometimes fatal, mistake is to limit a review of the relevant prior art to issued patents, published patent applications, and scientific journal articles. Equally, and often more relevant, prior art is found in commercial products, technical brochures, advertisements, and conference presentations. If a single prior art reference teaches each and every element of the patent claim of concern, that claim is said to be invalid as anticipated. If all of the elements in the patent claim are taught by a combination of two or more prior art references, and there was a motivation for making that combination at the time of the invention, then the patent claim is said to be invalid as obvious.

Step 4. Freedom to Operate Opinion

"Freedom to operate" can be based on noninfringement (Step 1) or invalidity based on anticipation or obviousness of the claimed idea in light of the prior art (Step 3). An opinion from patent counsel that a product or process under development does not infringe the claims of a valid patent provides more than peace of mind; it protects against potential treble damages for willful patent infringement. Also, it is increasingly common for both finished goods companies and suppliers to seek such an opinion.

Noninfringement opinions are often less time consuming (and less costly) to prepare. The reason, as discussed earlier, is that if a patent contains twenty claims—two independent and eighteen dependent—and both the independent claims are not infringed, the remaining eighteen dependent claims are not infringed as a matter of law. Anticipation and infringement are similar. According to a well-worn maxim of patent law, that which infringes if later, anticipates if before. However, unlike the independent/dependent claim noninfringement rule, there is no shortcut for opining that because an independent claim is invalid as anticipated so too are its dependent claims. For a claim to be invalid as anticipated or obvious, each claim element—irrespective of whether the claim is independent or dependent—must be shown to be present in the prior art.

Step 5. Licensing

There are times that a product, the process for making it, or methods of its use are claimed in a strong patent, one for which there is no practical and cost-effective design around and which is neither anticipated nor rendered obvious by the prior art. When this occurs, a different tack can be taken—licensing the right to use the process or make the product claimed in a "blocking patent." For a variety of reasons, not the least of which are large upfront and royalty payments, the holder of a strong patent may be willing to grant a license, even on an exclusive basis, enter into a joint venture or other R&D collaboration, or, in some instance, sell its patent rights outright.

Licenses are available on a wide range of terms: exclusive versus nonexclusive: by territory (i.e., market country): up-front, paid in full versus milestones + royalties. Licenses may be limited to field of use (personal care vs. plastics) or channel of distribution (prestige brick-and-mortar retail stores vs. medispas and doctors' offices).

For the biotech personal care industry, research tool patents are particularly of interest. The following two well-known examples are illustrative. The Cohen-Boyer technology for recombinant DNA developed at Stanford University and the UC was claimed in three patents. Those patents were broadly licensed on a nonexclusive basis for about a modest fee of $10,000 per year plus a royalty of 0.5–3% of sales. Stanford and UC granted hundreds of licenses and generated hundreds of millions of dollars in royalties for the universities.

The technology underlying polymerase chain reaction—specific, rapid amplification of targeted DNA or RNA sequences and Taq polymerase, the enzyme used in the amplification—was developed by Cetus Corp. and later sold to Roche. Roche recognized the value of the technology as more than a research tool and licensed the technology at higher royalty rates where the end use was diagnostic service applications.

Step 6. File a Patent Application

How do you know if your idea is patentable? Essentially by following the course laid out in Steps 1 to 3. If an idea is not claimed in an issued patent (Step 1) and is neither taught nor suggested in the prior art (Step 3), then the idea likely is novel and not obvious, two of the cornerstone criteria for receiving a patent under U.S. law. Serious consideration should then be given to protecting the idea by filing for a patent.

Prior to filing a patent application, a search of the nonpatent prior art is typically conducted. Why conduct a prior art search if no blocking patents have been identified? The simple answer is prudence. A motivated competitor intent on finding a way to copy your successful product might spare little expense to find prior art that invalidates the patent claim(s) protecting your product. The patentability search is not limited to claims of unexpired patent. It includes published, pending patent applications, expired patents in their entirety—not just the claims—journal articles, trade literature, internet postings, and so on.

Once a decision is made to pursue patent protection, the point(s) of novelty and nonobviousness of the invention need to be clearly articulated. Novelty may be a small improvement or a breakthrough advance. For example, a patent could be issued for a blemish concealer that combined two particular surfactants, both within narrow concentration ranges, to produce a stable emulsion with a specifically defined low viscosity. Similarly, a patent could be issued for the discovery that the appearance of facial wrinkles are reduced by topically applying a recombinantly produced active ingredient from a genus.

Once the patentable differences are identified, the inventor(s) and patent attorney work together to describe the permutations of the idea from broadest to most narrow. Strategic options, such as whether to file a U.S.-only application or an international application under the Patent Cooperation Treaty, are then considered, and an application is filed.

Approximately 18 to 24 months after a patent application is filed, the USPTO responds with an office action, typically containing one or more rejections. A rejection should be expected. A first action allowance is like a-hole-in-one in golf—perhaps a little more probable. A first action allowance likely means that the invention was claimed too narrowly. The most common rejection in cases involving personal care products is that the claimed idea is obvious in light of the teachings of the prior art. As discussed in section "Patentability," obviousness must be judged through the eyes of the hypothetical person of ordinary skill in the art at the time of the invention.

Responses to rejections range from attorney argument to narrowing the draft claims to distinguish the claimed invention from the prior art. Another type of response is for the inventor to submit a declaration demonstrating that the claimed invention is not obvious because of unexpected results.

There are two bites at the apple. If after a response to a nonfinal office action, the examiner maintains the rejection, the applicant generally has two choices—pay more fees and continue prosecuting the application or appeal the final rejection.

When a patent application is found by the examiner to be in condition for allowance, an interference search is ordered. Assuming no potentially competing pending applications or issued patents are found, formalities are addressed, fees paid, and a patent issued.

U.S. Provisional Application

For many reasons, filing for a provisional patent application is an increasingly common strategy for maximizing the protection of biotechnology inventions. First, cost savings (both in time in preparing the application and government fees); a provisional does not require the formalities of a nonprovisional application. Essentially, the provisional serves as a place holder, establishing an early effective filing date for a later-filed nonprovisional patent application. A provisional application also allows the term "Patent Pending" to be used in marketing and other sales materials.

The most common reason for filing a provisional patent application is the approaching one-year 102(b) bar. As discussed earlier in section "Novelty" page 392, under U.S. patent law, an inventor has up to one-year from the first public disclosure to file for a patent. The filing of the provisional stops the one-year clock and gives the inventor up to one additional year in which to file a nonprovisional application.

Two other typical scenarios where provisionals are used in the biotech arena both relate to the desire to disclose to others a potentially patentable idea while safeguarding the inventors' rights to the invention. One common circumstance is that an inventor is soon to submit a manuscript for publication or to make a public presentation. In Europe, however, there is an absolute novelty requirement. Under European patent law, any public disclosure destroys novelty and can be cited as evidence of "lack of inventive step" (the European equivalent of obviousness) against the inventor. A provisional patent application prevents the loss of novelty/inventive step.

Another reason why inventors, particularly in biotechnology, file provisional applications is to have laid down a marker that an invention is theirs prior to exploring the commercial viability of the idea with potential strategic partnership (e.g., cooperative research and development agreement). In the event of parting of the ways with a strategic partner along the bumpy road to commercialization, the inventors would have clearly articulated what was theirs and not the strategic partners'.

One further advantage of filing a provisional is that it extends the patent life by one-year. Remember, under the current U.S. patent law, the term of a utility patent is 20 years from the filing date of a nonprovisional application. Delaying filing of the nonprovisional by one year means one more year of exclusivity (and revenues) on the back end.

A few words of caution. A provisional application lasts 12 months from the filing date—not a second beyond midnight. If a nonprovisional application claiming priority to the provisional is not timely filed, that particular invention is no longer patentable. While provisionals are not required to contain claims, its written description (and drawings, if any) must adequately support the subject matter claimed in the later-filed nonprovisional application in order to benefit from the provisional filing date. A provisional must also comply with the enablement and best mode requirements of Section 112.

PCT Application

The United States is a signatory to the Patent Cooperation Treaty (PCT). The largest single advantage of filing a PCT application is deferring patent expenses (e.g., hiring local patent agents in each foreign country, preparing necessary translations, and paying national fees) for up to 30 months. By filing a single international patent application in English, under the PCT, it is possible to simultaneously seek protection for an invention in each of PCT contracting states, which include, for example, most of Europe, Japan, China, the Russian Federation, Korea, Australia, and Canada. A properly filed international application under the PCT cannot be rejected on formal grounds by any designated patent office during the national phase of examining the application.

Another advantage of the PCT is that the applicant is entitled to an international search report conducted by one of the major patent offices.[d] On that basis, the inventor can evaluate the probability that a patent will issue. The ability to assess the patentability of an invention early on is further enhanced by availability of preliminary examination report. During international preliminary examination, an applicant can amend the PCT application prior to examination by the designated national patent offices. One downside that must be weighed is that the overall cost of PCT is higher than pursuing separate national applications from the outset.

Biotechnology Patent Prosecution Strategy

On first blush, an inventor seeking to obtain the broadest protection for a biotechnology invention might consider filing a broad patent claim to a genus. However, if the genus claim is later amended and narrowed (e.g., for failure to meet the written description requirement of 35 USC §112, ¶1), inventors may obtain lesser protection had they claimed the invention narrowly and later attempted to broaden the protection by arguing infringement by equivalents. In order to understand this counterintuitive result, two series of court decisions, both relating to limitations on equivalents, must be discussed.

Festo: For more than a decade, the issue of prosecution history estoppel has made its way up and down and back up again the federal court system in the *Festo* line of cases (7). Most recently, this was the subject of decisions by the U.S. Supreme Court and the U.S. Court of Appeals for the Federal Circuit, in the spring 2002 and in late summer 2003.

---

[d]Australia, Austria, China, Japan, the Republic of Korea, the Russian Federation, Spain, Sweden, the United States of America, and the European Patent Office act as International Searching Authorities under the PCT.

Simplified, the 2002 Supreme Court decision held that where a patent claim has been narrowed by amendment during prosecution, a rebuttable presumption is created that the amendment was made for reasons relating to patentability (i.e., 35 USC Sections 102, 103, or 112). A narrowing amendment, in turn, would mean that the patentee was estopped from asserting infringement by equivalents for subject matter that had been given up resulting in the narrowing amendment. Put differently, a narrowing amendment is said to effect a surrender of all subject matter between the original and amended claims. Even a "voluntary" narrowing amendment—one not made in response to a specific rejection of otherwise required by the examiner—could create estoppel. The Supreme Court did not, however, go further; instead it left to the Federal Circuit the task of establishing standards for how a patentee could overcome the presumption, and continue to claim infringement by equivalents.

A year later, on remand from the Supreme Court, the Federal Circuit described three flexible criteria as "general guidance" for addressing whether the surrender of equivalents by amendment was complete: (*i*) foreseeability, (*ii*) tangentialness, and (*iii*) a catch-all "some other reason."

The foreseeability inquiry asks whether the alleged infringing equivalent was foreseeable to a person of ordinary skill in the art at the time of the amendment? In other words, could a skilled artisan have reasonably drafted a claim that would have literally encompassed the alleged equivalent. Examples of subject matter that should, in the words of the Federal Circuit, "usually" qualify as unforeseeable are later-developed technology or technology that was not known in the relevant art. In determining whether an alleged equivalent would have been foreseeable, expert testimony and other extrinsic evidence (i.e., documentary evidence, beyond the patent and its file wrapper) may be considered to ascertain both the scope of the relevant art and the level of the person of ordinary skill in the art. Both of these determinations are to be made at the time of the amendment, not in hindsight.

Alternatively, a patentee can rebut the presumption of surrender of equivalents by demonstrating that the reason for the amendment was only "tangentially" related to the equivalent later being asserted. The patentee must show that the reason for the narrowing amendment was not directly related to the equivalent being asserted. By way of example, an amendment to avoid prior art that encompassed an equivalent is not tangential. Unlike foreseeability, an inquiry into whether the amendment was tangential to the equivalent being claimed is limited to the intrinsic evidence (i.e., the patent itself and its prosecution history). The Federal Circuit did recognize that, in limited circumstances, a court could also consider the testimony from persons of ordinary skill in the relevant art to better understand the file wrapper.

Lastly, an "inferior design" known to the inventor, but purposefully not included when in the claims, cannot be recaptured by equivalents.

Johnson & Johnston: Another important facet of surrender by equivalents is set out in *Johnson & Johnston*. There, the Federal Circuit found a complete bar against asserting infringement by equivalents where subject matter had been disclosed in the specification but not claimed. A patentee may, however, attempt to obtain coverage of the disclosed subject matter by filing a reissue or continuation application.

Prosecution History Estoppel—Tying it Together: Where a genus claim is narrowed during prosecution, under *Festo* the narrowing amendment could be viewed as having been made for a reason related to patentability, and assertion of doctrine of equivalents would be foreclosed. A biotechnology prosecution strategy might limit the original claim to a species with the goal of not having to file a narrowing amendment. Once issued without amendment, the patentee could then seek to assert infringement by equivalents. Thus, where a patentee may be precluded from claiming broadly (i.e., the genus), by claiming narrowly (i.e., the species) the patentee could later seek to broaden the claim to cover the genus. The complexities of the interplay of *Festo* (7) and *Johnson & Johnston* (8) are further illustrated in the section "Patent Litigation."

POST-ISSUANCE CHALLENGES—U.S. RE-EXAMINATION AND EUROPEAN OPPOSITION

In the United States, the validity of an issued patent can be challenged after issuance through a reexamination—an administrative procedure in the USPTO. Typically, this is an ex parte, nonadversarial proceeding—only the patent examiner and the owner of the patent under reexamination are involved. A request for reexamination may be filed by anyone during the life of the patent, and six years thereafter (accounting for the statute of limitations for bringing a patent infringement lawsuit). The request, a detailed explanation of the art not previously considered by the PTO, including how the new reference bears on patentability, is submitted together with the required fee. The prior art that serves as the basis for the request must be a printed publication. This includes previously issued patents and published patent applications.

Within three months of the request—which may be submitted anonymously—the assigned examiner must determine whether the new reference raises a substantial new issue. If so, a reexamination is ordered and will proceed with "special dispatch." The examiner considers the new prior art as if it had been submitted to the PTO at the time the original application had been filed. Importantly, the scope of the claim under reexamination cannot be expanded by amendment.

Criticism was leveled at the ex parte nature of reexamination. Once a reference was submitted, the party requesting the reexamination had no further input into the examiner's deliberations. In response, as part of the American Inventors Protection Act of 1999, an inter partes reexamination was created. Limits on this new form of reexamination led to further criticisms. For example, the third-party requestor has limited opportunities for involvement. Also, adverse findings (i.e., reconfirming patentability) may not be appealed to court. Finally, perhaps the most far-reaching reason discouraging inter partes reexaminations is that the requester is precluded from later raising in litigation any questions of validity on grounds that were, or may have, been raised during the proceedings.

Europe, in contrast to the United States, has a full adversarial procedure following issuance of a patent. Under the European Patent Convention (EPC), any third party can institute an opposition proceeding to challenge a granted patent within nine months after the patent issues. The opposition is applicable to all of the EPC designated states; consequently, the opponent need not pursue legal proceedings in each of the European nations designated in the patent. Typical grounds for opposition are invalidity for failure to meet the standard requirements of patentability (e.g., lack of novelty or inventive step) as well as failure of the applicant to disclose the invention with sufficient clarity or completeness. In response to an opposition, the Opposition Division of the European Patent Office may reject the opposition, amend the patent, or revoke the patent entirely.

Despite its limitations (i.e., only printed prior art can be raised), the United States system does have one advantage over the European Opposition—timing. In Europe, a challenger must act with nine months. In contrast, in the United States, a party has the life of the patent, plus six years.

PATENT LITIGATION

Expensive. Disruptive. And for start-ups and not-so-small established businesses alike potentially "bet the company." The stakes and costs of biotech patent litigation are hard to quantify. In cases hard fought up and down the federal court system, attorneys' fees alone can soar into seven figures. (As attorneys' fees are awarded only in exceptional cases, the amount awarded is often substantially less than the plaintiff actually spent.) Damages are awarded based on lost profits, a reasonable royalty, or a combination of the two. There are, however, noneconomic factors that motivate biotech patent holders to bring suit—chief among them is establishing a reputation for toughness. The purpose of this section is to provide a snapshot of the litigation process and to highlight and reemphasize several of the key concepts discussed in the preceding sections.

Biotech litigation, like all patent litigations, begins with the filing of a complaint in a federal court, seeking a declaration of infringement, patent validity, injunctive relief (e.g., permanently enjoining the defendant from selling the product or practicing the method claimed in the patent-in-suit), treble damages, and attorneys' fees. The defendant then answers, commonly asserting as defenses noninfringement and invalidity (based on anticipation and/or obviousness) and, more and more frequently, lack of written description and lack of enablement. The defendant likely also counterclaims for a declaration of patent invalidity.

After a scheduling order is entered, written discovery (document requests, interrogatories, and requests to admit) is served. This is followed by depositions of fact witnesses. Thereafter, expert witnesses are designated who review the factual evidence and offer written opinions on issues of infringement and validity. As the plaintiff bears the burden of proving infringement, plaintiff's expert prepares an infringement opinion. In contrast, as patents are presumed valid, the burden of proving invalidity is on the defendant, whose expert opines on that issue. The experts then shift roles and prepare rebuttal reports. The exchange of reports is followed by expert depositions.

After the close of fact and expert discovery a court typically conducts a *Markman* hearing to determine the scope and meaning of the claims at issue. As a *Markman* ruling itself is not immediately appealable, the parties then generally make one or more motions for summary judgment. A summary judgment motion is one that does not involve any disputed facts and can therefore be decided by the court solely as a matter of law (i.e., applying the applicable legal standards to the undisputed facts). If a summary judgment is granted, that issue is resolved. If it is denied, the parties present argument on the issue at trial.

In patent cases, some have pointed to a trend that cases are being decided for the defendant based on summary judgment of noninfringement. If a defendant is found not to have infringed, the case is fully and finally over; issues of invalidity or failure to comply with the requirements of Section 112 are moot. The plaintiff may then appeal the finding of noninfringement together with the *Markman* ruling. The Federal Circuit reviews the district court's claim construction de novo. If the district court is found to err, the Federal Circuit will reverse, issue a claim construction, and remand the case for further proceedings (e.g., trial). In this manner, the district court trial judge can proceed to trial without being concerned that the Federal Circuit will reverse the lower court's claim construction and require yet another trial.

Trial is far from inevitable. Judges strongly encourage, and in some courts require, that the parties engage in some form of alternative dispute resolution. As the stakes are high—the plaintiff stands to lose a patent if found to be invalid while defendant may be liable for treble damages—the majority of cases settle, sometimes on the courthouse steps. Litigation is thus frequently used as a business tool to obtain leverage for the settlement endgame. Where both parties are accusing the other of patent infringement, as is often the case in biotech patent disputes, a common resolution is to grant cross licenses.

Although it is impossible to do justice to the strategic intricacies of biotech patent litigation in an introductory, overview chapter, three hypothetical litigation case studies are included with the goal of tying together key concepts that are frequently at issue in biotech patent cases.

Litigation Case Study 1—In a *Markman* hearing (in which a court is called upon to interpret the scope and meaning of the patent claims), a patentee argues for a broad claim construction under which a claim, literally construed, would cover the accused infringing product. In support of the argument, the patentee points to a particular example disclosed in the specification. Should the court construe the claim narrowly, so that there would be no literal infringement, the infringement analysis would turn to the doctrine of equivalents. The accused infringer would have a strong defense that under *Johnson & Johnston* (see Section VI F iii b; Ref. 8) the patentee should be barred from asserting infringement by equivalents based on examples that were disclosed but not claimed. In relying on a *Johnson & Johnston* bar, the accused infringer also faces strategic choices. By pointing to a disclosed but unclaimed example, the accused infringer could be viewed as conceding that the example worked and thus the enablement requirement was met.

Litigation Case Study 2—Company X obtains a patent claiming composition comprising A, B, and C_1. As originally filed, the patent claimed A, B, and C. During prosecution, X amended the claims from C to C_1. Company Y later receives a patent claiming a composition comprising A, B, C_2, and D. Y's invention was apparently viewed by the Patent Office as being novel and not obvious in light of X's invention. Although Y may have a patentable invention—an improvement on X's invention—X's patent could still be construed by a court to cover Y's product by equivalents (i.e., C_2 functions in substantially the same way to give substantially the same result as C_1). As Y's patent application was filed after X's, X has a defense—that it would not have been foreseeable at the time X filed its patent to claim A, B, C_2.

Litigation Case Study 3—Company A originally filed for a patent with a broad independent claim reciting "a DNA transfer vector comprising an inserted cDNA having a sequence coding for protein XYZ." The phrase "having" permitted inclusion of other sequences. When confronted with a rejection based on prior art, Company A amended the claim by changing "having" to "consisting essentially of." In a subsequent litigation alleging infringement of the independent claim, the defendant could mount a strong defense that the claim had been narrowed by amendment for a substantial reason related to patentability (i.e., to avoid a prior art rejection) and that Company A could not later assert that the surrendered subject matter is within the range of equivalents. Put differently, subject matter that was surrendered by the patentee during prosecution may not later be recaptured.

GAZING INTO THE CRYSTAL BALL

The face of personal care has changed—it involves biotech patents. Recombinant molecules that alter expression of genes and help reduce the signs and appearance of fine lines and wrinkles are genetically engineered products that treat and prevent skin disorders. DNA microarrays and other assays are being used to identify candidate molecules for a new generation of skin care, customized to the genetic makeup of individual users. Illustrative of this new frontier are the following recently issued U.S. patent and published U.S. patent applications.

At the top of the list of the hottest "anti-aging" treatments are Botox and short-chain peptides, such as Matrixyl. Two pending U.S. patent applications relating to the botulinum toxins rely on biotechnology. US Patent Application Serial No. 10/051,952 (filed January 2002 and assigned to Allergan) claims a method for expressing a recombinant DNA sequence encoding a Clostridium neurotoxin component in a cell of an animal in situ. The claimed method includes administering the DNA by injection. US Patent Application Serial No. 10/446562 (filed February 2003) claims a pharmaceutical composition comprising a botulinum neurotoxin formulated with a recombinant serum albumin. US Patent No. 6,620,419, claims methods for topical use of the Matrixyl (Pal-KTTKS) pentapeptide to inhibit the development of wrinkles associated with advancing age, or with sun-induced or pollution-induced skin aging as well as for inducing concommital synthesis of collagen and glyco-saminoglycans. The US Patent No. 6,620,419 specifically teaches that the claimed pentapeptide can be obtained by fermentation of a gentetically engi-neered strain of bacteria to produce the patented sequences or fragments of those sequences.

Techniques of biotechnology are beginning to be used to identify, isolate, and purify polypeptides useful in the treatment of skin conditions, as well as for posttranslational modifications of the polypeptides (e.g., formation of disul-phide bonds, specific proteolytic cleavages, glycosylation, combination with lipids). US Patent No. 6,645,509 (issued in November 2003 to L'Oréal), for example, claims a topically applied composition comprising corneodesmosine, a polypeptide that is naturally expressed in the horny layer of the epidermis and is involved in intercorneocyte cohesion. The corneodesmosine was claimed according to its amino acid sequence as well as by its uses (treating skin fragility, strengthening intercorneocyte cohesion). Like the US Patent No. 6,620,419, the enabling disclosure of US Patent No. 6,645,509 teaches that the amino acid sequence of the claimed polypeptide may be derived from synthetic DNA sequences that are defined to mean a sequence obtained by genetic engineering.

Other recent examples of genetically engineered molecules for use in personal care products are USPN 5,981,256 (recombinant stratum corneum chymotryptic enzyme, and its proteolytically active fragments, for the treatment or prophylaxis of dermatological conditions including acne and eczema) and US Patent Application Serial No. 10/097730 (carotenoid prep-aration comprising recombinant phytoene and recombinant phytofluene effec-tive in combined amounts to prevent oxidative damage from ultra violet (UV) exposure).

Patents that claim upregulation of gene expression in personal care pro-ducts are typified by U.S. Patent Application Serial No. 10/343,783 which claims a cosmetic/dermatological composition comprising as an active ingredi-ent, a specific acryl base copolymer having phosphorylcholine as a side chain or a pendant group, that inhibits or expression of β-glucocerebrosidase gene. Issued US Patent No. 6,399,580 also relates to enhancing the cosmetic appearance of skin and promoting healing of skin damaged from, among other causes, aging and UV exposure, by topical application of a composition comprising at least one inhibitor of β-glucocerebrosidase activity and a glycosphingolipid.

The inventors on the US Patent No. 6,399,580, Drs. Peter Elias and Walter Holleran, both of the Department of Dermatology, School of Medicine at the UC at San Francisco, presented quantitative evidence that inhibitors of β-glucocerebrosidase stimulated both the rate of DNA synthesis and the DNA content of mammalian skin. Related patents and patent applications to Drs. Elias and Holleran claim compositions comprising β-glucocerebrosidase inhibitors for stimulating tissue growth and epithelial moisturization. The Elias/Holleran patents are noteworthy for reasons other than their use of the tools of molecular biology to discover compositions with applications in personal care. They illustrate how research involving biotechnology, with applications in the personal care industry, was done at an academic institution with funding from the federal government. More and more, cutting edge university and/or government sponsored biotechnology research is available for licensing and commercialization into personal care products.

Private industry is also collaborating and funding academic research. A recent example is US Patent No. 6,379,887, jointly held by the Massachusetts General Hospital and Shiseido. The US Patent No. 6,379,887, relates to the discovery of a human protein, homologous to the rKr2 protein in rats, that binds to the human protein microphthalmia-associated transcription factor (MITF) and inhibits the activation of the tyrosinase and TRP1 genes. The patent broadly claims a human DNA fragment encoding a protein which binds to and inhibits the action of human MITF. When the claimed DNA fragment is inserted into a suitable vector and introduced into human melanocytes, the inventors claimed that production of melanin could be controlled.

Biotech patent developments in personal care are also extending to research tools. US Patent Application Serial No. 10/450,797 (with an earliest priority date of January 2001) relates to a process for the in vitro determination of skin stress and/or aging of the skin in humans, to test kits and biochips for determining the skin stress and/or aging of the skin and to the use of proteins, mRNA molecules or fragments of proteins or mRNA molecules as markers for skin stress and/or ageing of the skin. The patent application also relates to a test for screening and demonstrating the effectiveness of cosmetically active substances against skin stress and/or aging of the skin.

From this sampling, one need not look far into a crystal ball to see the importance of biotech patents in personal care—the future is already here.

REFERENCES

1. Rivette KG, Kline D. Discovering new value in intellectual property. Harvard Business Review. January–February 2000. 54–66.
2. Amgen v. Chugai, 927 F.2d 1200. (Fed. Cir. 1991).
3. Fiers v. Revel, 984 F.2d 1164. (Fed. Cir. 1993).

4. Regents of the Univ. of Calif. v. Eli Lilly & Co., 964 F.2d 1559. (Fed. Cir. 1997).
5. Enzo Biochem Inc. v. Gen-Probe Inc., 285 F.3d 1013. (Fed. Cir. 2002).
6. Enzo Biochem Inc. v. Gen-Probe Inc., 296 F.3d 1315. (Fed. Cir. 2002).
7. Festo Corp. v. Shoketsu Kinzoku Kogyo Kabushiki Co. Ltd., 535 U.S. 722. (2002), on remand, 344 F.3d 1359 (Fed. Cir. 2003).
8. Johnson & Johnson Assoc. Inc. v. R.E. Service Co., 285 F.3d 1046. (Fed. Cir. 2002).

17

Manufacturing Ingredients and Products by Fermentation

Gopal Chotani, Meng Heng, and Debbie Winetzky

Genencor International, a Danisco Company, Palo Alto, California, U.S.A.

INTRODUCTION

Fermentation, as the method of choice for manufacturing, has been used by mankind since the beginning of human history and is now recognized for its potential toward sustainable industrial development. Since discovery of the fermentative activity of microorganisms in the 18th century and its proof by the French scientist Louis Pasteur, fermentative production of alcohols, amino acids, enzymes (biocatalysts), organic acids, vitamins, and natural polymers for food, feed, and other industrial applications has become well established. Fermentative processes and enzymes can be applied to a wide variety of manufacturing processes in which renewable resource-based materials are used and produced, including health care, food processing, agriculture development, and waste treatment applications. Industrial biotechnology companies, such as Genencor International and Novozymes, sell enzymes for a wide variety of bioprocessing applications. The worldwide enzyme market is about U.S. $2 billion for such application areas as detergents, textiles, starch, baking, and animal feed (1).

Today, the use of microorganisms and cell-free enzymes as biocatalysts is growing and production of biochemicals by fermentation is replacing traditional chemically based processes. In the arena of personal care products, production of hyaluronic acid, xanthan, pigments, and carotenoids by fermentation is apparent. In the future, design and production of other specialty personal care ingredients by recombinant microorganisms is envisaged to become prevalent. Besides

419

enzymes and biochemicals, a fermentative approach is also attractive for manufacturing peptides, which have recently started to show their potential in personal care and cosmetic applications. A variety of organisms have been shown to express peptides as inactive fusion proteins comprising a highly expressed protein, joined by a cleavable linker. Microbial expression of peptides is especially advantageous when the number of amino acid residues in a peptide sequence has a dramatic influence on the production costs of peptides made by solid phase synthetic chemistry. Peptide expression could be made even more efficient if peptide polymers are produced, that is, monomers joined by cleavable linkers. It is anticipated that peptide production would become most economical when cell-free or in vitro transcription and translation systems become economically scalable.

Advances in genetic engineering in the 20th century are making use of diverse organisms and have provided more control over DNA recombination. With genetic manipulation becoming accurate and rapid and novel screening and selection methods leading to desired regulation in organisms, products with higher specific activity and specificity can be produced, making processes more economical. Through the availability of a wide range of gene sequences, genetic engineering is not limited to the production of enzymes and metabolites inherent to a given organism. Using a set of enabling technologies, today's scientists working in the multidisciplinary field of pathway engineering can manipulate a microorganism to use any carbon source to produce a range of desired biomolecules. By engineering a microbe, scientists can limit its growth, streamline the carbon flow, and focus energy into the production of the desired product. In short, scientists build nano-cell factories that can replicate under defined conditions with an operating system and software defined by the pathway engineer. The result is a new paradigm for the manufacture of materials by fermentation consistent with the demands for improved sustainability.

INGREDIENTS MANUFACTURING

As discussed by Vandamme and Soetaert (chap. 2), microbial catalysts are capable of synthesizing small molecules (hydroxyl acids), polymers (hyaluronic acid), peptides (Bowman-Birk inhibitor), proteins (silk-elastin), and enzymes. Figure 1 represents a cell factory model to produce personal care products via fermentation and biocatalysis as reviewed in chapter 2. For illustration of the fermentation-based manufacturing process, the following sections describe the major unit operations for secreted enzyme/protein/peptide as the model product.

Expression

As soon as the targeted molecule is identified and possibly engineered, its pathway gene(s) is (are) inserted into a suitable production organism. Even if

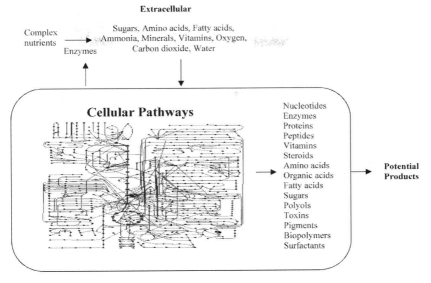

Figure 1 Fermentation-based cell factory for ingredients and products.

natural organisms could produce the targeted product, they are not usually productive or suitable for process development. It may be possible to improve the amount of product made by natural strains by optimizing the fermentation conditions. However, in almost all cases, strain improvement along with the process is necessary to achieve the desired productivity, purity, and economics of the final product. For safety reasons, production organisms are nonpathogenic and belong to a genus with a history of safe use. Moreover, the recombination techniques incorporate well-characterized gene sequences according to the regulatory guidelines.

A variety of different microorganisms are used for synthesizing the industrial bioproducts. They range from eukaryotic systems, such as yeasts and fungi, to prokaryotic systems (gram-negative and -positive bacteria). Biopharmaceutical production also employs mammalian and insect cell lines. Generally, production processes have been developed in the strains known to make the products of interest. Bacilli, aspergilli, and yeasts have been industrious cell factories for decades, based mainly upon their ability to secrete enzymes and excrete biochemicals of wide interest. These have the ability to: (*i*) produce and secrete large amounts of molecules, (*ii*) carry out proper folding and posttranslational modifications, and (*iii*) meet regulatory requirements. Most of the industrial strain types are capable of differentiation (sporulation), even though asporogenic type is preferred. This property also has positive effect on production and properties of the fermentation broth.

In the past, the strains have been improved through classical mutagenesis, screen, and selection. However, strain improvement has been rapid by the advent of genetic engineering. Manipulation of the host (base organism) genome or the addition of extrachromosomal DNA elements has greatly increased the speed of strain improvement. It is very efficient to manipulate DNA of the working host for production of differing products. As a result, most production strains are genetically engineered. The genetically modified microorganism (GMM) is generally well characterized and designed so that they will have limited survival in the general environment. As recombinant organisms can be grown under contained good industrial large-scale practices, safety issues relating to environmental release are minimized. Novel methods to improve strain performance include gene shuffling and directed evolution (2).

Fermentation

Once the host is selected, development of a culture, which can be used to inoculate the seed stage(s), begins with the process of correctly storing and maintaining the organism. Usual methods include making culture stocks in 10–20% glycerol or dimethylsulfoxide for long-term storage in liquid nitrogen temperature. Cultures can be stored for future use on solid media, in freeze-dried forms, or as spore suspensions. The process of reviving the stored culture, a typical seed train, is shown in Figure 2. For engineered strains, selection of culture storage conditions to maintain strain stability is vital. The objective of the seed train is also to adapt the cells for growth in the production media. Therefore, the seed medium must be designed based on the physiological needs of the organism.

All microorganisms have basic requirements, such as water, a source of energy, carbon, nitrogen, salts, trace metals, and in some cases growth factors. The fermentation medium is developed to supply the essential metal elements that make-up less than 5% of cell dry weight. Bulk elements, such as carbon, nitrogen, oxygen, and hydrogen elements, are generally fed via sugars and

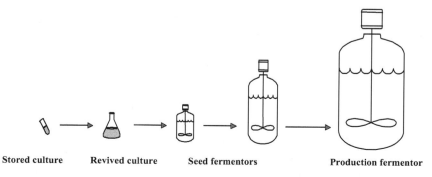

Stored culture   Revived culture   Seed fermentors   Production fermentor

Figure 2 Typical fermentation process train—stored cell to production scale.

ammonia. The challenge is to develop a medium and conditions that optimize growth by meeting the organism's essential needs, while economically producing the desired product. Many inexpensive nutrients provide good sources of the basic requirements and as inducers for product gene expression. The meal, concentrate, isolate, or flour form of soy, corn, cottonseed, wheat, peanut, potato, yeast, molasses, starch, cellulose, pectins, glucose, or oils are typically used to supply bulk of the carbon and nitrogen elements. Salts of ammonium, magnesium, potassium, phosphorus, sodium, iron, calcium, and so on are added separately if they are not sufficiently available in the complex raw materials.

After designing the medium, the next step is preparation of the fermentor. The method of sterilization, physical or chemical, is critical for inactivation or elimination of contaminants before the fermentation takes place. In addition, it is equally important to prevent contamination during the fermentation run. The lower the particulate matter in the medium, the more effective the sterilization procedure. Steam sterilization, as opposed to dry heat, is often preferred because it permits more efficient heat transfer and higher reactivity. This results in effective cell killing by rapid denaturization of cellular structure. Exposing all fermentor surfaces to saturated, but not superheated steam, for time periods of 10–60 minutes at 121°C, is sufficient to inactivate all organisms and heat-resistant bacterial spores (3). On the other hand, phage contaminants are difficult to contain and tend to spread rapidly throughout the plant. The only effective way to prevent phage contamination is to develop resistant cultures. The fermentation media are sometimes pretreated with enzymes or acid, before or after sterilization, to avoid mass transfer limitations. Besides sterilizing all liquids and surfaces in contact with fermenting cells, it is equally important to sterilize the air used for cultivation; such sterilization is primarily done by membrane filtration. Membranes are able to eliminate spores as well as cells. As the fermentor agitates and aerates the medium, the cells utilize nutrients, broth rheology starts to change, CO_2 is produced, and sometimes foaming occurs. Therefore, anti- or defoaming agents (surface-active compounds) are added initially or intermittently during the fermentation run. Avoiding nutrient and O_2 depletion is critical for an optimal fermentation run. Moreover, understanding the by-products formed is also important to avoid any negative effect on the fermentation process.

Because of its proven flexibility, the basic stirred tank reactor is still the workhorse of the fermentation industry. However, fermentation processes generally require large reactor vessels and high amount of air/oxygen; this in turn requires high amounts of electricity. Metabolism generates a large amount of heat, and thus efficient cooling systems are also required. During fermentation, high levels of CO_2 are released into the environment and only a portion of total batched and fed carbon is converted to product, which generally results in producing a dilute product stream, necessitating complex recovery schemes.

Many of the currently commercialized fermentation processes require de novo synthesis of biomass and the maintenance of other, sometimes unnecessary, cellular functions in addition to the production of the desired end product. As a consequence, in a number of processes, greater than 50% of the input carbon substrate, typically glucose, is expended for cell growth and maintenance. In addition, complex carbon and nitrogen sources are generally necessary as raw materials for cell growth, thereby complicating and adding costs to downstream processing of chemical products. For large-scale production, each of these biomass-building functions must be repeated with every new fermentation batch, thus wasting valuable raw materials. As a result, final titer (measure of product concentration), or yield (measure of efficiency of substrate conversion to product), or productivity (measure of volumetric rate of product formation), and sometimes all three are lower than expected. Thus, for building cost competitive commercial fermentation processes, it is essential to develop faster, better, and cheaper processes. Moreover, such manufacturing plants have to use regulatory approved microorganisms (2).

Downstream Processing

The isolation and purification of compounds from fermentation broth through a series of separation steps is often referred to as downstream processing. Figure 3 shows a typical downstream process train. A wide variety of conventional separation techniques are available, and further developments of these techniques continue, with a focus on making them more efficient and cost effective. A vast number of downstream schemes can be devised using a different order and permutation of these separation techniques. Table 1 shows the key downstream processing stages, the objectives, and the possible separation techniques for each stage that is used for large-scale protein production. The overall goal of the downstream processing is to develop a recovery scheme that satisfies product purity requirements in a cost effective manner.

Besides purity requirements, economic considerations constrain the separation processes that can be used for the manufacturing of personal care products. The cost of product recovery is not only tied to the final product purity requirement, but also to the starting feedstock characteristics (e.g., the host organism), target product concentration, and physiochemical properties. A lower starting feedstock concentration and purity, with a higher target product purity requirement, typically demands more processing steps. This in turn results in lower yields or higher cost. Multiple chromatographic steps, which are commonly

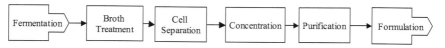

Figure 3 Typical downstream process train—fermentation to formulation.

Table 1 Key Downstream Process Stages, Objectives, and Techniques

Process stage	Objectives	Typical unit operations
Harvest and access to target protein	Access to target protein	Homogenization Treatment with lytic agents
Cell separation	Remove or collect cells, cell debris, or other particulates Reduce volume	Filtration Centrifugation Extraction
Concentration	Remove material having properties widely different from the desired product Reduce volume	Membrane filtration Precipitation
Purification	Remove remaining impurities (typically has similar chemical functionality and physical properties as the target product)	Crystallization Precipitation Chromatography

used in therapeutic production, generally would be too costly for economical production of personal care products. A combination of less expensive techniques, such as crystallization and precipitation, and perhaps a single chromatography step would offer a reasonable approach to accomplish purification. Typically, the final product produced using established recovery steps is tested for toxicological properties to show its safety for use in intended applications. Subsequent modifications to the established recovery strategy may require further toxicological studies, especially when the existing impurities levels are higher or new species arise. The common steps used in downstream processing are briefly described here.

Harvest and Access to Target Product

The first step in downstream processing is to gain access to the product from the fermentation broth. For extracellular expression, proteins are secreted by the cells and are readily accessible. Proteins associated with the cells or expressed intracellularly need to be released. This can be accomplished by lytic agents (e.g., enzyme or chemical), mechanical forces (e.g., homogenization or grinding with abrasive), or a combination of both. Some considerations that should be kept in mind when developing the process include: type of host organism/tissue, exact location of the protein, protein denaturation due to stress/shear, digestion by protease released from cells, and physical properties of the resulting suspension. The latter can have a significant impact on the subsequent solid–liquid separation step for cell separation.

Cell Separation

Cell separation is usually accomplished by means of either filtration or centrifugation. Filtration is the separation of solids present in a liquid by forcing the fluid through a porous barrier over a pressure differential. Filter press and rotary vacuum drum filter are two common types of filters used for large-scale cell separation. In centrifugation, separation of solids from liquid occurs by centrifugal force. Various types of designs are available for centrifugation in a large-scale operation: tubular, disk-stack, and scroll type.

Separation of cells or cell debris using either filtration or centrifugation can involve considerable difficulties due to the small size and physical properties of cells. The compressible nature of cells is the primary limiting factor for using filtration as a separation step to remove them. A typical cell cake has low permeability, resulting in a filtration rate that is often too slow. Filter aids, such as diatomaceous earth, are used to overcome this and work particularly well when fungal biomass needs to be separated using rotary drum vacuum filter. For cell removal by centrifugation, the small size and low density difference between the cells or cell debris and the medium results in a slow sedimentation rate. Flocculation of cell suspension to aid cell separation by both filtration, and centrifugation is a common practice. Cell flocculants are generally cationic and function by bridging the negative cell surface charges on neighboring cells to increase the particulate size and thereby facilitate filtration flux and clarity.

Product Concentration

Significant dilution of product may result from cell separation, especially when flocculation is used. Concentration of fermentation broth by membrane filtration to reduce the volume for subsequent processing is by far the most economical approach. Some purification steps, such as chromatography, precipitation, and crystallization can simultaneously purify and concentrate the product. However, the dilute nature of the feed may render these uneconomical. These technologies are more commonly used for purification and will be discussed in more detail in the following section.

A broad range of membranes from different materials fabricated into various configurations (e.g., tubular, flat-plate, hollow fiber, or spiral wound) and pore sizes are commercially available for concentration of fermentation broths. An ultra filtration membrane with average pore size of 0.001 to 0.02 μm is commonly used for concentrating macromolecules, such as proteins. For smaller molecules, nanofilters with an average pore size of 0.001 to 0.0001 μm can be used. Membrane selection largely depends on flux, product permeability, membrane life, and ease of cleaning. Removal of potential foulants, such as polysaccharides, antifoam, and other protein impurities, prior to concentration can significantly enhance fluxes and yields.

Purification

The product purity requirement for personal care products lies between the highly pure forms for therapeutic applications versus the relatively crude forms used in certain industrial applications. Methods employed for purifying therapeutic proteins can be applicable for manufacturing proteins for personal care, provided cost is not prohibitive. Chromatography has been the method of choice for therapeutic protein purification, and a vast amount of literature on the different chromatographic techniques is available (4). Thus, alternate cheaper purification methods will be discussed in the remainder of this section.

Precipitation is one of the oldest technologies and can be surprisingly effective for protein purification, especially when the protein of interest is only one of several proteins present in the fermentation broth. The tendency of a protein to precipitate is governed by the solvent environment, temperature, and the size, shape, charge, and hydrophobicity of the protein. The most common strategies to induce precipitation that have been practiced on a large-scale include addition of chaotropic salts, such as ammonium sulfate, or water-binding polymers, such as polyethylene glycol. This method is relatively straightforward to scale up and the protein precipitate can be recovered by centrifugation or filtration in a significantly concentrated form.

Crystallization, another approach for purification, can be viewed as a specialized case of precipitation in which formation of solid enzyme particles of defined shape and size occurs. Enzymes that have been crystallized for commercial production include a cellulase (5), glucose isomerase, and subtilisin (6). To the surprise of those unfamiliar with crystallization, the process is also highly scalable, reproducible, and a cost-effective technique. As in the case with precipitation, the crystals can be recovered by centrifugation or filtration in a significantly concentrated form. The purity attainable is comparable to what can be achieved with multiple chromatography steps. The challenge has been and will continue to be the search of suitable conditions for protein crystallization in large-scale manufacturing. Recently, development of high throughput screening approaches has lessened the laborious nature of the search and significantly increased the number of conditions screened. One challenge remains, however, because not all proteins can be crystallized.

Formulation

Formulation, for the purposes of this section, is the preparation of a saleable product ingredient made from the protein or peptide recovered during downstream processing. The formulation depends on how the product will be used and its ability to satisfy safety requirements. Product safety is an important consideration because proteins and peptides can generate immune responses in humans, namely sensitization and possibly allergy. Inhalation is the principal route of sensitization, and, therefore, a formulation that prevents direct contact of the protein or peptide with mucus membranes or lung tissue is needed.

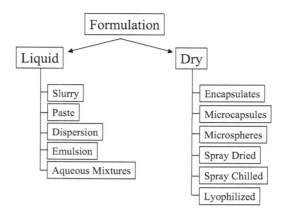

Figure 4 Formulation physical forms—liquid and dry.

As one can imagine, proteins or peptides can be formulated as solid granulates, particles, or encapsulates as a slurry or paste or as a liquid (Fig. 4). The product could also be sold as a frozen liquid, but this form is not commonly used in the personal care industry. The form to be chosen will depend on the inherent stability of the molecule, how it will be incorporated into personal care products, and its compatibility with formulation excipients in the final product. Some of the common product forms for proteins and peptides are discussed here (Table 2).

Solid Forms

In most industries, proteins (enzymes) are often supplied as encapsulated granules in order to satisfy safety requirements. These encapsulated granules may not be suitable for use in personal care products because of their large size and granulate ingredients, that is, stabilizers and coating, which may not be compatible with personal care product formulations. Other methods can be employed for the preparation of a solid product and include lyophilization, spray drying, or spray chilling. Alternatively, proteins can be incorporated into microspheres,

Table 2 Factors that Affect Selection of Formulation Form

	Liquid	Solid
Performance	Activity	Solubility/Release
Stability	Temperature, precipitation	Temperature, humidity
Safety	Aerosol	Dust
Compatibility	Precipitation	Polymer reaction
Appearance	Color and clarity, odor	Color, size, and shape
Handling	Viscosity, filterability	Flowability, segregation

microcapsules, or liposomes. Due to safety concerns, lyophilization or spray drying of pure proteins is not recommended. Spray chilling is the easiest and least expensive of the other methods. The major drawback of using this method, however, is finding a suitable carrier with the right melting characteristics and compatibility with a variety of finished products. Preparation methods for microspheres, microcapsules, or liposomes are well known, but they can be more expensive. There are several companies that specialize in preparing specialty liposomes for cosmetics, personal care products, and drug delivery. However, incorporating proteins into them would require special engineering and material handling training to ensure worker safety. Microspheres and microcapsules are used for medical diagnostics and medical devices and to deliver pharmaceuticals. These forms may offer some unique benefits over liposomes. They may be less "leaky" than liposomes, and, depending on their chemistry, they may assist in skin or hair penetration and/or targeting of the protein/peptide. The MML series on microspheres, microcapsules & liposomes (7) is an excellent reference for this technology.

Slurry or Paste Forms

Because nearly all proteins and peptides obtained by fermentation go through some type of recovery process, a slurry or paste from one of the recovery steps may be turned into the saleable product. For example, the concentrate from a polyethylene glycol (PEG) extraction step may be used if the protein is sufficiently pure and free of microbial contamination. In this case, the formulator must work closely with the recovery engineer to produce a clean, sterile formulation. Perhaps the addition of a sterile filtration step prior to a concentration step, in a clean, sterile tank, might be all that is necessary to obtain the final product. Another option is to force the precipitation or crystallization of the protein and then disperse it into a carrier system that is compatible with personal care products. The final step might be to determine a preservative system for the slurry or paste to ensure good shelf stability.

Liquid Forms

Liquid formulations of proteins or peptides may be prepared in a variety of ways, including aqueous high- or low-solids systems, dispersions, or emulsions. Many proteins reach a solubility limit somewhere between 20–30% solids, and some are even less soluble. Therefore, producing a liquid product with a high active payload may be very difficult.

Aqueous systems: The formulation of an aqueous system begins with characterizing the solubility of the protein or peptide. Determination of the maximum solubility concentration will be helpful in establishing the upper concentration limit for the formulated product. A solubility profile in a variety of solvents, such as butylene glycol, glycerol, polyethylene glycol, or cosmetic esters, should be created for evaluation of aqueous systems. Sometimes it may be necessary to solubilize the protein in water first and then dilute with the solvent. Glycols have the advantage of both stabilizing the three-dimensional structure of the protein and reducing the need for preservation. Additionally, the attachment or association of PEG to the protein may improve its stability.

Dispersions: Dispersions can be prepared from previously dried material or from a precipitate or crystal paste. The dried or partially dried material is suspended in a suitable solvent system and preserved if needed. One note of caution here is that salts are commonly used to force the precipitation or crystallization of proteins. It may be difficult to remove or reduce the salt concentration prior to formulation. As mentioned in the section earlier, glycols or glycol/water mixtures can be used for the solvent system. The dispersion may be visually clear or cloudy in appearance.

Emulsions: Proteins or peptides may be incorporated into emulsions. Peptides may be more suitable for this product form, especially if they have some surface activity. Proteins and peptides are typically hydrophilic in nature and would most likely reside in the aqueous phase of the emulsion. Proteins and peptides may be covalently attached to fatty acids, such as palmitic acid, that is, palmitoylated, which may partition them into the oil phase. The attachment of the fatty acids may improve the skin penetration or the "targeting" of the protein or peptide to specific structures or tissues in the skin.

No matter what delivery form is chosen, the components of the vehicle should be evaluated for their compatibility with the final personal care product formulation in which they will be incorporated and for their safety profiles. Moreover, components that are approved globally should be considered, especially if the product is to be sold worldwide, for example, butylene glycol versus propylene glycol. It is possible that certain components may be more suitable for particular applications, for instance, the salt level in the protein formulation may not be acceptable for incorporation into emulsions for skin care applications, but it may be acceptable for incorporation into hair-care products. Finally, increased concentrations of certain excipients may not be desirable given their properties. Personal care product formulators may not want to add a lot of extra glycols to their formulations due to unfavorable texture, smell and/or drying characteristics in the final personal care product formulation. Having chosen a desired delivery system, all protein and peptide formulations should be evaluated for their shelf stability as stand-alone products and in some targeted personal care products. Stability evaluations should encompass activity and phase stability after several freeze/thaw cycles, at elevated temperatures, and long-term stability at ambient and cold temperatures.

Process Integration

The goal of most fermentation processes is to produce a final formulated product and will likely include many postfermentation unit operations as already discussed. Total process integration is clearly necessary to realize operating and capital cost, as well as overcome any commercialization barrier. For the entire process, maximum production rate could still be the most important metric. However, lowest unit production cost could also be an important driver. Optimization of each individual unit operation will not always lead to the optimal overall process performance, especially when there are strong interactions between unit operations. Understanding these interactions is crucial to overall process optimization. For instance, product concentration or purity in the fermentation broth can significantly impact downstream purification unit operation. If the fermentation is optimized for productivity, without taking into account its effect on the purification step, the overall process productivity can be negatively affected. The use of antifoaming agents in the fermentation process is another example of such a trade-off. By reducing foaming in the fermentation, a higher working volume can be used to optimize the fermentation unit operation. However, many antifoaming agents negatively impact ultrafiltration membranes and final formulation.

The key to overcoming many of the biotechnology barriers is in rational biocatalyst design. Through control of cellular metabolic processes, we can not only optimize product formation but also control waste product generation and other accessory processes, such as simpler recovery steps, thereby shrinking the size of the factory necessary to complete the synthesis of the targeted product.

Product quality assurance methods are part of the process transfer package sent to the manufacturing plant. Regulatory and environmental compliance is based on the validated quality control assays. The EPA, FDA, and other agencies throughout the world are all involved in regulation of microorganism-derived products. Regulatory requirements dictate appropriate waste containment that is related to the risk presented by the organism. Most of the processes are subject to existing guidelines for industrial applications of recombinant DNA. Containment is generally achieved on the basis of inherent properties of the organisms, that is, nonpathogenic, safe organism with limited survival in the open environment. Also operating procedures and manufacturing plant design minimize potential releases of the recombinant organism to the environment. The degree of physical containment is matched to the risk presented by the organism.

SUMMARY

Besides economic benefits, bioprocess-based manufacturing has a favorable environmental impact potential for production of desired materials. Some of the major challenges to consider en route to bioprocess development are noteworthy. Regardless of the nature of the production organism, fermentation and recovery processes should be able to produce high quality product. The main goal in process development is to meet product specifications and minimize costs. Also, the process must meet all safety and quality assurance requirements. Ideally, the strain development and fermentation development efforts should be highly interactive. The strain development program must be aware of the limitations associated with various fermentation process options. In turn, the fermentation development effort needs to be in conjunction with the recovery efforts because the nature of the fermentation broth exerts a large impact on downstream processes, such as cell separation and product recovery. The fermentation and recovery processes together must generate a concentrated liquid product that can be formulated as a stable liquid or dry product without significant cost.

REFERENCES

1. Ho L, Edward Lee S, Humphrey AE. Industrial fermentation: principles, processes, and products. In: Kent JA, ed. Riegel's Handbook of Industrial Chemistry. 10th ed. Kluwer Academic/Plenum Press, 2003:963–1045.
2. Aehle W. Enzymes. In: Ullmann's Encyclopedia of Industrial Chemistry, Wiley-VCH Verlag GmbH & Co, 2003.
3. Atkinson B, Mavituna F. Biochemical Engineering and Biotechnology Handbook. New York: The Nature Press, 1983.
4. Ganapathy Subramanian. Bioseparations and Bioprocessing. Vol I: Biochromatography, Membrane Separation, Modeling, and Validation. Wiley-VCH Verlag GmbH, 1998.
5. Becker NT, Braunstein EL, Fewkes R, Meng H. US Pat. 6190898 Crystalline Cellulase and Method for Producing Same, 2001.
6. Becker T, Lawlis VB Jr. Subtilisin Crystallization Process. U.S. Patent 5,041,377, 1991.
7. Arshady R. Microspheres, Microcapsules & Liposomes. The MML Series. London: Citus Books, 1999.

Index

Editor's Biography

Pushkaraj (Raj) Lad, Ph.D., is Sr. Director of Consumer Markets at Genencor International, a Danisco Company. He obtained his B.S. in biology from Bombay University, Bombay, India in 1970 and his masters degree in biology in 1972 from Pittsburg State University, Kansas. He obtained his Ph.D. in biochemistry from University of Missouri, Columbia, in 1976. Lad did his post-doctoral training in cell biology and enzymology at The Salk Institute in La Jolla, California, and University of Missouri, Columbia. Subsequently, he held research faculty positions at University of California, San Diego, and University of Missouri.

Dr. Lad's research efforts have covered many disciplines like Biochemistry, Cell Biology, Pharmacology, Immunochemistry, and Molecular Biology. He has characterized various enzymes from bacterial and mammalian sources and studied their implications in health and consumer applications.

Since joining the R&D group at Genencor in 1984, he has held many technical and business management positions. He is at present responsible for business development and development of products and technologies for the Personal Care Business.

He has published more than 30 research articles in scientific journals and coauthored more than 10 chapters in books. He has 11 U.S. granted patents to his credit.